P9-BJT-476

Depression

SOURCEBOOK

Fourth Edition

Health Reference Series

Fourth Edition

Depression
SOURCEBOOK

Basic Consumer Health Information about the Symptoms, Causes, and Types of Depression, Including Major Depression, Dysthymia, Atypical Depression, Bipolar Disorder, Depression during and after Pregnancy, Premenstrual Dysphoric Disorder, Schizoaffective Disorder, and Seasonal Affective Disorder

Along with Facts about Depression and Chronic Illness, Treatment-Resistant Depression and Suicide, Mental Health Medications, Therapies, and Treatments, Tips for Improving Self-Esteem, Resilience, and Quality of Life while Living with Depression, a Glossary of Related Terms, and Resources for Additional Help and Information

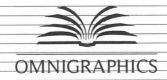

OMNIGRAPHICS

615 Griswold, Ste. 901, Detroit, MI 48226

Bibliographic Note
Because this page cannot legibly accommodate all the copyright notices, the Bibliographic
Note portion of the Preface constitutes an extension of the copyright notice.

* * *

Health Reference Series
Keith Jones, *Managing Editor*
***

OMNIGRAPHICS
A PART OF RELEVANT INFORMATION
***

Copyright © 2017 Omnigraphics
ISBN 978-0-7808-1498-1
E-ISBN 978-0-7808-1499-8

Library of Congress Cataloging-in-Publication Data

Names: Omnigraphics, Inc.

Title: Depression sourcebook: basic consumer health information about the
symptoms, causes, and types of depression, including major depression,
dysthymia, atypical depression, bipolar disorder, depression during and after
pregnancy, premenstrual dysphoric disorder, schizoaffective disorder, and
seasonal affective disorder; along with facts about depression and chronic illness,
treatment-resistant depression and suicide, mental health medications, therapies,
and treatments, tips for improving self-esteem, resilience, and quality of life while
living with depression, a glossary of related terms, and resources for additional
help and information. *61020839 2/17*

Description: Fourth edition. | Detroit, MI: Omnigraphics, [2017] | Series: Health
reference series | Includes bibliographical references and index.

Identifiers: LCCN 2016052760 (print) | LCCN 2016053552 (ebook) | ISBN
9780780814981 (hardcover: alk. paper) | ISBN 9780780814998 (ebook) | ISBN
9780780814998 (eBook))

Subjects: LCSH: Depression, Mental--Popular works.

Classification: LCC RC537.D4455 2017 (print) | LCC RC537 (ebook) | DDC
616.85/27--dc23

LC record available at https://lccn.loc.gov/2016052760

Table of Contents

Part III: Who Develops Depression?

Part IV: Causes and Risk Factors for Depression

Part VI: Diagnosis and Treatment of Depression

Part VIII: Suicide

Part IX: Additional Help and Information

Preface

About This Book

Depression, which is characterized by persistent sadness, hopelessness, trouble concentrating, fatigue, and changes in appetite and sleep
habits, is one of the most disabling health problems in the world. It is
also one of the most common. Recent statistics indicate around 15.7
million adults age 18 or older in the United States have experienced at
least one major depressive episode in the last year, which represents
6.7 percent of all American adults. At any point in time, 3 to 5 percent
of adults suffer from major depression. A variety of factors, including
genetics, biology, and environment, may contribute to the development
of depression, but prompt diagnosis and treatment helps those who
suffer manage their symptoms and develop strategies for living with
this chronic disease.

Depression Sourcebook, Fourth Edition, offers basic information about the prevalence, symptoms, and types of depressive mood
disorders, including major depression, dysthymia, atypical depression, bipolar disorder, depression during and after pregnancy, depression with psychosis, and seasonal affective disorder. It discusses
genetic, biological, and environmental risk factors for depression and
examines the impact of depression among the chronically ill, minority
populations, children, adolescents, college students, men, women, and
older adults. Information about depression's diagnosis and treatment—
including therapies, medications, and brain stimulation techniques—is

provided, along with facts about alternative and complementary therapies used to improve depression symptoms. Strategies for managing depression are also discussed, along with information about the warning signs and prevalence of suicide. The book concludes with a glossary of related terms and a directory of resources for additional help and information.

How to Use This Book

This book is divided into parts and chapters. Parts focus on broad areas of interest. Chapters are devoted to single topics within a part.

Part I: Introduction to Mental Health Disorders and Depression defines depression and discusses how brain function and chemistry play a role in the development and severity of mental health disorders. It discusses various myths and facts around mental health disorders, and provides information on potential reasons for depression. The part concludes with statistical reports on depression and other related mental health disorders.

Part II: Types of Depression gives an overview of the most common types of depression and related mental health disorders including; major depression, dysthymia, atypical depression, bipolar disorder, premenstrual syndrome, psychotic depression, and seasonal affective disorder.

Part III: Who Develops Depression? provides information about gender, age, and racial disparities in the diagnosis of depression. Facts about depression in men, women, children, adolescents, college students, pregnant women, and seniors are discussed. Information about the prevalence of depression in minority population, LGBTs, employees, prison inmates, and caregivers is also provided.

Part IV: Causes and Risk Factors for Depression highlights genetic, environmental, and situational factors that can predispose a person to developing depression. The impact of stress, trauma, unemployment, and substance use and addiction on the development of depression is also included.

Part V: Depression and Chronic Illness discusses chronic illnesses often linked to depression, such as autoimmune diseases, brain injury, cancer, diabetes, heart disease, human immunodeficiency virus (HIV), multiple sclerosis, Alzheimer disease, Parkinson disease, and stroke.

Part VI: Diagnosis and Treatment of Depression describes the process of receiving a depression diagnosis, paying for mental healthcare, and finding and choosing a mental healthcare provider. It also identifies mental health medications and therapies used to treat depression, including psychotherapy (talk therapy) and cognitive processing therapy. Other forms of treatment, including light therapy for seasonal affective disorder and brain stimulation therapies, are also discussed. The part ends with a discussion of alternative and complementary depression therapies, treatments for adolescents and children with depression, and strategies for treating severe or relapsed forms of depression.

Part VII: Strategies for Managing Depression discusses strategies for maintaining emotional wellness in people who have depression. People with depression will find information on developing resilience, avoiding depression triggers, and improving self-esteem, as well as tips on managing workplace depression, dealing with trauma, and coping with grief, bereavement, and loss.

Part VIII: Suicide offers information about the prevalence of suicide. It describes the warning signs of suicide and suggests next steps if you or a loved one expresses thoughts about suicide. It also provides information on how to recover from a suicide attempt.

Part IX: Additional Help and Information provides a glossary of important terms related to depression and a directory of organizations that help people with depression and suicidal thoughts.

Bibliographic Note

This volume contains documents and excerpts from publications issued by the following U.S. government agencies:

Centers for Disease Control and Prevention (CDC); Centers for Medicare and Medicaid Services (CMS); Federal Bureau of Prisons (BOP); National Cancer Institute (NCI); National Center for Complementary and Integrative Health (NCCIH); National Human Genome Research Institute (NHGRI); National Institute of Arthritis and Musculoskeletal and Skin Diseases (NIAMS); National Institute of Mental Health (NIMH); National Institute of Neurological Disorders and Stroke (NINDS); National Institute on Aging (NIA); National Institute on Drug Abuse (NIDA); National Institutes of Health (NIH); *NIH News in Health*; Office of Disease Prevention and Health Promotion (ODPHP); Office of Minority Health (OMH); Office on Women's Health (OWH); Substance Abuse and Mental Health Services Administration (SAMHSA); U.S. Department of Health and

Human Services (HHS); U.S. Department of Justice (DOJ); U.S. Department of Veterans Affairs (VA); and U.S. Food and Drug Administration (FDA).

In addition, this volume contains copyrighted documents from the following organization: The Nemours Foundation

It may also contain original material produced by Omnigraphics and reviewed by medical consultants.

About the Health Reference Series

The *Health Reference Series* is designed to provide basic medical information for patients, families, caregivers, and the general public. Each volume takes a particular topic and provides comprehensive coverage. This is especially important for people who may be dealing with a newly diagnosed disease or a chronic disorder in themselves or in a family member. People looking for preventive guidance, information about disease warning signs, medical statistics, and risk factors for health problems will also find answers to their questions in the *Health Reference Series.* The *Series*, however, is not intended to serve as a tool for diagnosing illness, in prescribing treatments, or as a substitute for the physician/patient relationship. All people concerned about medical symptoms or the possibility of disease are encouraged to seek professional care from an appropriate healthcare provider.

A Note about Spelling and Style

Health Reference Series editors use *Stedman's Medical Dictionary* as an authority for questions related to the spelling of medical terms and the *Chicago Manual of Style* for questions related to grammatical structures, punctuation, and other editorial concerns. Consistent adherence is not always possible, however, because the individual volumes within the *Series* include many documents from a wide variety of different producers, and the editor's primary goal is to present material from each source as accurately as is possible. This sometimes means that information in different chapters or sections may follow other guidelines and alternate spelling authorities.

Medical Review

Omnigraphics contracts with a team of qualified, senior medical professionals who serve as medical consultants for the *Health Reference*

Series. As necessary, medical consultants review reprinted and originally written material for currency and accuracy. Citations including the phrase, "Reviewed (month, year)" indicate material reviewed by this team. Medical consultation services are provided to the *Health Reference Series* editors by:

Dr. Senthil Selvan, MBBS, DCH, MD
Dr. K. Sivanandham, MBBS, DCH, MS (Research), PhD

Our Advisory Board

We would like to thank the following board members for providing initial guidance on the development of this series:

- Dr. Lynda Baker, Associate Professor of Library and Information Science, Wayne State University, Detroit, MI

- Nancy Bulgarelli, William Beaumont Hospital Library, Royal Oak, MI

- Karen Imarisio, Bloomfield Township Public Library, Bloomfield Township, MI

- Karen Morgan, Mardigian Library, University of Michigan-Dearborn, Dearborn, MI

- Rosemary Orlando, St. Clair Shores Public Library, St. Clair Shores, MI

Health Reference Series *Update Policy*

The inaugural book in the *Health Reference Series* was the first edition of *Cancer Sourcebook* published in 1989. Since then, the *Series* has been enthusiastically received by librarians and in the medical community. In order to maintain the standard of providing high-quality health information for the layperson the editorial staff at Omnigraphics felt it was necessary to implement a policy of updating volumes when warranted.

Medical researchers have been making tremendous strides, and it is the purpose of the *Health Reference Series* to stay current with the most recent advances. Each decision to update a volume is made on an individual basis. Some of the considerations include how much new information is available and the feedback we receive from people who use the books. If there is a topic you would like to see added to the update list, or an area of medical concern you feel has not been adequately addressed, please write to:

Managing Editor
Health Reference Series
Omnigraphics
615 Griswold, Ste. 901
Detroit, MI 48226

Part One

Introduction to Mental Health Disorders and Depression

Chapter 1

What Are Mental Health Disorders?

What Is Mental Health?

Mental health includes our emotional, psychological, and social well-being. It affects how we think, feel, and act. It also helps determine how we handle stress, relate to others, and make choices. Mental health is important at every stage of life, from childhood and adolescence through adulthood.

Over the course of your life, if you experience mental health problems, your thinking, mood, and behavior could be affected. Many factors contribute to mental health problems, including:

- Biological factors, such as genes or brain chemistry

- Life experiences, such as trauma or abuse

- Family history of mental health problems

This chapter contains text excerpted from the following sources: Text beginning with the heading "What Is Mental Health?" is excerpted from "What Is Mental Health?" MentalHealth.gov, U.S. Department of Health and Human Services (HHS), May 31, 2013. Reviewed November 2016; Text under the heading "Mental Illness" is excerpted from "Mental Health Basics," Centers for Disease Control and Prevention (CDC), August 11, 2016; Text under the heading "Categories of Mental Disorders" is excerpted from "Mental Disorders," Substance Abuse and Mental Health Services Administration (SAMHSA), October 27, 2015.

Mental health problems are common but help is available. People with mental health problems can get better and many recover completely.

Mental Health and Wellness

Positive mental health allows people to:

- Realize their full potential
- Cope with the stresses of life
- Work productively
- Make meaningful contributions to their communities

Ways to maintain positive mental health include:

- Getting professional help if you need it
- Connecting with others
- Staying positive
- Getting physically active
- Helping others
- Getting enough sleep
- Developing coping skills

Early Warning Signs

Not sure if you or someone you know is living with mental health problems? Experiencing one or more of the following feelings or behaviors can be an early warning sign of a problem:

- Eating or sleeping too much or too little
- Pulling away from people and usual activities
- Having low or no energy
- Feeling numb or like nothing matters
- Having unexplained aches and pains
- Feeling helpless or hopeless
- Smoking, drinking, or using drugs more than usual
- Feeling unusually confused, forgetful, on edge, angry, upset, worried, or scared

- Yelling or fighting with family and friends

- Experiencing severe mood swings that cause problems in relationships

- Having persistent thoughts and memories you can't get out of your head

- Hearing voices or believing things that are not true

- Thinking of harming yourself or others

- Inability to perform daily tasks like taking care of your kids or getting to work or school

Mental Illness

Mental illnesses refer to disorders generally characterized by dysregulation of mood, thought, and/or behavior, as recognized by the *Diagnostic and Statistical Manual, 4th edition*, of the American Psychiatric Association (DSM-IV). Mood disorders are among the most pervasive of all mental disorders and include major depression, in which the individual commonly reports feeling, for a time period of two weeks or more, sad or blue, uninterested in things previously of interest, psychomotor retardation or agitation, and increased or decreased appetite since the depressive episode ensued.

Categories of Mental Disorders

The following are descriptions of the most common categories of mental illness in the United States.

Anxiety Disorders

Anxiety disorders are characterized by excessive fear or anxiety that is difficult to control and negatively and substantially impacts daily functioning. Fear refers to the emotional response to a real or perceived threat while anxiety is the anticipation of a future threat. These disorders can range from specific fears (called phobias), such as the fear of flying or public speaking, to more generalized feelings of worry and tension. Anxiety disorders typically develop in childhood and persist to adulthood. Specific anxiety disorders include generalized anxiety disorder (GAD), panic disorder, separation anxiety disorder, and social anxiety disorder (social phobia).

National prevalence data indicate that nearly 40 million people in the United States (18%) experience an anxiety disorder in any given year. According to Substance Abuse and Mental Health Services Administration (SAMHSA) report, Behavioral Health, United States-2012, lifetime phobias and generalized anxiety disorders are the most prevalent among adolescents between the ages of 13 and 18 and have the earliest median age of first onset, around age 6. Phobias and generalized anxiety usually first appear around age 11, and they are the most prevalent anxiety disorders in adults.

Evidence suggests that many anxiety disorders may be caused by a combination of genetics, biology, and environmental factors. Adverse childhood experiences may also contribute to risk for developing anxiety disorders.

Attention Deficit Hyperactivity Disorder

Attention deficit hyperactivity disorder (ADHD) is defined by a persistent pattern of inattention (for example, difficulty keeping focus) and/or hyperactivity-impulsivity (for example, difficulty controlling behavior, excessive and inappropriate motor activity). Children with ADHD have difficulty performing well in school, interacting with other children, and following through on tasks. Adults with ADHD are often extremely distractible and have significant difficulties with organization. There are three sub-types of the disorder:

• Predominantly hyperactive/impulsive

• Predominantly inattentive

• Combined hyperactive/inattentive

ADHD is one of the more common mental disorders diagnosed among children. Data from the 2011 National Health Interview Survey (NHIS) indicate that parents of 8.4% of children aged 3 to 17 years had been informed that their child had ADHD. For youth ages 13 to 18, the prevalence rate is 9%. The disorder occurs four times as often among boys than girls. It is estimated that the prevalence of ADHD among adults is 2.5%.

Current research suggests that ADHD has a high degree of heritability, however, the exact gene or constellation of genes that give rise to the disorder are not known. Environmental risk factors may include low birth weight, smoking and alcohol use during pregnancy, exposure to lead, and history of child maltreatment.

The three overarching features of ADHD include inattention, hyperactivity, and impulsivity. Inattentive children may have trouble paying close attention to details, make careless mistakes in schoolwork, are easily distracted, have difficulty following through on tasks, such as homework assignments, or quickly become bored with a task. Hyperactivity may be defined by fidgeting or squirming, excessive talking, running about, or difficulty sitting still. Finally, impulsive children may be impatient, may blurt out answers to questions prematurely, have trouble waiting their turn, may frequently interrupt conversations, or intrude on others' activities.

Bipolar and Related Disorders

People with bipolar and related disorders experience atypical, dramatic swings in mood, and activity levels that go from periods of feeling intensely happy, irritable, and impulsive to periods of intense sadness and feelings of hopelessness. Individuals with this disorder experience discrete mood episodes, characterized as either a:

- **Manic episode**: Abnormally elevated, expansive, or irritable mood accompanied by increased energy or activity that substantially impairs functioning

- **Hypomanic episode**: Similar to a manic episode, however not severe enough to cause serious social or occupational problems

- **Major depressive episode**: Persistent depressed mood or loss of interest or pleasure

- **Mixed state**: Includes symptoms of both a manic episode and a major depressive episode

People exhibiting these symptoms are most frequently identified as having one of two types of bipolar disorders: bipolar I disorder or bipolar II disorder. The bipolar I diagnosis is used when there has been at least one manic episode in a person's life. The bipolar II diagnosis is used when there has been a more regular occurrence of depressive episodes along with a hypomanic episode, but not a full-blown manic episode. Cyclothymic disorder, or cyclothymia, is a diagnosis used for a mild form of bipolar disorder.

The combined prevalence of bipolar I disorder, bipolar II disorder and cyclothymia is estimated at 2.6% of the U.S. adult population and 11.2% for 13 to 18 year olds.

7

A family history of bipolar disorder is the strongest risk factor for the condition, and the level of risk increases with the degree of kinship.

As mentioned previously, bipolar disorders are characterized by manic and depressive episodes. In children, manic episodes may present as an excessively silly or joyful mood that is unusual for the child or an uncharacteristically irritable temperament and are accompanied by unusual behavioral changes, such as decreased need for sleep, risk-seeking behavior, and distractibility. Depressive episodes may present as a persistent, sad mood, feelings of worthlessness or guilt, and loss of interest in previously enjoyable activities. Behavioral changes associated with depressive episodes may include fatigue or loss of energy, gaining or losing a significant amount of weight, complaining about pain, or suicidal thoughts or plans.

Depressive Disorders (Including Major Depressive Disorder)

Depressive disorders are among the most common mental health disorders in the United States. They are characterized by a sad, hopeless, empty, or irritable mood, and somatic and cognitive changes that significantly interfere with daily life. Major depressive disorder (MDD) is defined as having a depressed mood for most of the day and a marked loss of interest or pleasure, among other symptoms present nearly every day for at least a two-week period. In children and adolescents, MDD may manifest as an irritable rather than a sad disposition. Suicidal thoughts or plans can occur during an episode of major depression, which can require immediate attention (to be connected to a skilled, trained counselor at a local crisis center, people can call 1-800-272-TALK (8255) anytime 24/7).

Based on the 2014 The National Survey on Drug Use and Health (NSDUH) data, 6.6% of adults aged 18 or older had a major depressive episode (MDE) in 2014, which was defined by the 4th edition of the *Diagnostic and Statistical Manual of Mental Disorders* (DSM-IV). The NSDUH data also show that the prevalence of MDE among adolescents aged 12 to 17 was 11.4% in 2014, while female youths were about three times as likely as male youths to experience a MDE.

MDD is thought to have many possible causes, including genetic, biological, and environmental factors. Adverse childhood experiences and stressful life experiences are known to contribute to risk for MDD. In addition, those with closely related family members (for example, parents or siblings) who are diagnosed with the disorder are at increased risk.

A diagnosis for MDD at a minimum requires that symptoms of depressed mood (for example, feelings of sadness, emptiness, hopelessness) and loss of interest or pleasure in activities are present. Additional symptoms may include significant weight loss or gain, insomnia or hypersomnia, feelings of restlessness, lethargy, feelings of worthlessness or excessive guilt, distractibility, and recurrent thoughts of death, including suicidal ideation. Symptoms must be present for at least two-weeks and cause significant impairment or dysfunction in daily life.

Disruptive, Impulse Control, and Conduct Disorders

This class of disorders is characterized by problems with self-control of emotions or behaviors that violate the rights of others and/or bring a person into conflict with societal norms or authority figures. Oppositional defiant disorder and conduct disorder are the most prominent of this class of disorders in children.

Oppositional Defiant Disorder

Children with oppositional defiant disorder (ODD) display a frequent and persistent pattern of angry or irritable mood, argumentative/defiant behavior, or vindictiveness. Symptoms are typically first seen in the preschool years, and often precede the development of conduct disorder.

The average prevalence of ODD is estimated at 3.3%, and occurs more often in boys than girls.

Children who experienced harsh, inconsistent, or neglectful child-rearing practices are at increased risk for developing ODD.

Symptoms of ODD include angry/irritable mood, argumentative/defiant behavior, or vindictiveness. A child with an angry/irritable mood may often lose their temper, be frequently resentful, or easily annoyed. Argumentative or defiant children are frequently combative with authority figures or adults and often refuse to comply with rules. They may also deliberately annoy others or blame others for their mistakes or misbehavior. These symptoms must be evident for at least six months and observed when interacting with at least one individual who is not a sibling.

Conduct Disorder

Occurring in children and teens, conduct disorder is a persistent pattern of disruptive and violent behaviors that violate the basic rights of others or age-appropriate social norms or rules, and causes significant impairment in the child or family's daily life.

An estimated 8.5% of children and youth meet criteria for conduct disorder at some point in their life. Prevalence increases from childhood to adolescence and is more common among males than females.

Conduct disorder may be preceded by temperamental risk factors, such as behavioral difficulties in infancy and below-average intelligence. Similar to ODD, environmental risk factors may include harsh or inconsistent child-rearing practices and/or child maltreatment. Parental criminality, frequent changes of caregivers, large family size, familial psychopathology, and early institutional living may also contribute to risk for developing the disorder. Community-level risk factors may include neighborhood exposure to violence, peer rejection, and association with a delinquent peer group. Children with a parent or sibling with conduct disorder or other behavioral health disorders (for example, ADHD, schizophrenia, severe alcohol use disorder) are more likely to develop the condition. Children with conduct disorder often present with other disorders as well, including ADHD, learning disorders, and depression.

The primary symptoms of conduct disorder include aggression to people and animals (for example, bullying or causing physical harm), destruction of property (for example, fire-setting), deceitfulness or theft (for example, breaking and entering), and serious violations of rules (for example, truancy, elopement). Symptoms must be present for 12 months and fall into one of three subtypes depending on the age at onset (childhood, adolescent, or unspecified).

Obsessive-Compulsive and Related Disorders

Obsessive-compulsive disorder (OCD) is defined by the presence of persistent thoughts, urges, or images that are intrusive and unwanted (obsessions), or repetitive and ritualistic behaviors that a person feels are necessary in order to control obsessions (compulsions). OCD tends to begin in childhood or adolescence, with most individuals being diagnosed by the age of 19.

In the United States, the 12-month prevalence rate of OCD is estimated at 1.2% or nearly 2.2 million American adults.

The causes of OCD are largely unknown, however there is some evidence that it runs in families and is associated with environmental risk factors, such as child maltreatment or traumatic childhood events.

Prerequisites for OCD include the presence of obsessions, compulsions, or both. Obsessions may include persistent thoughts (for example, of contamination), images (for example, of horrific scenes), or urges (for example, to jump from a window) and are perceived as unpleasant and involuntary. Compulsions include repetitive behaviors that the person is compelled to carry out ritualistically in response to an obsession or according to a rigid set of rules. Compulsions are carried out in an effort to prevent or reduce anxiety or distress, and yet are clearly excessive or unrealistic. A common example of an OCD symptom is a person who is obsessed with germs and feels compelled to wash their hands excessively. OCD symptoms are time-consuming and cause significant dysfunction in daily life.

Schizophrenia Spectrum and Other Psychotic Disorders

The defining characteristic of schizophrenia and other psychotic disorders is abnormalities in one or more of five domains: delusions, hallucinations, disorganized thinking, grossly disorganized or abnormal motor behavior, and negative symptoms, which include diminished emotional expression and a decrease in the ability to engage in self-initiated activities. Disorders in this category include schizotypal disorder, schizoaffective disorder, and schizophreniform disorder. The most common diagnosis in this category is schizophrenia.

Schizophrenia

Schizophrenia is a brain disorder that impacts the way a person thinks (often described as a "thought disorder"), and is characterized by a range of cognitive, behavioral, and emotional experiences that can include: delusions, hallucinations, disorganized thinking, and grossly disorganized or abnormal motor behavior. These symptoms are chronic and severe, significantly impairing occupational and social functioning.

The lifetime prevalence of schizophrenia is estimated to be about 1% of the population. Childhood-onset schizophrenia (defined as onset before age 13) is much rarer, affecting approximately 0.01% of children. Symptoms of schizophrenia typically manifest between the ages of 16 and 30.

While family history of psychosis is often not predictive of schizophrenia, genetic predisposition correlates to risk for developing the disease. Physiological factors, such as certain pregnancy and birth complications and environmental factors, such as season of birth (late winter/early spring) and growing up in an urban environment may be associated with increased risk for schizophrenia.

People with schizophrenia can experience what are termed positive or negative symptoms. Positive symptoms are psychotic behaviors including:

- Delusions of false and persistent beliefs that are not part of the individual's culture. For example, people with schizophrenia may believe that their thoughts are being broadcast on the radio.

- Hallucinations that include hearing, seeing, smelling, or feeling things that others cannot. Most commonly, people with the disorder hear voices that talk to them or order them to do things.

- Disorganized speech that involves difficulty organizing thoughts, thought-blocking, and making up nonsensical words.

- Grossly disorganized or catatonic behavior.

Negative symptoms may include flat affect, disillusionment with daily life, isolating behavior, lack of motivation, and infrequent speaking, even when forced to interact. As with other forms of serious mental illness, schizophrenia is related to homelessness, involvement with the criminal justice system, and other negative outcomes.

Trauma- and Stressor-Related Disorders

The defining characteristic of trauma- and stressor-related disorders is previous exposure to a traumatic or stressful event. The most common disorder in this category is posttraumatic stress disorder (PTSD).

Posttraumatic Stress Disorder (PTSD)

PTSD is characterized as the development of debilitating symptoms following exposure to a traumatic or dangerous event. These can include re-experiencing symptoms from an event, such as flashbacks or nightmares, avoidance symptoms, changing a personal routine to escape having to be reminded of an event, or being hyper-aroused (easily startled or tense) that makes daily tasks nearly impossible to complete. PTSD was first identified as a result of symptoms experienced by soldiers and those in war; however, other traumatic events, such as rape, child abuse, car accidents, and natural disasters have also been shown to give rise to PTSD.

It is estimated that more than 7.7 million people in the United States could be diagnosed as having a PTSD with women being more likely to have the disorder when compared to men.

Risk for PTSD is separated into three categories, including pretraumatic, peritraumatic, and posttraumatic factors.

- Pretraumatic factors include childhood emotional problems by age 6, lower socioeconomic status, lower education, prior exposure to trauma, childhood adversity, lower intelligence, minority racial/ethnic status, and a family psychiatric history. Female gender and younger age at exposure may also contribute to peritraumatic risk.

- Posttraumatic factors include the severity of the trauma, perceived life threat, personal injury, interpersonal violence, and dissociation during the trauma that persists afterwards.

- Posttraumatic risk factors include negative appraisals, ineffective coping strategies, subsequent exposure to distressing reminders, subsequent adverse life events, and other trauma-related losses.

Diagnosis of PTSD must be preceded by exposure to actual or threatened death, serious injury, or violence. This may entail directly experiencing or witnessing the traumatic event, learning that the traumatic event occurred to a close family member or friend, or repeated exposure to distressing details of the traumatic event. Individuals diagnosed with PTSD experience intrusive symptoms (for example, recurrent upsetting dreams, flashbacks, distressing memories, intense psychological distress), avoidance of stimuli associated with the traumatic event, and negative changes in cognition and mood corresponding with the traumatic event (for example, dissociative amnesia, negative beliefs about oneself, persistent negative affect, feelings of detachment or estrangement). They also experience significant changes in arousal and reactivity associated with the traumatic events, such as hypervigilance, distractibility, exaggerated startle response, and irritable or self-destructive behavior.

Chapter 2

Brain Function and Mental Health

Understanding the Human Brain

The brain is the most complex part of the human body. This three-pound organ is the seat of intelligence, interpreter of the senses, initiator of body movement, and controller of behavior. Lying in its bony shell and washed by protective fluid, the brain is the source of all the qualities that define our humanity. The brain is the crown jewel of the human body.

For centuries, scientists and philosophers have been fascinated by the brain, but until recently they viewed the brain as nearly incomprehensible. Now, however, the brain is beginning to relinquish its secrets. Scientists have learned more about the brain in the last 10 years than in all previous centuries because of the accelerating pace of research in neurological and behavioral science and the development

This chapter contains text excerpted from the following sources: Text beginning with the heading "Understanding the Human Brain" is excerpted from "Brain Basics: Know Your Brain," National Institute of Neurological Disorders and Stroke (NINDS), April 17, 2015; Text beginning with the heading "Some Key Neurotransmitters at Work" is excerpted from "Brain Basics," National Institute of Mental Health (NIMH), May 6, 2011. Reviewed November 2016. Text under the heading "Disruption in Neural Circuits and Mental Illness" is excerpted from "Mental Illness Defined as Disruption in Neural Circuits," National Institute of Mental Health (NIMH), August 12, 2011. Reviewed November 2016.

of new research techniques. As a result, Congress named the 1990s the Decade of the Brain. At the forefront of research on the brain and other elements of the nervous system is the National Institute of Neurological Disorders and Stroke (NINDS), which conducts and supports scientific studies in the United States and around the world.

This chapter may help you understand how the healthy brain works, how to keep it healthy, and what happens when the brain is diseased or dysfunctional.

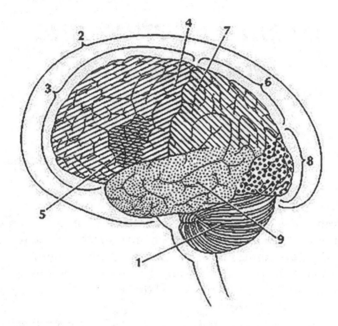

Figure 2.1. *The Human Brain*

The Architecture of the Brain

The brain is like a committee of experts. All the parts of the brain work together, but each part has its own special properties. The brain can be divided into three basic units: the forebrain, the midbrain, and the hindbrain.

The hindbrain includes the upper part of the spinal cord, the brain stem, and a wrinkled ball of tissue called the cerebellum (1). The hindbrain controls the body's vital functions such as respiration and heart rate. The cerebellum coordinates movement and is involved in learned rote movements. When you play the piano or hit a tennis ball you are activating the cerebellum. The uppermost part of the brainstem is the midbrain, which controls some reflex actions and is part of the circuit involved in the control of eye movements and other voluntary movements. The forebrain is the largest and most highly developed part of the human brain: it consists primarily of the cerebrum (2) and the structures hidden beneath it.

When people see pictures of the brain it is usually the cerebrum that they notice. The cerebrum sits at the topmost part of the brain and is the source of intellectual activities. It holds your memories, allows you to plan, enables you to imagine and think. It allows you to recognize friends, read books, and play games.

The cerebrum is split into two halves (hemispheres) by a deep fissure. Despite the split, the two cerebral hemispheres communicate with each other through a thick tract of nerve fibers that lies at the base of this fissure. Although the two hemispheres seem to be mirror images of each other, they are different. For instance, the ability to form words seems to lie primarily in the left hemisphere, while the right hemisphere seems to control many abstract reasoning skills.

For some as-yet-unknown reason, nearly all of the signals from the brain to the body and vice-versa cross over on their way to and from the brain. This means that the right cerebral hemisphere primarily controls the left side of the body and the left hemisphere primarily controls the right side. When one side of the brain is damaged, the opposite side of the body is affected. For example, a stroke in the right hemisphere of the brain can leave the left arm and leg paralyzed.

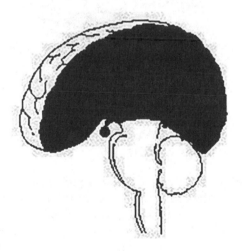

Figure 2.2. *The Forebrain*

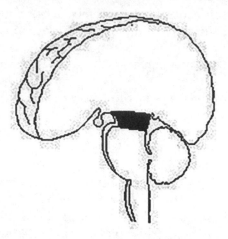

Figure 2.3. *The Midbrain*

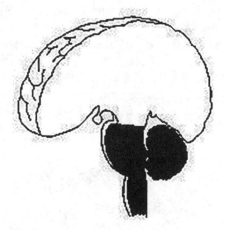

Figure 2.4. *The Hindbrain*

The Geography of Thought

Each cerebral hemisphere can be divided into sections, or lobes, each of which specializes in different functions. To understand each lobe and its specialty we will take a tour of the cerebral hemispheres, starting with the two frontal lobes (3), which lie directly behind the forehead. When you plan a schedule, imagine the future, or use reasoned arguments, these two lobes do much of the work. One of the ways the frontal lobes seem to do these things is by acting as short-term storage sites, allowing one idea to be kept in mind while other ideas are considered. In the rearmost portion of each frontal lobe is a motor area (4), which helps control voluntary movement. A nearby place on the left frontal lobe called Broca's area (5) allows thoughts to be transformed into words.

When you enjoy a good meal—the taste, aroma, and texture of the food—two sections behind the frontal lobes called the parietal lobes (6) are at work. The forward parts of these lobes, just behind the motor areas, are the primary sensory areas (7). These areas receive information about temperature, taste, touch, and movement from the rest of the body. Reading and arithmetic are also functions in the repertoire of each parietal lobe.

As you look at the words and pictures on this page, two areas at the back of the brain are at work. These lobes, called the occipital lobes (8), process images from the eyes and link that information with images stored in memory. Damage to the occipital lobes can cause blindness.

The last lobes on our tour of the cerebral hemispheres are the temporal lobes (9), which lie in front of the visual areas and nest under the parietal and frontal lobes. Whether you appreciate symphonies or rock music, your brain responds through the activity of these lobes. At the top of each temporal lobe is an area responsible for receiving information from the ears. The underside of each temporal lobe plays a crucial role in forming and retrieving memories, including those associated with music. Other parts of this lobe seem to integrate memories and sensations of taste, sound, sight, and touch.

The Cerebral Cortex

Coating the surface of the cerebrum and the cerebellum is a vital layer of tissue the thickness of a stack of two or three dimes. It is called the cortex, from the Latin word for bark. Most of the actual information processing in the brain takes place in the cerebral cortex. When people talk about "gray matter" in the brain they are talking about this thin rind. The cortex is gray because nerves in this area lack the insulation that makes most other parts of the brain appear to be white. The folds in the brain add to its surface area and therefore increase the amount of gray matter and the quantity of information that can be processed.

The Inner Brain

Deep within the brain, hidden from view, lie structures that are the gatekeepers between the spinal cord and the cerebral hemispheres.

These structures not only determine our emotional state, they also modify our perceptions and responses depending on that state, and allow us to initiate movements that you make without thinking about them. Like the lobes in the cerebral hemispheres, the structures described below come in pairs: each is duplicated in the opposite half of the brain.

The hypothalamus (10), about the size of a pearl, directs a multitude of important functions. It wakes you up in the morning, and gets the adrenaline flowing during a test or job interview. The hypothalamus is also an important emotional center, controlling the molecules that make you feel exhilarated, angry, or unhappy. Near the hypothalamus lies the thalamus (11), a major clearinghouse for information going to and from the spinal cord and the cerebrum.

An arching tract of nerve cells leads from the hypothalamus and the thalamus to the hippocampus (12). This tiny nub acts as a memory indexer—sending memories out to the appropriate part of the cerebral hemisphere for long-term storage and retrieving them when necessary. The basal ganglia (not shown) are clusters of nerve cells surrounding the thalamus. They are responsible for initiating and integrating movements. Parkinson disease, which results in tremors, rigidity, and a stiff, shuffling walk, is a disease of nerve cells that lead into the basal ganglia.

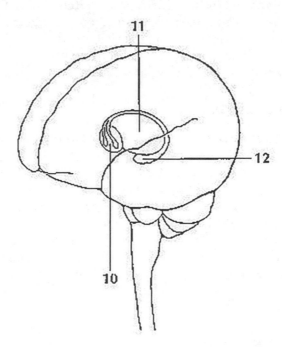

Figure 2.5. *The Inner Brain*

Making Connections

The brain and the rest of the nervous system are composed of many different types of cells, but the primary functional unit is a cell called the neuron. All sensations, movements, thoughts, memories, and feelings are the result of signals that pass through neurons. Neurons consist of three parts. The cell body (13) contains the nucleus, where most of the molecules that the neuron needs to survive and function are manufactured. Dendrites (14) extend out from the cell body like the branches of a tree and receive messages from other nerve cells. Signals then pass from the dendrites through the cell body and may travel away from the cell body down an axon (15) to another neuron, a muscle cell, or cells in some other organ. The neuron is usually surrounded by many support cells. Some types of cells wrap around the axon to form an insulating sheath (16). This sheath can include a fatty molecule called myelin, which provides insulation for the axon and helps nerve signals travel faster and farther. Axons may be very short, such as those that carry signals from one cell in the cortex to another cell less than a hair's width away. Or axons may be very long, such as those that carry messages from the brain all the way down the spinal cord.

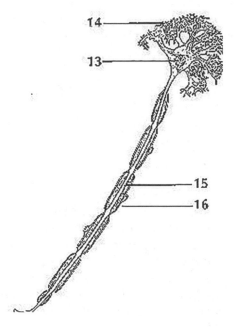

Figure 2.6. *Neuron*

- Scientists have learned a great deal about neurons by studying the synapse—the place where a signal passes from the neuron to another cell. When the signal reaches the end of the axon it stimulates the release of tiny sacs (17). These sacs release chemicals known as neurotransmitters (18) into the synapse (19). The neurotransmitters cross the synapse and attach to receptors (20) on the neighboring cell. These receptors can change the properties of the receiving cell. If the receiving cell is also a neuron, the signal can continue the transmission to the next cell.

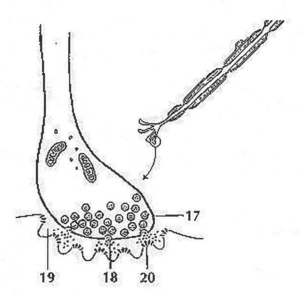

Figure 2.7. *Axon*

Some Key Neurotransmitters at Work

Everything we do relies on neurons communicating with one another. Electrical impulses and chemical signals carrying messages across different parts of the brain and between the brain and the rest of the nervous system. When a neuron is activated a small difference in electrical charge occurs. This unbalanced charge is called an action potential and is caused by the concentration of ions (atoms or molecules with unbalanced charges) across the cell membrane. The action potential travels very quickly along the axon, like when a line of dominoes falls.

When the action potential reaches the end of an axon, most neurons release a chemical message (a neurotransmitter) which crosses the synapse and binds to receptors on the receiving neuron's dendrites and starts the process over again. At the end of the line, a neurotransmitter may stimulate a different kind of cell (like a gland cell), or may trigger a new chain of messages.

Neurotransmitters send chemical messages between neurons. Mental illnesses, such as depression, can occur when this process does not work correctly. Communication between neurons can also be electrical, such as in areas of the brain that control movement. When electrical signals are abnormal, they can cause tremors or symptoms found in Parkinson disease.

- **Serotonin** helps control many functions, such as mood, appetite, and sleep. Research shows that people with depression often have lower than normal levels of serotonin. The types of medications most commonly prescribed to treat depression act by blocking the recycling, or reuptake, of serotonin by the sending neuron. As a result, more serotonin stays in the synapse for the receiving neuron to bind onto, leading to more normal mood functioning.

- **Dopamine** mainly involved in controlling movement and aiding the flow of information to the front of the brain, which is linked to thought and emotion. It is also linked to reward systems in the brain. Problems in producing dopamine can result in Parkinson's disease, a disorder that affects a person's ability to move as they want to, resulting in stiffness, tremors or shaking, and other symptoms. Some studies suggest that having too little dopamine or problems using dopamine in the thinking and feeling regions of the brain may play a role in disorders like schizophrenia or attention deficit hyperactivity disorder (ADHD).

- **Glutamate**—the most common neurotransmitter, glutamate has many roles throughout the brain and nervous system. Glutamate is an excitatory transmitter: when it is released it increases the chance that the neuron will fire. This enhances the electrical flow among brain cells required for normal function and plays an important role during early brain development. It may also assist in learning and memory. Problems in making or using glutamate have been linked to many mental disorders, including autism, obsessive compulsive disorder (OCD), schizophrenia, and depression.

Brain Regions

Just as many neurons working together form a circuit, many circuits working together form specialized brain systems. We have many specialized brain systems that work across specific brain regions to help us talk, help us make sense of what we see, and help us to solve a problem. Some of the regions most commonly studied in mental health research are listed below.

- **Amygdala**: The brain's "fear hub," which activates our natural "fight-or-flight" response to confront or escape from a dangerous situation. The amygdala also appears to be involved in learning to fear an event, such as touching a hot stove, and learning not to fear, such as overcoming a fear of spiders. Studying how the amygdala helps create memories of fear and safety may help improve treatments for anxiety disorders like phobias or Posttraumatic stress disorder (PTSD).

- **Prefrontal cortex (PFC)**: Seat of the brain's executive functions, such as judgment, decision making, and problem solving. Different parts of the PFC are involved in using short-term or "working" memory and in retrieving long-term memories. This area of the brain also helps to control the amygdala during stressful events. Some research shows that people who have PTSD or ADHD have reduced activity in their PFCs.

- **Anterior cingulate cortex (ACC)**: The ACC has many different roles, from controlling blood pressure and heart rate to responding when we sense a mistake, helping us feel motivated and stay focused on a task, and managing proper emotional reactions. Reduced ACC activity or damage to this brain area has been linked to disorders such as ADHD, schizophrenia, and depression.

- **Hippocampus**: Helps create and file new memories. When the hippocampus is damaged, a person can't create new memories, but can still remember past events and learned skills, and carry on a conversation, all which rely on different parts of the brain. The hippocampus may be involved in mood disorders through its control of a major mood circuit called the hypothalamic-pituitary-adrenal (HPA) axis.

Disruption in Neural Circuits and Mental Illness

It has become an National Institute of Mental Health (NIMH) mantra to describe mental disorders as brain disorders. What does this mean? Is it accurate to group schizophrenia, depression, and ADHD together with Alzheimer disease, Parkinson disease, and Huntington disease? Is a neurologic approach to mental disorders helpful or does this focus on the brain lead to less attention to the mind?

First, mental disorders appear to be disorders of brain circuits, in contrast to classical neurological disorders in which focal lesions are apparent. By analogy, heart disease can involve arrhythmias or infarction (death) of heart muscle. Both can be fatal, but the arrhythmia may not have a demonstrable lesion. In past decades, there was little hope of finding abnormal brain circuitry beyond the coarse approach of an EEG, which revealed little detail about regional cortical function. With the advent of imaging techniques like PET, fMRI, MEG, and high resolution EEG, we can map the broad range of cortical function with high spatial and temporal resolution. For the first time, we can study the mind via the brain. Mapping patterns of cortical activity reveals mechanisms of mental function that are just not apparent by observing behavior.

Has brain imaging been useful for understanding mental disorders? While we are still in the early days of using these powerful technologies, a recent survey of the literature reveals some excellent examples of how studying the brain forces us to "re-think" mental disorders. For instance, studies of brain development demonstrate delays in cortical maturation in children with attention deficit hyperactivity disorder. How curious that this disorder, which is defined by cognitive (attention) and behavioral (hyperactivity) symptoms, increasingly appears to be a disorder of cortical development. Viewing ADHD as a brain disorder raises new, important questions: What causes delayed maturation? What treatments might accelerate cortical development?

A brain disorder approach also may transform the way we diagnose mental disorders. The NIMH Research Domain Criteria (R-DoC) project is involved in re-thinking diagnosis based on understanding the underlying brain changes. As an example, what we now call "major depressive disorder" probably represents many unique syndromes, responding to different interventions. Neuroimaging is beginning to yield biomarkers, that is, patterns that predict response to treatment or possibly reflect changes in physiology prior to changes in behavior or mood. And studies with deep brain stimulation addressing depression as a "brain arrhythmia" are demonstrating how changing the activity of specific circuits leads to remission of otherwise treatment refractory depressive episodes.

An important implication of this new approach is that abnormal behavior and cognition (e.g., mood, attention) may be late and convergent outcomes of altered brain development. This is a familiar lesson from neurodegenerative disorders: the symptoms of Alzheimer's, Parkinson's, and Huntington's diseases emerge years after changes in the brain. Could the same be true of these circuit disorders that appear early in life? If so, could imaging allow earlier detection and preemption of the behavioral and cognitive changes—from the social isolation of autism to the psychosis of schizophrenia? This preemptive approach, which has transformed outcomes in heart disease and cancer, could also transform psychiatry, by focusing on prevention for those at risk rather than the partial amelioration of symptoms late in the process.

But we need to recognize the range of unknowns that remain. In truth, we still do not know how to define a circuit. Where does a circuit begin or end? How do the patterns of "activity" on imaging scans actually translate to what is happening in the brain? What is the direction of information flow? In fact, the metaphor of a circuit in the sense of flow of electricity may be woefully inadequate for describing how mental activity emerges from neuronal activity in the brain. Hence the need for continuing research into fundamental neuroscience. The advent of new tools, such as optogenetics, which uses light for precise manipulation of cells in awake, behaving animals will take us a long way towards understanding the characteristics of a neuronal circuit.

While the neuroscience discoveries are coming fast and furious, one thing we can say already is that earlier notions of mental disorders as chemical imbalances or as social constructs are beginning to look antiquated. Much of what we are learning about the neural basis of mental illness is not yet ready for the clinic, but there can be little doubt that clinical neuroscience will soon be helping people with mental disorders to recover.

Chapter 3

Myths and Facts about Mental Health Disorders

Mental Health Problems Affect Everyone

Myth: Mental health problems don't affect me.

Fact: Mental health problems are actually very common. In 2014, about:

- One in five American adults experienced a mental health issue

- One in 10 young people experienced a period of major depression

- One in 25 Americans lived with a serious mental illness, such as schizophrenia, bipolar disorder, or major depression

Suicide is the 10th leading cause of death in the United States. It accounts for the loss of more than 41,000 American lives each year, more than double the number of lives lost to homicide.

Myth: Children don't experience mental health problems.

Fact: Even very young children may show early warning signs of mental health concerns. These mental health problems are often clinically diagnosable, and can be a product of the interaction of biological, psychological, and social factors.

This chapter includes text excerpted from "Mental Health Myths and Facts," MentalHealth.gov, U.S. Department of Health and Human Services (HHS), May 31, 2013. Reviewed November 2016.

Half of all mental health disorders show first signs before a person turns 14 years old, and three quarters of mental health disorders begin before age 24.

Unfortunately, less than 20% of children and adolescents with diagnosable mental health problems receive the treatment they need. Early mental health support can help a child before problems interfere with other developmental needs.

Myth: People with mental health problems are violent and unpredictable.

Fact: The vast majority of people with mental health problems are no more likely to be violent than anyone else. Most people with mental illness are not violent and only 3%–5% of violent acts can be attributed to individuals living with a serious mental illness. In fact, people with severe mental illnesses are over 10 times more likely to be victims of violent crime than the general population. You probably know someone with a mental health problem and don't even realize it, because many people with mental health problems are highly active and productive members of our communities.

Myth: People with mental health needs, even those who are managing their mental illness, cannot tolerate the stress of holding down a job.

Fact: People with mental health problems are just as productive as other employees. Employers who hire people with mental health problems report good attendance and punctuality as well as motivation, good work, and job tenure on par with or greater than other employees.

When employees with mental health problems receive effective treatment, it can result in:

- Lower total medical costs
- Increased productivity
- Lower absenteeism
- Decreased disability costs

Myth: Personality weakness or character flaws cause mental health problems. People with mental health problems can snap out of it if they try hard enough.

Fact: Mental health problems have nothing to do with being lazy or weak and many people need help to get better. Many factors contribute to mental health problems, including:

- Biological factors, such as genes, physical illness, injury, or brain chemistry

- Life experiences, such as trauma or a history of abuse

- Family history of mental health problems

People with mental health problems can get better and many recover completely.

Helping Individuals with Mental Health Problems

Myth: There is no hope for people with mental health problems. Once a friend or family member develops mental health problems, he or she will never recover.

Fact: Studies show that people with mental health problems get better and many recover completely. Recovery refers to the process in which people are able to live, work, learn, and participate fully in their communities. There are more treatments, services, and community support systems than ever before, and they work.

Myth: Therapy and self-help are a waste of time. Why bother when you can just take a pill?

Fact: Treatment for mental health problems varies depending on the individual and could include medication, therapy, or both. Many individuals work with a support system during the healing and recovery process.

Myth: I can't do anything for a person with a mental health problem.

Fact: Friends and loved ones can make a big difference. Only 44% of adults with diagnosable mental health problems and less than 20% of children and adolescents receive needed treatment. Friends and family can be important influences to help someone get the treatment and services they need by:

- Reaching out and letting them know you are available to help

- Helping them access mental health services

- Learning and sharing the facts about mental health, especially if you hear something that isn't true

- Treating them with respect, just as you would anyone else

- Refusing to define them by their diagnosis or using labels such as "crazy"

Myth: Prevention doesn't work. It is impossible to prevent mental illnesses.

Fact: Prevention of mental, emotional, and behavioral disorders focuses on addressing known risk factors such as exposure to trauma that can affect the chances that children, youth, and young adults will develop mental health problems. Promoting the social-emotional well-being of children and youth leads to:

- Higher overall productivity
- Better educational outcomes
- Lower crime rates
- Stronger economies
- Lower healthcare costs
- Improved quality of life
- Increased lifespan
- Improved family life

Chapter 4

Depression: What You Need to Know

Depression Is a Real Illness

Sadness is something we all experience. It is a normal reaction to difficult times in life and usually passes with a little time. When a person has depression, it interferes with daily life and normal functioning. It can cause pain for both the person with depression and those who care about him or her. Doctors call this condition "depressive disorder," or "clinical depression." It is a real illness. It is not a sign of a person's weakness or a character flaw. You can't "snap out of" clinical depression. Most people who experience depression need treatment to get better.

Signs and Symptoms

Sadness is only a small part of depression. Some people with depression may not feel sadness at all. Depression has many other symptoms, including physical ones. If you have been experiencing any of the following signs and symptoms for at least 2 weeks, you may be suffering from depression:

- Persistent sad, anxious, or "empty" mood

This chapter includes text excerpted from "Depression: What You Need to Know," National Institute of Mental Health (NIMH), November 2015.

- Feelings of hopelessness, pessimism

- Feelings of guilt, worthlessness, helplessness

- Loss of interest or pleasure in hobbies and activities

- Decreased energy, fatigue, being "slowed down"

- Difficulty concentrating, remembering, making decisions

- Difficulty sleeping, early-morning awakening, or oversleeping

- Appetite and/or weight changes

- Thoughts of death or suicide, suicide attempts

- Restlessness, irritability

- Persistent physical symptoms

Factors That Play a Role in Depression

Many factors may play a role in depression, including genetics, brain biology and chemistry, and life events such as trauma, loss of a loved one, a difficult relationship, an early childhood experience, or any stressful situation.

Depression can happen at any age, but often begins in the teens or early 20s or 30s. Most chronic mood and anxiety disorders in adults begin as high levels of anxiety in children. In fact, high levels of anxiety as a child could mean a higher risk of depression as an adult.

Depression can co-occur with other serious medical illnesses such as diabetes, cancer, heart disease, and Parkinson disease. Depression can make these conditions worse and vice versa. Sometimes medications taken for these illnesses may cause side effects that contribute to depression. A doctor experienced in treating these complicated illnesses can help work out the best treatment strategy.

Research on depression is ongoing, and one day these discoveries may lead to better diagnosis and treatment.

Types of Depression

There are several types of depressive disorders.

Major depression: Severe symptoms that interfere with the ability to work, sleep, study, eat, and enjoy life. An episode can occur only once in a person's lifetime, but more often, a person has several episodes.

Persistent depressive disorder: A depressed mood that lasts for at least 2 years. A person diagnosed with persistent depressive disorder may have episodes of major depression along with periods of less severe symptoms, but symptoms must last for 2 years.

Some forms of depression are slightly different, or they may develop under unique circumstances. They include: Psychotic depression, which occurs when a person has severe depression plus some form of psychosis, such as having disturbing false beliefs or a break with reality (delusions), or hearing or seeing upsetting things that others cannot hear or see (hallucinations).

Postpartum depression, which is much more serious than the "baby blues" that many women experience after giving birth, when hormonal and physical changes and the new responsibility of caring for a newborn can be overwhelming. It is estimated that 10 to 15 percent of women experience postpartum depression after giving birth.

Seasonal affective disorder (SAD), which is characterized by the onset of depression during the winter months, when there is less natural sunlight. The depression generally lifts during spring and summer. SAD may be effectively treated with light therapy, but nearly half of those with SAD do not get better with light therapy alone. Antidepressant medication and psychotherapy can reduce SAD symptoms, either alone or in combination with light therapy.

Bipolar disorder is different from depression. The reason it is included in this list is because someone with bipolar disorder experiences episodes of extreme low moods (depression). But a person with bipolar disorder also experiences extreme high moods (called "mania").

Depression Affects People in Different Ways

Not everyone who is depressed experiences every symptom. Some people experience only a few symptoms. Some people have many. The severity and frequency of symptoms, and how long they last, will vary depending on the individual and his or her particular illness. Symptoms may also vary depending on the stage of the illness.

Women

Women with depression do not all experience the same symptoms. However, women with depression typically have symptoms of sadness, worthlessness, and guilt.

Depression is more common among women than among men. Biological, lifecycle, hormonal, and psychosocial factors that are unique to women may be linked to their higher depression rate.

For example, women are especially vulnerable to developing postpartum depression after giving birth, when hormonal and physical changes and the new responsibility of caring for a newborn can be overwhelming.

Men

Men often experience depression differently than women. While women with depression are more likely to have feelings of sadness, worthlessness, and excessive guilt, men are more likely to be very tired, irritable, lose interest in once-pleasurable activities, and have difficulty sleeping.

Men may turn to alcohol or drugs when they are depressed. They also may become frustrated, discouraged, irritable, angry, and sometimes abusive. Some men may throw themselves into their work to avoid talking about their depression with family or friends, or behave recklessly. And although more women attempt suicide, many more men die by suicide in the United States.

Children

Before puberty, girls and boys are equally likely to develop depression. A child with depression may pretend to be sick, refuse to go to school, cling to a parent, or worry that a parent may die. Because normal behaviors vary from one childhood stage to another, it can be difficult to tell whether a child is just going through a temporary "phase" or is suffering from depression. Sometimes the parents become worried about how the child's behavior has changed, or a teacher mentions that "your child doesn't seem to be himself." In such a case, if a visit to the child's pediatrician rules out physical symptoms, the doctor will probably suggest that the child be evaluated, preferably by a mental health professional who specializes in the treatment of children. Most chronic mood disorders, such as depression, begin as high levels of anxiety in children.

Teens

The teen years can be tough. Teens are forming an identity apart from their parents, grappling with gender issues and emerging sexuality, and making independent decisions for the first time in their lives. Occasional bad moods are to be expected, but depression is different. Older children and teens with depression may sulk, get into trouble at school, be negative and irritable, and feel misunderstood. If you're unsure if an adolescent in your life is depressed or just "being a teenager," consider how long the symptoms have been present, how severe they are, and how different the teen is acting from his or her usual self. Teens with depression may also have other disorders such as anxiety, eating disorders, or substance abuse. They may also be at higher risk for suicide.

Children and teenagers usually rely on parents, teachers, or other caregivers to recognize their suffering and get them the treatment they need. Many teens don't know where to go for mental health treatment or believe that treatment won't help. Others don't get help because they think depression symptoms may be just part of the typical stress of school or being a teen. Some teens worry what other people will think if they seek mental healthcare.

Depression often persists, recurs, and continues into adulthood, especially if left untreated. If you suspect a child or teenager in your life is suffering from depression, speak up right away.

Older People

Having depression for a long period of time is not a normal part of growing older. Most older adults feel satisfied with their lives, despite having more illnesses or physical problems. But depression in older adults may be difficult to recognize because they may show different, less obvious symptoms.

Sometimes older people who are depressed appear to feel tired, have trouble sleeping, or seem grumpy and irritable. Confusion or attention problems caused by depression can sometimes look like Alzheimer disease or other brain disorders. Older adults also may have more medical conditions such as heart disease, stroke, or cancer, which may cause depressive symptoms. Or they may be taking medications with side effects that contribute to depression.

Some older adults may experience what doctors call vascular depression, also called arteriosclerotic depression or subcortical ischemic depression. Vascular depression may result when blood vessels become less flexible and harden over time, becoming constricted. The hardening of vessels prevents normal blood flow to the body's organs, including the brain. Those with vascular depression may have or be at risk for heart disease or stroke.

Sometimes it can be difficult to distinguish grief from major depression. Grief after loss of a loved one is a normal reaction and generally does not require professional mental health treatment. However, grief that is complicated and lasts for a very long time following a loss may require treatment.

Older adults who had depression when they were younger are more at risk for developing depression in late life than those who did not have the illness earlier in life.

Depression Is Treatable

Depression, even the most severe cases, can be treated. The earlier treatment begins, the more effective it is. Most adults see an improvement in their symptoms when treated with antidepressant drugs, talk therapy (psychotherapy), or a combination of both.

If you think you may have depression, start by making an appointment to see your doctor or healthcare provider. This could be your primary doctor or a health provider who specializes in diagnosing and treating mental health conditions (psychologist or psychiatrist). Certain medications, and some medical conditions, such as viruses or a thyroid disorder, can cause the same symptoms as depression. A doctor can rule out these possibilities by doing a physical exam, interview, and lab tests. If the doctor can find no medical condition that may be causing the depression, the next step is a psychological evaluation.

Talking to Your Doctor

How well you and your doctor talk to each other is one of the most important parts of getting good healthcare. But talking to your doctor isn't always easy. It takes time and effort on your part as well as your doctor's.

To prepare for your appointment, make a list of:

- Any symptoms you've had, including any that may seem unrelated to the reason for your appointment

- When did your symptoms start?

- How severe are your symptoms?

- Have the symptoms occurred before?

- If the symptoms have occurred before, how were they treated?

- Key personal information, including any major stresses or recent life changes

- All medications, vitamins, or other supplements that you're taking, including how much and how often

- Questions to ask your health provider

If you don't have a primary doctor or are not at ease with the one you currently see, now may be the time to find a new doctor. Whether you just moved to a new city, changed insurance providers, or had a bad experience with your doctor or medical staff, it is worthwhile to spend time finding a doctor you can trust.

Tests and Diagnosis

Your doctor or healthcare provider will examine you and talk to you at the appointment. Your doctor may do a physical exam and ask questions about your health and symptoms.

There are no lab tests that can specifically diagnose depression, but your doctor may also order some lab tests to rule out other conditions.

Ask questions if the doctor's explanations or instructions are unclear, bring up problems even if the doctor doesn't ask, and let the doctor know if you have concerns about a particular treatment or change in your daily life.

Your doctor may refer you to a mental health professional, such as a psychiatrist, psychologist, social worker, or mental health counselor, who should discuss with you any family history of depression or other mental disorder, and get a complete history of your symptoms. The mental health professional may also ask if you are using alcohol or drugs, and if you are thinking about death or suicide.

Treatment

Depression is treated with medicines, talk therapy (where a person talks with a trained professional about his or her thoughts and feelings; sometimes called "psychotherapy"), or a combination of the two.

Medications

Antidepressants are medicines that treat depression. They may help improve the way your brain uses certain chemicals that control mood or stress.

There are several types of antidepressants:

- Selective serotonin reuptake inhibitos (SSRI)

- Serotonin and norepinephrine reuptake inhibitors (SNRI)

- Tricyclic antidepressants (TCA)

- Monoamine oxidase inhibitors (MAOI)

There are other antidepressants that don't fall into any of these categories and are considered unique, such as Mirtazapine and Bupropion. Although all antidepressants can cause side effects, some are more likely to cause certain side effects than others. You may need to try several different antidepressant medicines before finding the one that improves your symptoms and has side effects that you can manage.

Most antidepressants are generally safe, but the U.S. Food and Drug Administration (FDA) requires that all antidepressants carry black box warnings, the strictest warnings for prescriptions. In some cases, children, teenagers, and young adults under age 25 may experience an increase in suicidal thoughts or behavior when taking antidepressants, especially in the first few weeks after starting or when the dose is changed. The warning also says that patients of all ages taking antidepressants should be watched closely, especially during the first few weeks of treatment.

Common side effects listed by the FDA for antidepressants are:

- Nausea and vomiting

- Weight gain

- Diarrhea

- Sleepiness

- Sexual problems

Other more serious but much less common side effects listed by the FDA for antidepressant medicines can include seizures, heart problems, and an imbalance of salt in your blood, liver damage, suicidal thoughts, or serotonin syndrome (a life-threatening reaction where your body makes too much serotonin). Serotonin syndrome can cause shivering, diarrhea, fever, seizures, and stiff or rigid muscles.

Chapter 5

Why Do People Get Depressed?

Depression affects people of every age, economic situation, and race. Even though depression is common—especially in teens—some people get depressed but others don't. Why?

There's No One Reason for Depression

Lots of things influence whether a person gets depressed. Some of it is biology—things like our genes, brain chemistry, and hormones. Some is environment, including daylight and seasons, or social and family situations we face. And some is personality, like how we react to life events or the support systems we create for ourselves. All these things can help shape whether or not a person becomes depressed.

Genes

Research shows that depression runs in families. Some people inherit genes that contribute to depression. But not everyone who has a family member with depression will develop it too. And many people with no family history of depression still get depressed. So genes are one factor, but they aren't the only reason for depression.

Brain Chemistry

Chemicals called neurotransmitters help send messages between nerve cells in the brain. Some neurotransmitters regulate mood. When a person is depressed, these neurotransmitters might be in low supply or not effective enough. Genes and brain chemistry can be connected: Having the genes for depression may make a person more likely to have the neurotransmitter problem that is part of depression.

Stress, Health, and Hormones

Things like stress, using alcohol or drugs, and hormone changes also affect the brain's delicate chemistry and mood. Some health conditions may cause depression-like symptoms. For example, hypothyroidism is known to cause a depressed mood in some people. Mono can drain a person's energy. When health conditions are diagnosed and treated by a doctor, the depression-like symptoms usually disappear. Getting enough sleep and regular exercise often has a positive effect on neurotransmitter activity and mood.

Daylight and Seasons

Daylight affects how the brain produces melatonin and serotonin. These neurotransmitters help regulate a person's sleep–wake cycles, energy, and mood. When there is less daylight, the brain produces more melatonin. When there is more daylight, the brain makes more serotonin.

Shorter days and longer hours of darkness in fall and winter may lead the body to have more melatonin and less serotonin. This imbalance is what creates the conditions for depression in some people—a condition known as seasonal affective disorder (SAD). Exposure to light can help improve mood for people affected by SAD.

Life Events

The death of a family member, friend, or pet sometimes goes beyond normal grief and leads to depression. Other difficult life events—such as when parents' divorce, separate, or remarry—can trigger depression.

Whether or not difficult life situations lead to depression can depend a lot on how well a person is able to cope, stay positive, and receive support.

Family and Social Environment

For some people, a negative, stressful, or unhappy family atmosphere can lead to depression. Other high-stress living situations—such as poverty, homelessness, or violence—can contribute, too. Dealing with bullying, harassment, or peer pressure leaves some people feeling isolated, victimized, or insecure.

Situations like these don't necessarily lead to depression, but facing them without relief or support can make it easier to become depressed.

Reacting to Life Situations

Life is full of ups and downs. Stress, hassles, and setbacks happen (but hopefully not too often). How we react to life's struggles matters a lot. A person's outlook can contribute to depression—or it can help guard against it.

Research shows that a positive outlook acts as a protection against depression, even for people who have the genes, brain chemistry, or life situations that put them at risk for developing it. The opposite is also true: People who tend to think more negatively may be more at risk for developing depression.

We can't control our genes, brain chemistry, or some of the other things that contribute to depression. But we do have control over how we see situations and how we cope.

Making an effort to think positively—like believing there's a way around any problem—helps ward off depression. So does developing coping skills and a support system of positive relationships. These things help build resilience (the quality that helps people bounce back and do well, even in difficult situations).

Here are three ways to build resilience:

- Try thinking of change as a challenging and normal part of life. When a problem crops up, take action to solve it.

- Remind yourself that setbacks and problems are temporary and solvable. Nothing lasts forever.

- Build a support system. Ask friends and family for help (or just a shoulder to cry on) when you need it. Offer to help when they need it. This kind of give and take creates strong relationships that help people weather life's storms.

Being positive and resilient isn't a magic shield that automatically protects us from depression. But these qualities can help offset the other factors that might lead to trouble.

Chapter 6

Statistics on Depression and Related Mental Health Disorders

Chapter Contents

Section 6.1

Statistics on Depression

This section contains text excerpted from the following sources:
Text under the heading "Depression—A Public Health Concern" is
excerpted from "Mental Illness," Centers for Disease Control and
Prevention (CDC), March 30, 2016; Text beginning with the heading
"Prevalence of Depression" is excerpted from "Key Substance Use and
Mental Health Indicators in the United States: Results from the 2015
National Survey on Drug Use and Health," Substance Abuse and
Mental Health Services Administration (SAMHSA), September 2016.

Depression—A Public Health Concern

Depression is a serious medical illness and an important public
health issue. Depression is characterized by persistent sadness and
sometimes irritability (particularly in children) and is one of the leading causes of disease or injury worldwide for both men and women.
Depression can cause suffering for depressed individuals and can also
have negative effects on their families and the communities in which
they live. The economic burden of depression, including workplace
costs, direct costs and suicide-related costs, has been estimated to be
$210.5 billion. Depression is associated with significant healthcare
needs, school problems, loss of work, and earlier mortality.

Prevalence of Depression

Major Depressive Episode (MDE) and MDE with Severe Impairment among Adults

National Survey on Drug Use and Health (NSDUH) provides estimates of having a past year major depressive episode (MDE) among
adults. MDE is defined using the diagnostic criteria from the DSM-IV.
Adults were defined as having an MDE if they had a period of 2 weeks
or longer in the past 12 months when they experienced a depressed
mood or loss of interest or pleasure in daily activities, and they had at
least some additional symptoms, such as problems with sleep, eating,
energy, concentration, and self-worth. Adults were defined as having

44

an MDE with severe impairment if their depression caused severe problems with their ability to manage at home, manage well at work, have relationships with others, or have a social life.

In 2015, 6.7 percent of adults aged 18 or older (16.1 million adults) had at least one MDE in the past year, and 4.3 percent of adults (10.3 million adults) had an MDE with severe impairment in the past year. Adults in 2015 who had an MDE with severe impairment represent nearly two thirds (64.0 percent) of adults who had a past year MDE.

The percentage of adults who had a past year MDE remained stable between 2005 and 2015. The percentage of adults with a past year MDE with severe impairment also remained stable between 2009 and 2015.

Aged 18 to 25

In 2015, an estimated 3.6 million young adults aged 18 to 25 had a past year MDE, or 10.3 percent of young adults. The percentage of young adults with a past year MDE was greater in 2015 than in 2005 to 2014.

In 2015, an estimated 2.2 million young adults aged 18 to 25 had a past year MDE with severe impairment, or 6.5 percent of young adults. The percentage of young adults with a past year MDE with severe impairment was greater in 2015 than in 2009 to 2013, but it was similar to the percentage in 2014.

Aged 26 to 49

In 2015, an estimated 7.3 million adults aged 26 to 49 had a past year MDE, or 7.5 percent of adults in this age group. The percentage of adults aged 26 to 49 in 2015 who had a past year MDE was similar to the corresponding percentages in 2005 to 2014.

In 2015, an estimated 4.8 million adults aged 26 to 49 had a past year MDE with severe impairment, or 4.9 percent of adults in this age group. The percentage of adults aged 26 to 49 in 2015 who had a past year MDE with severe impairment was similar to the percentages in 2009 to 2014.

Aged 50 or Older

In 2015, an estimated 5.2 million adults aged 50 or older had a past year MDE, or 4.8 percent of adults in this age group. The percentage of adults aged 50 or older in 2015 who had a past year MDE was similar to the corresponding percentages in 2005 to 2014.

In 2015, an estimated 3.2 million adults aged 50 or older had a past year MDE with severe impairment, or 3.0 percent of adults in this age group. The percentage of adults aged 50 or older in 2015 who had a past year MDE with severe impairment was similar to the percentages in 2009 to 2014.

Treatment for Depression among Adults

Adults who had met the criteria for having a past year MDE were asked whether they had received treatment for their depression in the past year. Treatment for depression in adults is defined as seeing or talking to a health professional or other professional or using prescription medication for depression in the past year.

In 2015, an estimated 67.2 percent of adults aged 18 or older who had a past year MDE received treatment for depression. This percentage represents 10.8 million adults with a past year MDE who received treatment for depression. The percentage of adults with a past year MDE who received treatment for depression remained stable between 2009 and 2015. Among adults who had a past year MDE with severe impairment, 7.5 million, or 72.7 percent, received treatment for depression. The percentage of adults with an MDE with severe impairment in 2015 who received treatment for depression was similar to the percentages in most years from 2009 to 2014.

Aged 18 to 25

In 2015, 1.7 million young adults aged 18 to 25 with a past year MDE received treatment for depression in the past year. Among young adults, the percentage of adults with MDE in 2015 who received treatment for depression (46.8 percent) was similar to the percentages in 2009 to 2014.

In 2015, 1.2 million young adults aged 18 to 25 with a past year MDE with severe impairment received treatment for depression in the past year. Among young adults, the percentage of adults with MDE with severe impairment in 2015 who received treatment for depression (52.0 percent) was similar to the percentages in 2009 to 2014.

Aged 26 to 49

In 2015, 4.9 million adults aged 26 to 49 with a past year MDE received treatment for depression in the past year. Among adults aged 26 to 49, the percentage of adults with MDE in 2015 who received treatment for depression (67.4 percent) was similar to the percentages in 2009 to 2014.

In 2015, 3.4 million adults aged 26 to 49 with a past year MDE with severe impairment received treatment for depression in the past year. Among adults aged 26 to 49, the percentage of adults with MDE with severe impairment in 2015 who received treatment for depression (72.0 percent) was similar to the percentages in 2009 to 2014.

Aged 50 or Older

In 2015, 4.2 million adults aged 50 or older with a past year MDE received treatment for depression in the past year. Among adults aged 50 or older, the percentage of adults with MDE in 2015 who received treatment for depression (80.9 percent) was similar to the percentages in 2009 to 2014.

In 2015, 2.8 million adults aged 50 or older with a past year MDE with severe impairment received treatment for depression in the past year. Among adults aged 50 or older, the percentage of adults with MDE with severe impairment in 2015 who received treatment for depression (87.9 percent) was similar to the percentages in 2009 to 2014.

MDE and MDE with Severe Impairment among Adolescents

Although NSDUH does not have an overall measure of mental illness among adolescents aged 12 to 17, the survey provides estimates of having a past year MDE for this age group. MDE is defined using the diagnostic criteria from DSM-IV. Similar to adults, adolescents were defined as having an MDE if they had a period of 2 weeks or longer in the past 12 months when they experienced a depressed mood or loss of interest or pleasure in daily activities, and they had at least some additional symptoms, such as problems with sleep, eating, energy, concentration, and self-worth. However, some wordings to the questions for adolescents were designed to make them more developmentally appropriate for youths. Adolescents were defined as having an MDE with severe impairment if their depression caused severe problems with their ability to do chores at home, do well at work or school, get along with their family, or have a social life.

In 2015, 12.5 percent of adolescents aged 12 to 17 (3.0 million adolescents) had an MDE during the past year, and 8.8 percent of adolescents (2.1 million adolescents) had a past year MDE with severe impairment. Adolescents in 2015 who had an MDE with severe impairment represent more than two thirds (70.7 percent) of adolescents who had a past year MDE.

The percentage of adolescents aged 12 to 17 in 2015 who had a past year MDE was higher than the percentages in 2004 to 2014. The percentage of adolescents in 2015 who had a past year MDE with severe impairment was higher than the percentages in 2006 to 2013, which ranged from 5.5 to 7.7 percent. However, the 2015 estimate was similar to the estimate in 2014.

Treatment for Depression among Adolescents

Adolescents who had met the criteria for having a past year MDE were asked whether they had received treatment for their depression in the past year. Adolescents were defined as having received treatment for their depression in the past year if they reported seeing or talking to a health professional or taking prescribed medication for their depression.

An estimated 1.2 million youth aged 12 to 17 in 2015 who had a past year MDE received treatment for depression, or 39.3 percent of youths who had a past year MDE. This 2015 percentage was similar to the percentages in most years from 2004 to 2014. Among youths who had a past year MDE with severe impairment, 945,000 (44.6 percent) received treatment for depression. The percentage of adolescents with MDE with severe impairment in 2015 who received treatment for depression was similar to the percentages in most years from 2006 to 2014.

Section 6.2

Statistics on Other Common Mental Illnesses

This chapter contains text excerpted from the following sources: Text under the heading "Serious Mental Illness (SMI) among U.S. Adults" is excerpted from "Serious Mental Illness (SMI) among U.S. Adults," National Institute of Mental Health (NIMH), December 15, 2015; Text under the heading "Any Mental Illness (AMI) among U.S. Adults" is excerpted from "Any Mental Illness (AMI) among U.S. Adults," National Institute of Mental Health (NIMH), December 15, 2015; Text beginning with the heading "Alzheimer Disease" is excerpted from "Burden of Mental Illness," Centers for Disease Control and Prevention (CDC), July 1, 2011. Reviewed November 2016.

Serious Mental Illness (SMI) among U.S. Adults

- While mental disorders are common in the United States, their burden of illness is particularly concentrated among those who experience disability due to serious mental illness (SMI).

- The data presented here are from the National Survey on Drug Use and Health (NSDUH), which defines SMI as:

  - A mental, behavioral, or emotional disorder (excluding developmental and substance use disorders);

- Diagnosable currently or within the past year;

- Of sufficient duration to meet diagnostic criteria specified within the 4th edition of the *Diagnostic and Statistical Manual of Mental Disorders* (DSM-IV); and,

- Resulting in serious functional impairment, which substantially interferes with or limits one or more major life activities.

- In 2014, there were an estimated 9.8 million adults aged 18 or older in the United States with SMI. This number represented 4.2% of all U.S. adults.

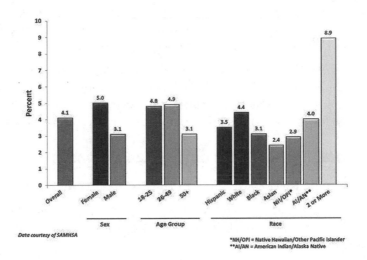

Figure 6.1. *Prevalence of Serious Mental Illness among U.S. Adults (2014)*

Population

- The entirety of NSDUH respondents for the SMI estimates is the civilian, non-institutionalized population aged 18 years old or older residing within the United States.

- The survey covers residents of households (persons living in houses/townhouses, apartments, condominiums; civilians living in housing on military bases, etc.) and persons in non-institutional group quarters (e.g., shelters, rooming/boarding houses, college dormitories, migratory workers' camps, and halfway houses).

- The survey does not cover persons who, for the entire year, had no fixed address (e.g., homeless and/or transient persons not in shelters); were on active military duty; or who resided in institutional group quarters (e.g., correctional facilities, nursing homes, mental institutions, long-term hospitals).

- Some people in these excluded categories have SMI, but they are not accounted for in the NSDUH SMI estimates.

Survey Non-Response

- In 2014, 28.8% of the selected NSDUH sample did not complete the interview.

- Reasons for non-response to interviewing include: refusal to participate (21%); respondent unavailable or no one at home/not answering the door (3.2%); and other reasons such as physical/mental incompetence or language barriers (4.6%).

- People with SMI may disproportionately fall into these non-response categories. While NSDUH weighting includes non-response adjustments to reduce bias, these adjustments may not fully account for differential non-response by mental illness status.

Any Mental Illness (AMI) among U.S. Adults

- Mental illnesses are common in the United States.

- The data presented here are from the National Survey on Drug Use and Health (NSDUH), which defines any mental illness (AMI) as:

  - A mental, behavioral, or emotional disorder (excluding developmental and substance use disorders);

  - Diagnosable currently or within the past year; and,

  - Of sufficient duration to meet diagnostic criteria specified within the 4th edition of the *Diagnostic and Statistical Manual of Mental Disorders* (DSM-IV).

- AMI can range in impact from no or mild impairment to significantly disabling impairment, such as in individuals with serious mental illness (SMI), defined as individuals with a mental disorder with serious functional impairment which substantially interferes with or limits one or more major life activities.

- As noted, these estimates of AMI do not include substance use disorders, such as drug- or alcohol-related disorders. For statistics and other information about drug- and alcohol-related disorders, please visit the statistics pages of the National Institute on Drug Abuse (NIDA), the National Institute on Alcohol Abuse and Alcoholism (NIAAA), and the Substance Abuse and Mental Health Services Administration (SAMHSA).

- In 2014, there were an estimated 43.6 million adults aged 18 or older in the United States with AMI in the past year. This number represented 18.1% of all U.S. adults.

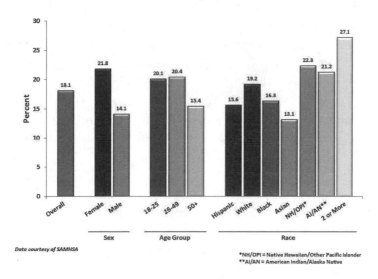

Figure 6.2. *Prevalence of Any Mental Illness (AMI) among U.S. Adults*

Population

- The entirety of NSDUH respondents for the AMI estimates is the civilian, non-institutionalized population aged 18 years old or older residing within the United States.

- The survey covers residents of households (persons living in houses/townhouses, apartments, condominiums; civilians living in housing on military bases, etc.) and persons in non-institutional group quarters (e.g., shelters, rooming/boarding houses, college dormitories, migratory workers' camps, and halfway houses).

- The survey does not cover persons who, for the entire year, had no fixed address (e.g., homeless and/or transient persons not in shelters); were on active military duty; or who resided in institutional group quarters (e.g., correctional facilities, nursing homes, mental institutions, long-term hospitals).

- Some people in these excluded categories have AMI, but they are not accounted for in the NSDUH AMI estimates.

Survey Non-Response

- In 2014, 28.8% of the selected NSDUH sample did not complete the interview.

- Reasons for non-response to interviewing include: refusal to participate (21%); respondent unavailable or no one at home/not answering the door (3.2%); and other reasons such as physical/ mental incompetence or language barriers (4.6%).

- People with mental illness may disproportionately fall into these non-response categories. While NSDUH weighting includes non-response adjustments to reduce bias, these adjustments may not fully account for differential non-response by mental illness status.

Alzheimer Disease

- Alzheimer disease is the sixth leading cause of death in the United States and is the fifth leading cause among persons age 65 years and older.

- Up to 5.3 million Americans currently have Alzheimer disease.

- By 2050, the number is expected to more than double due to the aging of the population.

Anxiety

- Anxiety disorders, which include panic disorder, generalized anxiety disorder, posttraumatic stress disorder, phobias, and separation anxiety disorder, are the most common class of mental disorders present in the general population.

- The estimated lifetime prevalence of any anxiety disorder is over 15%, while the 12-month prevalence is more than 10%.

- Prevalence estimates of anxiety disorders are generally higher in developed countries than in developing countries.

- Most anxiety disorders are more prevalent in women than in men.

- One study estimated the annual cost of anxiety disorders in the United States to be approximately $42.3 billion in the 1990s, a majority of which was due to non-psychiatric medical treatment costs. This estimate focused on short-term effects and did not include the effect of outcomes such as the increased risk of other disorders.

Bipolar Disorder

- The National Comorbidity Study reported a lifetime prevalence of nearly 4% for bipolar disorder. Bipolar disorder is more common in women than men, with a ratio of approximately 3:2. The median age of onset for bipolar disorder is 25 years, with men having an earlier age of onset than women.

- In an insured population, 7.5% of all claimants with behavioral healthcare coverage filed a claim, of which 3.0% had bipolar disorder. Persons with bipolar disorder incurred $568 in annual out-of-pocket expenses—more than double the expenses incurred by all claimants. Annual insurance payments were greater for medical services for persons with bipolar disorder than for patients with other behavioral healthcare diagnoses.

- The inpatient hospitalization rate of bipolar patients (39.1%) was greater than the 4.5% characterizing all other patients with behavioral healthcare diagnoses.

- Bipolar disorder has been deemed the most expensive behavioral healthcare diagnosis, costing more than twice as much as depression per affected individual. Total costs largely arise from indirect costs and are attributable to lost productivity, in turn arising from absenteeism and presenteeism.

- For every dollar allocated to outpatient care for persons with bipolar disorder, $1.80 is spent on inpatient care, suggesting early intervention and improved prevention management could decrease the financial impact of this illness.

Schizophrenia

- Worldwide prevalence estimates range between 0.5% and 1%. Age of first episode is typically younger among men (about 21 years of age) than women (27 years). Of persons with schizophrenia, by age 30, 9 out of 10 men, but only 2 out of 10 women, will manifest the illness.

- Persons with schizophrenia pose a high risk for suicide. Approximately one-third will attempt suicide and, eventually, about 1 out of 10 will take their own lives.

- A Canadian study found that the direct healthcare and non-healthcare costs of schizophrenia were estimated to be 2.02 billion Canadian dollars in 2004. This, combined with a high unemployment rate due to schizophrenia and an added productivity and morbidity and mortality loss of 4.83 billion Canadian dollars, yielded a total cost estimate of 6.85 billion in U.S. and Canadian dollars.

- The economic burden of schizophrenia is particularly great during the first year following the index episode, relative to the third year onwards. This finding suggests the need for improved monitoring of persons with schizophrenia upon initial diagnosis.

Frequent Mental Distress

Frequent mental distress is defined based on the response to the following quality of life question, "Now thinking about your mental health, which includes stress, depression, and problems with emotions, for how many days during the past 30 days was your mental health not good?" Frequent mental distress is identified as a report of 14 or more days of poor mental health in the past 30 days.

- 9.4% of U.S. adults experienced Frequent Mental Distress (FMD) for the combined periods 1993–2001 and 2003–2006.

- The Appalachian and the Mississippi Valley regions had high and increasing FMD prevalence, and the upper Midwest had low and decreasing FMD prevalence during this same time period.

Part Two

Types of Depression

Chapter 7

Major Depression

What Is Major Depression?

Major depression is a medical condition distinguished by one or more major depressive episodes. A major depressive episode is characterized by at least two weeks of depressed mood or loss of interest (pleasure) and accompanied by at least four more symptoms of depression. Such symptoms can include changes in appetite, weight, difficulty in thinking and concentrating, and recurrent thoughts of death or suicide. Depression differs from feeling "blue" in that it causes severe enough problems to interfere with a person's day-to-day functioning.

People's experience with major depression varies. Some people describe it as a total loss of energy or enthusiasm to do anything. Others may describe it as constantly living with a feeling of impending doom. There are treatments that help improve functioning and relieve many symptoms of depression. Recovery is possible!

Prevalence

Major depression is a common psychiatric disorder. It is more common in adolescent and adult women than in adolescent and adult men. In between 15 to 20 out of every 100 people experience an episode of major depression during their lifetime. Prevalence has not been found to be related to ethnicity, income, education, or marital status.

This chapter includes text excerpted from "What Is Major Depression?" U.S. Department of Veterans Affairs (VA), March 15, 2012. Reviewed November 2016.

Diagnosis

Major depression cannot be diagnosed with a blood test, CAT–scan, or any other laboratory test. The only way to diagnose major depression is with a clinical interview. The interviewer checks to see if the person has experienced severe symptoms for at least two weeks. If the symptoms are less severe, but last over long periods of time, the person may be diagnosed with persistent depressive disorder. The clinician must also check to be sure there are no physical problems that could cause symptoms like those of major depression, such as a brain tumor or a thyroid problem.

Course of Illness

The average age of onset is in the mid-20s, however, major depression can begin at any age in life. The frequency of episodes varies from person to person. Some people have isolated episodes over many years, while others suffer from frequent episodes clustered together. The number of episodes generally increases as the person grows older. The severity of the initial episode of major depression seems to indicate persistence. Episodes also seem to follow major stressors, such as the death of a loved one or a divorce. Chronic medical conditions and substance abuse may further exacerbate depressive episodes.

Causes

There is no simple answer to what causes depression because several factors play a part in the onset of the disorder. These include a genetic or family history of depression, environmental stressors, life events, biological factors, and psychological vulnerability to depression.

Research shows that the risk for depression results from the influence of multiple genes acting together with environmental factors. This is called the stress vulnerability model. A family history of depression does not necessarily mean children or other relatives will develop major depression. However, those with a family history of depression have a slightly higher chance of becoming depressed at some stage in their lives. Although genetic research suggests that depression can run in families, genetics alone are unlikely to cause depression. Environmental factors, such as a traumatic childhood or adult life events, may act as triggers. Studies show that early childhood trauma and losses, such as the death or separation of parents, or adult life events, such as the death of a loved one, divorce, loss of a job, retirement, serious financial problems, and family conflict, can lead to the onset of depression. Subsequent episodes are usually caused by more mild stressors or even none at all.

Many scientists believe the cause is biological, such as an imbalance in brain chemicals, specifically serotonin and norepinephrine. There are also theories that physical changes to the body may play a role in depression. Such physical changes can include viral and other infections, heart attack, cancer, or hormonal disorders.

Personality style may also contribute to the onset of depression. People are at a greater risk of becoming depressed if they have low self-esteem, tend to worry a lot, are overly dependent on others, are perfectionists, or expect too much from themselves and others.

Symptoms of Depression

To meet criteria for major depressive disorder, a person must meet at least five symptoms of depression for at least a two week period. Social, occupational, and other areas of functioning must be significantly impaired, or at least require increased effort. Depressed mood caused by substances (such as drugs, alcohol, or medications) or related to another medical condition is not considered to be major depressive disorder. Major depressive disorder also cannot be diagnosed if a person has a history of manic, hypomanic, or mixed episodes (e.g., bipolar disorder) or if the depressed mood is better accounted for by schizoaffective disorder.

Not all symptoms must be present for a person to be diagnosed with depression. Five (or more) of the following symptoms have to be present during the same 2-week period and represent a change from previous functioning. At least one of the symptoms must be either (1) depressed mood or (2) loss of interest or pleasure.

1. Depressed mood most of the day, nearly every day, as indicated by either subjective report (e.g., feels sad or empty) or observation made by others (e.g., appears tearful). In children and adolescents, this may be characterized as irritable mood rather than sad mood.

2. Markedly diminished interest or pleasure in all, or almost all, activities most of the day, nearly every day. This includes activities that were previously found enjoyable.

3. Significant weight loss when not dieting or weight gain (e.g., a change of more than 5% of body weight in a month), or a decrease or increase in appetite nearly every day.

4. Insomnia or hypersomnia nearly every day. The person may have difficulty falling asleep, staying asleep, or waking early in the morning and not being able to get back to sleep. Alternatively, the person may sleep excessively (such as over 12 hours per night) and spend much of the day in bed.

5. Psychomotor agitation (e.g., inability to sit still or pacing) or psychomotor retardation (e.g., slowed speech, thinking, and body movements) nearly every day. Changes in activity level are common in depression. The person may feel agitated, "on edge," and restless. Alternatively, they may experience decreased activity level reflected by slowness and lethargy, both in terms of the person's behavior and thought processes.

6. Fatigue or loss of energy nearly every day.

7. Feelings of worthlessness or excessive or inappropriate guilt nearly every day. Depressed people may feel they are worthless or that there is no hope for improving their lives. Feelings of guilt may be present about events with which the person had no involvement, such as a catastrophe, a crime, or an illness.

8. Diminished ability to think or concentrate, or indecisiveness, nearly every day. A significant decrease in the ability to concentrate makes it difficult to pay attention to others or contemplate simple tasks. The person may be quite indecisive about even minor things.

9. Recurrent thoughts of death (not just fear of dying), recurrent suicidal ideation without a specific plan, a specific plan for committing suicide, or a suicide attempt.

There are other psychiatric symptoms that depressed people often experience. They might complain of bodily aches and pains rather than feelings of sadness. They might report or exhibit persistent anger, angry outbursts, and an exaggerated sense of frustration over seemingly minor events. Symptoms of anxiety are also very common among people with depression. Other symptoms include hallucinations (false perceptions, such as hearing voices) and delusions (false beliefs, such as paranoid delusions). These symptoms usually disappear when the symptoms of depression have been controlled.

Common symptoms of depression include:

*   Depressed mood

*   Loss of interest/pleasure

- Change in appetite/weight
- Change in sleep, energy, and activity level
- Feelings of worthlessness, hopelessness, and helplessness
- Guilt
- Recurrent thoughts of death

Treatment

There are a variety of antidepressant medications and therapies available to those suffering from depression. Antidepressant medications help to stabilize mood. People can also learn to manage their symptoms with psychotherapy. People with a milder form of depression may benefit from psychotherapy alone, while those with more severe symptoms and episodes may benefit from antidepressants. A combination of both types of treatment is often most helpful to people. The treatments listed here are ones which research have shown to be effective for people with depression.

Medication

There are five different classes of antidepressant medications.

Cognitive Behavioral Therapy (CBT)

Cognitive behavioral therapy (CBT) is a well established treatment for people with depression. CBT is a blend of two therapies: cognitive therapy and behavioral therapy. Cognitive therapy focuses on a person's thoughts and beliefs, and how they influence a person's mood and actions, and aims to change a person's thinking to be more adaptive and healthy. Behavioral therapy focuses on a person's actions and aims to change unhealthy behavior patterns.

CBT helps a person focus on his or her current problems and how to solve them. Both patient and therapist need to be actively involved in this process. The therapist helps the patient learn how to identify and correct distorted thoughts or negative self-talk often associated with depressed feelings, recognize and change inaccurate beliefs, engage in more enjoyable activities, relate to self and others in more positive ways, learn problem-solving skills, and change behaviors. Another focus of CBT is behavioral activation (i.e., increasing activity levels and helping the patient take part in rewarding activities which can improve mood). CBT is a structured, weekly intervention. Weekly homework assignments help the individual apply the learned techniques.

Family Psychoeducation

Mental illness affects the whole family. Family treatment can play an important role to help both the person with depression and his or her relatives. Family psychoeducation is one way families can work together towards recovery. The family and clinician will meet together to discuss the problems they are experiencing. Families will then attend educational sessions where they will learn basic facts about mental illness, coping skills, communication skills, problem-solving skills, and ways to work together toward recovery.

Assertive Community Treatment (ACT)

Assertive community treatment (ACT) is an approach that is most effective with individuals with the greatest service needs, such as those with a history of multiple hospitalizations. In ACT, the person receives treatment from an interdisciplinary team of usually 10 to 12 professionals, including case managers, a psychiatrist, several nurses and social workers, vocational specialists, substance abuse treatment specialists, and peer specialists. The team provides coverage 24 hours a day, 7 days a week, and utilizes small caseloads, usually one staff for every 10 clients. Services provided include case management, comprehensive treatment planning, crisis intervention, medication management, individual supportive therapy, substance abuse treatment, rehabilitation services (i.e., supported employment), and peer support.

Electroconvulsive Therapy (ECT)

Electroconvulsive therapy (ECT) is a procedure used to treat severe or life-threatening depression. It is used when other treatments such as psychotherapy and antidepressant medications have not worked. Electrical currents are briefly sent to the brain through electrodes placed on the head. The electrical current can last up to 8 seconds, producing a short seizure. It is believed this brain stimulation helps relieve symptoms of depression by altering brain chemicals, including neurotransmitters like serotonin and natural pain relievers called endorphins. ECT treatments are usually done two to three times a week for two to three weeks. Maintenance treatments may be done one time each week, tapering down to one time each month. They may continue for several months to a year, to reduce the risk of relapse. eCT is usually given in combination with medication, psychotherapy, family therapy, and behavioral therapy.

The family environment is important to the recovery of people who are depressed. Even though depression can be a frustrating illness, family members can help the process of recovering from depression in many ways.

Chapter 8

Dysthymia: Chronic Depression

Persistent Depressive Disorder

Persistent depressive disorder (also called dysthymia) is a depressed mood that lasts for at least two years. A person diagnosed with persistent depressive disorder may have episodes of major depression along with periods of less severe symptoms, but symptoms must last for two years to be considered persistent depressive disorder.

Dysthymic Disorder among Children

Dysthymic disorder is characterized by chronic low-level depression. While the depression is not as severe as that characterizing major depressive disorder, a diagnosis of dysthymia requires having

This chapter contains text excerpted from the following sources: Text under the heading "Persistent Depressive Disorder" is excerpted from "Depression," National Institute of Mental Health (NIMH), October 2016; Text under the heading "Dysthymic Disorder among Children" is excerpted from "Dysthymic Disorder among Children," National Institute of Mental Health (NIMH), October 15, 2014; Text under the heading "Dysthymic Disorder among Adults," is excerpted from "Dysthymic Disorder among Adults," National Institute of Mental Health (NIMH), October 15, 2014; Text beginning with the heading "Diagnosis and Relation to Major Depression" is excerpted from "Management of Major Depressive Disorder (MDD)," U.S. Department of Veterans Affairs (VA), May 2009. Reviewed November 2016.

experienced a combination of depressive symptoms for two years or more.

The National Comorbidity Survey–Adolescent Supplement (NCS–A) examines both dysthymic disorder and major depressive disorder together. These depressive disorders have affected approximately 11.2 percent of 13 to 18 year olds in the United States at some point during their lives. Girls are more likely than boys to experience depressive disorders. Additionally, 3.3 percent of 13 to 18 year olds have experienced a seriously debilitating depressive disorder.

Dysthymic Disorder among Adults

Dysthymic disorder is characterized by chronic low-level depression. While the depression is not as severe as that characterizing major depressive disorder, a diagnosis of dysthymia requires having experienced a combination of depressive symptoms for two years or more. Dysthymic disorder affects approximately 1.5 percent of the adult population in the United States.

Diagnosis and Relation to Major Depression

Dysthymia is a chronic mood disorder. To be diagnosed with dysthymia, an individual must report at least a two-year period during which, for most days, the individual experiences depressed mood for more than half of the day, along with at least two of the following symptoms:

- Increased or decreased appetite
- Insomnia or hypersomnia
- Fatigue or low energy
- Poor self-image
- Reduced concentration or indecisiveness
- Hopelessness

Dysthymia is distinct from major depression due to the longer course (a minimum of two years as opposed to 2 weeks of symptoms) and lower severity (3 or more symptoms, most days, most of the time, versus 5 or more symptoms nearly every day). However, the two disorders are often difficult to distinguish in clinical settings. Some specific areas of differential diagnosis are chronic depression, double depression, and depression in partial remission. Depressive episodes lasting more than two years are defined as chronic depression. In this case, the higher severity of symptoms indicates a diagnosis of major depression rather than dysthymia. Double depression refers to comorbid diagnoses of both dysthymia and major depression. In this situation, a patient initially meets criteria for dysthymia (i.e., two years of symptoms that do not meet MDD criteria), and then develops an episode of major depression in the context of the dysthymic disorder.

For diagnostic purposes, a separate dysthymic disorder is not diagnosed if a patient initially experiences a depressive episode, and continues to experience subsyndromal symptoms following recovery, even if those symptoms last more than two years. In this case, a diagnosis of major depression in partial remission is appropriate.

Treatment of Dysthymia

There is limited evidence regarding treatment for dysthymia, and treatment studies of dysthymia often include other disorders as well (e.g., chronic depression, minor depression). Most studies have examined the same interventions that have been studied for major depression.

- Reviews of psychotherapy and pharmacotherapy indicate that there is good evidence that antidepressant medications are efficacious for reducing dysthymia, and there is some evidence that psychotherapy is beneficial as well, although it appears that the benefits of psychotherapy, and possibly pharmacotherapy, are lower than those found in treatment of major depression.

- Studies of combined pharmacotherapy and psychotherapy found that combined sertraline and interpersonal psychotherapy (IPT) was not superior to sertraline alone, and either medication was superior to IPT alone. A comparison of sertraline with or without group cognitive behavioral therapy (CBT) found some evidence that combined treatment may improve functioning over medication alone, but did not find group CBT alone superior to placebo. In the context of major depression, some studies suggest that combined treatment may lead to better treatment response for double depression. These results suggest that either medication or psychotherapy may be beneficial for patients with dysthymia, and combined treatment may be of value in patients with major depression and comorbid dysthymia. However, the variability in findings and limited number of studies prevent definitive conclusions.

- In contrast, a meta-analysis of later life major depression treatments found that in studies that included patients with either minor depression or dysthymia, psychotherapy had a greater effect than pharmacotherapy.

- In general, the course of dysthymia appears to be relatively stable, and individuals who recover from dysthymic episodes had a 71.4 percent likelihood of recurrence of some depressive disorder. Patients with a dysthymic disorder had a slower rate of symptom recovery over time, and had higher rates of depression after 10 years when compared to patients with nonchronic major depression.

Chapter 9

Atypical Depression

Atypical depression is a subtype of major depressive disorder. Although the name suggests otherwise, it is actually quite common. According to the *Diagnostic and Statistical Manual of Mental Disorders*, the main symptoms of atypical depression include moods that react strongly to environmental circumstances, overeating, oversleeping, and a sensation of heavy limbs or being weighed down. These symptoms contrast with—or are atypical of—the symptoms of another subtype, melancholic depression. Melancholic depression is usually characterized by a lack of mood reactivity, loss of appetite, insomnia, and a diminished ability to experience pleasure.

Causes and Symptoms

Researchers believe that depression, or dysthymic / persistent disorder, is caused by differences in brain circuits that transmit signal-carrying chemicals called neurotransmitters. These chemicals—such as dopamine, norepinephrine, and serotonin—help regulate mood. When the brain circuits are impaired or the chemical signals are abnormal, mood disorders can result. Although the exact cause of depression remains unknown, some of the known risk factors include a family history, a significant loss or traumatic life event, interpersonal conflicts, social isolation, or serious illness.

People with common depression often feel sad, hopeless, dejected, and unable to enjoy themselves. In people with melancholic depression, these feelings are persistent and do not change in response to

---

"Atypical Depression," © 2017 Omnigraphics. Reviewed November 2016.

environmental circumstances. People with atypical depression, on the other hand, usually experience significant changes in mood in response to pleasurable experiences or positive events. In addition to mood reactivity, the diagnostic criteria for atypical depression requires patients to present at least two of the following symptoms:

- increased appetite, overeating (hyperphagia), or significant weight gain

- excessive fatigue, sleepiness, or hypersomnia (sleeping more than ten hours per day)

- a sensation of weakness, heaviness, or being weighed down (leaden paralysis)

- extreme sensitivity to interpersonal rejection that affects workplace and social relationships

The risk of atypical depression is two times higher in women than in men. People with bipolar disorder and seasonal affective disorder are also more likely to experience atypical depression symptoms. On average, it tends to have an earlier onset than melancholic depression, and it is also associated with an increased risk of anxiety disorders and suicidal ideation.

Diagnosis and Treatment

The first step in diagnosing atypical depression involves a complete medical examination to determine whether the patient's symptoms may have a physical cause. Hypothyroidism, for instance, may cause symptoms such as mood changes, fatigue, and weight gain due to low levels of thyroid hormones. If a physical examination and blood tests fail to reveal an underlying health condition, the doctor may recommend a psychological evaluation. A mental health professional will typically ask questions about the patient's symptoms, recent experiences, feelings, and behavior patterns and compare that information to the diagnostic criteria for atypical depression.

The treatment for atypical depression usually involves a combination of psychotherapy (talk therapy) and medications. Both treatment methods have proven to be effective, depending on the patient's condition and symptoms. Psychotherapy involves meeting with a mental health professional to identify unhealthy thoughts or behaviors, explore problematic relationships and experiences, and develop new coping and problem-solving methods.

A number of prescription medications have also proven effective in treating atypical depression. These antidepressant medications work by improving the function of brain circuits and neurotransmitters that help regulate mood. Research suggests that many patients with atypical depression respond well to monoamine oxidase inhibitors (MAOIs), whereas fewer patients experience good results with tricyclic antidepressants. All patients are different, however, so it may be necessary to try several different types or combinations of medications to find the option that works best.

References

1. "Atypical Depression," WebMD, 2016.

2. Lieber, Arnold. "Atypical Depression: An Overview of Depression with Atypical Symptoms," PsyCom, n.d.

3. Moran, Mark. "Atypical Depression: What's in a Name?" Psychiatric News, October 17, 2003.

Chapter 10

Bipolar Disorder (Manic-Depressive Illness)

Chapter Contents

Section 10.1

What Is Bipolar Disorder?

This section includes text excerpted from "Bipolar Disorder,"
National Institute of Mental Health (NIMH), April 2016.

Definition

Bipolar disorder, also known as manic-depressive illness, is a brain disorder that causes unusual shifts in mood, energy, activity levels, and the ability to carry out day-to-day tasks.

There are four basic types of bipolar disorder; all of them involve clear changes in mood, energy, and activity levels. These moods range from periods of extremely "up," elated, and energized behavior (known as manic episodes) to very sad, "down," or hopeless periods (known as depressive episodes). Less severe manic periods are known as hypomanic episodes.

- **Bipolar I Disorder:** Defined by manic episodes that last at least 7 days, or by manic symptoms that are so severe that the person needs immediate hospital care. Usually, depressive episodes occur as well, typically lasting at least 2 weeks. Episodes of depression with mixed features (having depression and manic symptoms at the same time) are also possible.

- **Bipolar II Disorder:** Defined by a pattern of depressive episodes and hypomanic episodes, but not the full-blown manic episodes described above.

- **Cyclothymic Disorder (also called cyclothymia):** Defined by numerous periods of hypomanic symptoms as well numerous periods of depressive symptoms lasting for at least 2 years (1 year in children and adolescents). However, the symptoms do not meet the diagnostic requirements for a hypomanic episode and a depressive episode.

- **Other Specified and Unspecified Bipolar and Related Disorders:** Defined by bipolar disorder symptoms that do not match the three categories listed above.

Signs and Symptoms

People with bipolar disorder experience periods of unusually intense emotion, changes in sleep patterns and activity levels, and unusual behaviors. These distinct periods are called "mood episodes." Mood episodes are drastically different from the moods and behaviors that are typical for the person. Extreme changes in energy, activity, and sleep go along with mood episodes.

Sometimes a mood episode includes symptoms of both manic and depressive symptoms. This is called an episode with mixed features. People experiencing an episode with mixed features may feel very sad, empty, or hopeless, while at the same time feeling extremely energized.

Bipolar disorder can be present even when mood swings are less extreme. For example, some people with bipolar disorder experience hypomania, a less severe form of mania. During a hypomanic episode, an individual may feel very good, be highly productive, and function well. The person may not feel that anything is wrong, but family and friends may recognize the mood swings and/or changes in activity levels as possible bipolar disorder. Without proper treatment, people with hypomania may develop severe mania or depression.

People having a manic episode may:

- feel very "up," "high," or elated
- have a lot of energy
- have increased activity levels
- feel "jumpy" or "wired"
- have trouble sleeping
- become more active than usual
- talk really fast about a lot of different things
- be agitated, irritable, or "touchy"
- teel like their thoughts are going very fast
- think they can do a lot of things at once
- do risky things, like spend a lot of money or have reckless sex

People having a depressive episode may:

- feel very sad, down, empty, or hopeless
- have very little energy

- have decreased activity levels

- have trouble sleeping, they may sleep too little or too much

- feel like they can't enjoy anything

- feel worried and empty

- have trouble concentrating

- forget things a lot

- eat too much or too little

- feel tired or "slowed down"

- think about death or suicide

Bipolar Disorder and Other Illnesses

Some bipolar disorder symptoms are similar to other illnesses, which can make it hard for a doctor to make a diagnosis. In addition, many people have bipolar disorder along with another illness such as anxiety disorder, substance abuse, or an eating disorder. People with bipolar disorder are also at higher risk for thyroid disease, migraine headaches, heart disease, diabetes, obesity, and other physical illnesses.

Psychosis: Sometimes, a person with severe episodes of mania or depression also has psychotic symptoms, such as hallucinations or delusions. The psychotic symptoms tend to match the person's extreme mood. For example:

- Someone having psychotic symptoms during a manic episode may believe she is famous, has a lot of money, or has special powers.

- Someone having psychotic symptoms during a depressive episode may believe he is ruined and penniless, or that he has committed a crime.

As a result, people with bipolar disorder who also have psychotic symptoms are sometimes misdiagnosed with schizophrenia.

Anxiety and ADHD: Anxiety disorders and attention-deficit hyperactivity disorder (ADHD) are often diagnosed among people with bipolar disorder.

Substance Abuse: People with bipolar disorder may also misuse alcohol or drugs, have relationship problems, or perform poorly in school or at work. Family, friends and people experiencing symptoms may not recognize these problems as signs of a major mental illness such as bipolar disorder.

Risk Factors

Scientists are studying the possible causes of bipolar disorder. Most agree that there is no single cause. Instead, it is likely that many factors contribute to the illness or increase risk.

Brain Structure and Functioning: Some studies show how the brains of people with bipolar disorder may differ from the brains of healthy people or people with other mental disorders. Learning more about these differences, along with new information from genetic studies, helps scientists better understand bipolar disorder and predict which types of treatment will work most effectively.

Genetics: Some research suggests that people with certain genes are more likely to develop bipolar disorder than others. But genes are not the only risk factor for bipolar disorder. Studies of identical twins have shown that even if one twin develops bipolar disorder, the other twin does not always develop the disorder, despite the fact that identical twins share all of the same genes.

Family History: Bipolar disorder tends to run in families. Children with a parent or sibling who has bipolar disorder are much more likely to develop the illness, compared with children who do not have a family history of the disorder. However, it is important to note that most people with a family history of bipolar disorder will not develop the illness.

Section 10.2

Bipolar Disorder in Children and Teens

This section includes text excerpted from "Bipolar
Disorder in Children and Teen," National Institute of
Mental Health (NIMH), 2015.

Does your child go through intense mood changes? Does your child
have extreme behavior changes? Does your child get much more excited
and active than other kids his or her age? Do other people say your
child is too excited or too moody? Do you notice he or she has highs
and lows much more often than other children? Do these mood changes
affect how your child acts at school or at home?

Some children and teens with these symptoms may have bipolar
disorder, a serious mental illness.

What Is Bipolar Disorder?

Bipolar disorder is a serious brain illness. It is also called manic-depressive illness or manic depression. Children with bipolar
disorder go through unusual mood changes. Sometimes they feel
very happy or "up," and are much more energetic and active than
usual, or than other kids their age. This is called a manic episode.
Sometimes children with bipolar disorder feel very sad and "down,"
and are much less active than usual. This is called depression or a
depressive episode.

Bipolar disorder is not the same as the normal ups and downs every
kid goes through. Bipolar symptoms are more powerful than that. The
mood swings are more extreme and are accompanied by changes in
sleep, energy level, and the ability to think clearly. Bipolar symptoms
are so strong, they can make it hard for a child to do well in school
or get along with friends and family members. The illness can also
be dangerous. Some young people with bipolar disorder try to hurt
themselves or attempt suicide.

Children and teens with bipolar disorder should get treatment.
With help, they can manage their symptoms and lead successful
lives.

Who Develops Bipolar Disorder?

Anyone can develop bipolar disorder, including children and teens. However, most people with bipolar disorder develop it in their late teen or early adult years. The illness usually lasts a lifetime.

Why Does Someone Develop Bipolar Disorder?

Doctors do not know what causes bipolar disorder, but several things may contribute to the illness. Family genes may be one factor because bipolar disorder sometimes runs in families. However, it is important to know that just because someone in your family has bipolar disorder, it does not mean other members of the family will have it as well.

Another factor that may lead to bipolar disorder is the brain structure or the brain function of the person with the disorder. Scientists are finding out more about the disorder by studying it. This research may help doctors do a better job of treating people. Also, this research may help doctors to predict whether a person will get bipolar disorder. One day, doctors may be able to prevent the illness in some people.

What Are the Symptoms of Bipolar Disorder?

Bipolar "mood episodes" include unusual mood changes along with unusual sleep habits, activity levels, thoughts, or behavior. In a child, these mood and activity changes must be very different from their usual behavior and from the behavior of other children. A person with bipolar disorder may have manic episodes, depressive episodes, or "mixed" episodes. A mixed episode has both manic and depressive symptoms. These mood episodes cause symptoms that last a week or two or sometimes longer. During an episode, the symptoms last every day for most of the day.

Children and teens having a manic episode may:

- Feel very happy or act silly in a way that's unusual for them and for other people their age
- Have a very short temper
- Talk really fast about a lot of different things
- Have trouble sleeping but not feel tired
- Have trouble staying focused

- Talk and think about sex more often
- Do risky things

Children and teens having a depressive episode may:

- Feel very sad
- Complain about pain a lot, such as stomachaches and headaches
- Sleep too little or too much
- Feel guilty and worthless
- Eat too little or too much
- Have little energy and no interest in fun activities
- Think about death or suicide

How Is Bipolar Disorder Diagnosed?

An experienced doctor will carefully examine your child. There are no blood tests or brain scans that can diagnose bipolar disorder. Instead, the doctor will ask questions about your child's mood and sleeping patterns. The doctor will also ask about your child's energy and behavior. Sometimes doctors need to know about medical problems in your family, such as depression or alcoholism. The doctor may use tests to see if something other than bipolar disorder is causing your child's symptoms.

Can Children and Teens with Bipolar Disorder Have Other Problems?

Young people with bipolar disorder can have several problems at the same time. These include:

- **Substance abuse.** Both adults and kids with bipolar disorder are at risk of drinking or taking drugs.
- **Attention deficit hyperactivity disorder (ADHD).** Children who have both bipolar disorder and ADHD may have trouble staying focused.
- **Anxiety disorders,** like separation anxiety.

Sometimes behavior problems go along with mood episodes. Young people may take a lot of risks, such as driving too fast or spending too much money. Some young people with bipolar disorder think about suicide. Watch for any signs of suicidal thinking. Take these signs seriously and call your child's doctor.

How Can I Help My Child or Teen?

Help begins with the right diagnosis and treatment. If you think your child may have bipolar disorder, make an appointment with your family doctor to talk about the symptoms you notice.

If your child has bipolar disorder, here are some basic things you can do:

- Be patient.
- Encourage your child to talk, and listen to your child carefully.
- Be understanding about mood episodes.
- Help your child have fun.
- Help your child understand that treatment can make life better.

How Does Bipolar Disorder Affect Parents and Family?

Taking care of a child or teenager with bipolar disorder can be stressful for you, too. You have to cope with the mood swings and other problems, such as short tempers and risky activities. This can challenge any parent. Sometimes the stress can strain your relationships with other people, and you may miss work or lose free time.

If you are taking care of a child with bipolar disorder, take care of yourself too. Find someone you can talk to about your feelings. Talk with the doctor about support groups for caregivers. If you keep your stress level down, you will do a better job. It might help your child get better too.

Where Do I Go for Help?

If you're not sure where to get help, call your family doctor. You can also check the phone book for mental health professionals. Hospital doctors can help in an emergency.

I Know Someone Who Is in Crisis. What Do I Do?

If you know someone who might be thinking about hurting himself or herself or someone else, get help quickly.

- Do not leave the person alone.

- Call your doctor.

- Call 911 or go to the emergency room.

- Call National Suicide Prevention Lifeline, toll-free: 1-800-273-TALK (8255). The TTY number is 1-800-799-4TTY (4889).

Chapter 11

Premenstrual Syndrome

What Is Premenstrual Syndrome (PMS)?

Premenstrual syndrome (PMS) is a group of symptoms linked to the menstrual cycle. PMS symptoms occur 1 to 2 weeks before your period (menstruation or monthly bleeding) starts. The symptoms usually go away after you start bleeding. PMS can affect menstruating women of any age and the effect is different for each woman. For some people, PMS is just a monthly bother. For others, it may be so severe that it makes it hard to even get through the day. PMS goes away when your monthly periods stop, such as when you get pregnant or go through menopause.

What Causes PMS?

The causes of PMS are not clear, but several factors may be involved. Changes in hormones during the menstrual cycle seem to be an important cause. These changing hormone levels may affect some women more than others. Chemical changes in the brain may also be involved. Stress and emotional problems, such as depression, do not seem to cause PMS, but they may make it worse. Some other possible causes include:

- low levels of vitamins and minerals

This chapter includes text excerpted from "Premenstrual Syndrome (PMS) Fact Sheet," Office on Women's Health (OWH), U.S. Department of Health and Human Services (HHS), December 23, 2014.

- eating a lot of salty foods, which may cause you to retain (keep) fluid

- drinking alcohol and caffeine, which may alter your mood and energy level

What Are the Symptoms of PMS?

PMS often includes both physical and emotional symptoms, such as:

- Acne

- Swollen or tender breasts

- Feeling tired

- Trouble sleeping

- Upset stomach, bloating, constipation, or diarrhea

- Headache or backache

- Appetite changes or food cravings

- Joint or muscle pain

- Trouble with concentration or memory

- Tension, irritability, mood swings, or crying spells

- Anxiety or depression
  Symptoms vary from woman to woman.

How Do I Know If I Have PMS?

Your doctor may diagnose PMS based on which symptoms you have, when they occur, and how much they affect your life. If you think you have PMS, keep track of which symptoms you have and how severe they are for a few months. Record your symptoms each day on a calendar or PMS symptom tracker. Take this form with you when you see your doctor about your PMS.

Your doctor will also want to make sure you don't have one of the following conditions that shares symptoms with PMS:

- Depression

- Anxiety

- Menopause

- Chronic fatigue syndrome (CFS)

- Irritable bowel syndrome (IBS)
- Problems with the endocrine system, which makes hormones

How Common Is PMS?

There's a wide range of estimates of how many women suffer from PMS. The American College of Obstetricians and Gynecologists (ACOG) estimates that at least 85 percent of menstruating women have at least 1 PMS symptom as part of their monthly cycle. Most of these women have fairly mild symptoms that don't need treatment. Others (about 3 to 8 percent) have a more severe form of PMS, called premenstrual dysphoric disorder (PMDD).

PMS occurs more often in women who:

- are between their late 20s and early 40s
- have at least 1 child
- have a family history of depression
- have a past medical history of either postpartum depression or a mood disorder

What Is Premenstrual Dysphoric Disorder (PMDD)?

A brain chemical called serotonin may play a role in Premenstrual Dysphoric Disorder (PMDD), a severe form of PMS. The main symptoms, which can be disabling, include:

- feelings of sadness or despair, or even thoughts of suicide
- feelings of tension or anxiety
- panic attacks
- mood swings or frequent crying
- lasting irritability or anger that affects other people
- lack of interest in daily activities and relationships
- trouble thinking or focusing
- tiredness or low energy
- food cravings or binge eating
- trouble sleeping

- feeling out of control

- physical symptoms, such as bloating, breast tenderness, head-aches, and joint or muscle pain

You must have 5 or more of these symptoms to be diagnosed with PMDD. Symptoms occur during the week before your period and go away after bleeding starts.

Chapter 12

Psychotic Depression

Chapter Contents

Section 12.1

Psychosis

This section includes text excerpted from "Recovery After an Initial Schizophrenia Episode (RAISE)," National Institute of Mental Health (NIMH), October 7, 2015.

What Is Psychosis?

The word *psychosis* is used to describe conditions that affect the mind, where there has been some loss of contact with reality. When someone becomes ill in this way it is called a psychotic episode. During a period of psychosis, a person's thoughts and perceptions are disturbed and the individual may have difficulty understanding what is real and what is not. Symptoms of psychosis include delusions (false beliefs) and hallucinations (seeing or hearing things that others do not see or hear). Other symptoms include incoherent or nonsense speech, and behavior that is inappropriate for the situation. A person in a psychotic episode may also experience depression, anxiety, sleep problems, social withdrawal, lack of motivation and difficulty functioning overall.

What Causes Psychosis?

There is not one specific cause of psychosis. Psychosis may be a symptom of a mental illness, such as schizophrenia or bipolar disorder, but there are other causes, as well. Sleep deprivation, some general medical conditions, certain prescription medications, and the abuse of alcohol or other drugs, such as marijuana, can cause psychotic symptoms. Because there are many different causes of psychosis, it is important to see a qualified healthcare professional (e.g., psychologist, psychiatrist, or trained social worker) in order to receive a thorough assessment and accurate diagnosis. A mental illness, such as schizophrenia, is typically diagnosed by excluding all of these other causes of psychosis.

How Common Is Psychosis?

Approximately 3 percent of the people in the United States (3 out of 100 people) will experience psychosis at some time in their lives. About

100,000 adolescents and young adults in the United States experience first episode psychosis each year.

What Is the Connection between Psychosis and Schizophrenia?

Schizophrenia is a mental illness characterized by periods of psychosis. An individual must experience psychotic symptoms for at least six months in order to be diagnosed with schizophrenia. However, a person may experience psychosis and never be diagnosed with schizophrenia, or any other mental health condition. This is because there are many different causes of psychosis, such as sleep deprivation, general medical conditions, the use of certain prescription medications, and the abuse of alcohol or other drugs.

What Are the Early Warning Signs of Psychosis?

Typically, a person will show changes in their behavior before psychosis develops. The list below includes behavioral warning signs for psychosis.

- Worrisome drop in grades or job performance
- New trouble thinking clearly or concentrating
- Suspiciousness, paranoid ideas or uneasiness with others
- Withdrawing socially, spending a lot more time alone than usual
- Unusual, overly intense new ideas, strange feelings or having no feelings at all
- Decline in self-care or personal hygiene
- Difficulty telling reality from fantasy
- Confused speech or trouble communicating

Any one of these items by itself may not be significant, but someone with several of the items on the list should consult a mental health professional. A qualified psychologist, psychiatrist or trained social worker will be able to make a diagnosis and help develop a treatment plan. Early treatment of psychosis increases the chance of a successful recovery. If you notice these changes in behavior and they begin to intensify or do not go away, it is important to seek help.

What Does "Duration of Untreated Psychosis" Mean?

The length of time between the start of psychotic symptoms and the beginning of treatment is called the duration of untreated psychosis or DUP. In general, research has shown that treatments for psychosis work better when they are delivered closer to the time when symptoms first appear. This was the case in the RAISE-ETP study. Individuals who had a shorter DUP when they started treatment showed much greater improvement in symptoms, functioning, and quality of life than those with longer DUP. The RAISE-ETP project also found that average DUP in the United States is typically longer than what is considered acceptable by international standards. Future RAISE-related efforts are working to find ways of decreasing DUP so that individuals receive care as early as possible after symptoms appear.

Do People Recover from Psychosis?

With early diagnosis and appropriate treatment, it is possible to recover from psychosis. Many people who receive early treatment never have another psychotic episode. For other people, recovery means the ability to live a fulfilling and productive life, even if psychotic symptoms return sometimes.

What Should I Do If I Think Someone Is Having a Psychotic Episode?

If you think someone you know is experiencing psychosis, encourage the person to seek treatment as early as possible. Psychosis can be treated effectively, and early intervention increases the chance of a successful outcome. To find a qualified treatment program, contact your healthcare professional. If someone having a psychotic episode is in distress or you are concerned about their safety, consider taking them to the nearest emergency room, or calling 911.

Section 12.2

Schizophrenia

This section includes text excerpted from "Schizophrenia," National
Institute of Mental Health (NIMH), December 4, 2015.

What Is Schizophrenia?

Schizophrenia is a chronic and severe disorder that affects how a
person thinks, feels, and acts. Although schizophrenia is not as common as other mental disorders, it can be very disabling. Approximately
7 or 8 individuals out of 1,000 will have schizophrenia in their lifetime.

People with the disorder may hear voices or see things that aren't
there. They may believe other people are reading their minds, controlling their thoughts, or plotting to harm them. This can be scary
and upsetting to people with the illness and make them withdrawn
or extremely agitated. It can also be scary and upsetting to the people
around them.

People with schizophrenia may sometimes talk about strange or
unusual ideas, which can make it difficult to carry on a conversation.
They may sit for hours without moving or talking. Sometimes people
with schizophrenia seem perfectly fine until they talk about what they
are really thinking.

Families and society are impacted by schizophrenia too. Many people with schizophrenia have difficulty holding a job or caring for themselves, so they may rely on others for help. Stigmatizing attitudes and
beliefs about schizophrenia are common and sometimes interfere with
people's willingness to talk about and get treatment for the disorder.

People with schizophrenia may cope with symptoms throughout
their lives, but treatment helps many to recover and pursue their life
goals. Researchers are developing more effective treatments and using
new research tools to understand the causes of schizophrenia. In the
years to come, this work may help prevent and better treat the illness.

What Are the Symptoms of Schizophrenia?

The symptoms of schizophrenia fall into three broad categories:
positive, negative, and cognitive symptoms.

Positive Symptoms

Positive symptoms are psychotic behaviors not generally seen in healthy people. People with positive symptoms may "lose touch" with some aspects of reality. For some people, these symptoms come and go. For others, they stay stable over time. Sometimes they are severe, and at other times hardly noticeable. The severity of positive symptoms may depend on whether the individual is receiving treatment. Positive symptoms include the following:

Hallucinations are sensory experiences that occur in the absence of a stimulus. These can occur in any of the five senses (vision, hearing, smell, taste, or touch). "Voices" (auditory hallucinations) are the most common type of hallucination in schizophrenia. Many people with the disorder hear voices. The voices can either be internal, seeming to come from within one's own mind, or they can be external, in which case they can seem to be as real as another person speaking. The voices may talk to the person about his or her behavior, command the person to do things, or warn the person of danger. Sometimes the voices talk to each other, and sometimes people with schizophrenia talk to the voices that they hear. People with schizophrenia may hear voices for a long time before family and friends notice the problem.

Other types of hallucinations include seeing people or objects that are not there, smelling odors that no one else detects, and feeling things like invisible fingers touching their bodies when no one is near.

Delusions are strongly held false beliefs that are not consistent with the person's culture. Delusions persist even when there is evidence that the beliefs are not true or logical. People with schizophrenia can have delusions that seem bizarre, such as believing that neighbors can control their behavior with magnetic waves. They may also believe that people on television are directing special messages to them, or that radio stations are broadcasting their thoughts aloud to others. These are called "delusions of reference."

Sometimes they believe they are someone else, such as a famous historical figure. They may have paranoid delusions and believe that others are trying to harm them, such as by cheating, harassing, poisoning, spying on, or plotting against them or the people they care about. These beliefs are called "persecutory delusions."

Thought disorders are unusual or dysfunctional ways of thinking. One form is called "disorganized thinking." This is when a person has trouble organizing his or her thoughts or connecting them logically. He or she may talk in a garbled way that is hard to understand. This is often called "word salad." Another form is called "thought blocking." This is when a person stops speaking abruptly in the middle of a thought. When asked why he or she stopped talking, the person may say that it felt as if the thought had been taken out of his or her head. Finally, a person with a thought disorder might make up meaningless words, or "neologisms."

Movement disorders may appear as agitated body movements. A person with a movement disorder may repeat certain motions over and over. In the other extreme, a person may become catatonic. Catatonia is a state in which a person does not move and does not respond to others. Catatonia is rare today, but it was more common when treatment for schizophrenia was not available.

Negative Symptoms

Negative symptoms are associated with disruptions to normal emotions and behaviors. These symptoms are harder to recognize as part of the disorder and can be mistaken for depression or other conditions. These symptoms include the following:

- "Flat affect" (reduced expression of emotions via facial expression or voice tone)
- Reduced feelings of pleasure in everyday life
- Difficulty beginning and sustaining activities
- Reduced speaking

People with negative symptoms may need help with everyday tasks. They may neglect basic personal hygiene. This may make them seem lazy or unwilling to help themselves, but the problems are symptoms caused by schizophrenia.

Cognitive Symptoms

For some people, the cognitive symptoms of schizophrenia are subtle, but for others, they are more severe and patients may notice changes in their memory or other aspects of thinking. Similar to negative symptoms, cognitive symptoms may be difficult to recognize as part of the disorder. Often, they are detected only when specific tests are performed. Cognitive symptoms include the following:

- poor "executive functioning" (the ability to understand information and use it to make decisions)

- trouble focusing or paying attention

- problems with "working memory" (the ability to use information immediately after learning it)

Poor cognition is related to worse employment and social outcomes and can be distressing to individuals with schizophrenia.

When Does Schizophrenia Start, and Who Gets It?

Schizophrenia affects slightly more males than females. It occurs in all ethnic groups around the world. Symptoms such as hallucinations and delusions usually start between ages 16 and 30. Males tend to experience symptoms a little earlier than females. Most commonly, schizophrenia occurs in late adolescence and early adulthood. It is uncommon to be diagnosed with schizophrenia after age 45. Schizophrenia rarely occurs in children, but awareness of childhood-onset schizophrenia is increasing.

It can be difficult to diagnose schizophrenia in teens. This is because the first signs can include a change of friends, a drop in grades, sleep problems, and irritability—behaviors that are common among teens. A combination of factors can predict schizophrenia in up to 80 percent of youth who are at high risk of developing the illness. These factors include isolating oneself and withdrawing from others, an increase in unusual thoughts and suspicions, and a family history of psychosis. This pre-psychotic stage of the disorder is called the "prodromal" period.

Are People with Schizophrenia Violent?

Most people with schizophrenia are not violent. In fact, most violent crimes are not committed by people with schizophrenia. People with schizophrenia are much more likely to harm themselves than others. Substance abuse may increase the chance a person will become violent. The risk of violence is greatest when psychosis is untreated and decreases substantially when treatment is in place.

Schizophrenia and Suicide

Suicidal thoughts and behaviors are very common among people with schizophrenia. People with schizophrenia die earlier than people without a mental illness, partly because of the increased suicide risk.

It is hard to predict which people with schizophrenia are more likely to die by suicide, but actively treating any co-existing depressive symptoms and substance abuse may reduce suicide risk. People who take their antipsychotic medications as prescribed are less likely to attempt suicide than those who do not. If someone you know is talking about or has attempted suicide, help him or her find professional help right away or call 911.

Schizophrenia and Substance Use Disorders

Substance use disorders occur when frequent use of alcohol and/or drugs interferes with a person's health, family, work, school, and social life. Substance use is the most common co-occurring disorder in people with schizophrenia, and the complex relationships between substance use disorders and schizophrenia have been extensively studied. Substance use disorders can make treatment for schizophrenia less effective, and individuals are also less likely to engage in treatment for their mental illness if they are abusing substances. It is commonly believed that people with schizophrenia who also abuse substances are trying to "self-medicate" their symptoms, but there is little evidence that people begin to abuse substances in response to symptoms or that abusing substances reduces symptoms.

Nicotine is the most common drug abused by people with schizophrenia. People with schizophrenia are much more likely to smoke than people without a mental illness, and researchers are exploring whether there is a biological basis for this. There is some evidence that nicotine may temporarily alleviate a subset of the cognitive deficits commonly observed in schizophrenia, but these benefits are outweighed by the detrimental effects of smoking on other aspects of cognition and general health. Bupropion has been found to be effective for smoking cessation in people with schizophrenia. Most studies find that reducing or stopping smoking does not make schizophrenia symptoms worse.

Cannabis (marijuana) is also frequently abused by people with schizophrenia, which can worsen health outcomes. Heavy cannabis use is associated with more severe and earlier onset of schizophrenia symptoms, but research has not yet definitively determined whether cannabis directly causes schizophrenia. Drug abuse can increase rates of other medical illnesses (such as hepatitis, heart disease, and infectious disease) as well as suicide, trauma, and homelessness in people with schizophrenia.

It is generally understood that schizophrenia and substance use disorders have strong genetic risk factors. While substance use disorder and a family history of psychosis have individually been identified as risk factors for schizophrenia, it is less well understood if and how these factors are related. When people have both schizophrenia and a substance abuse disorder, their best chance for recovery is a treatment program that integrates the schizophrenia and substance abuse treatment.

What Causes Schizophrenia?

Research has identified several factors that contribute to the risk of developing schizophrenia.

Genes and Environment

Scientists have long known that schizophrenia sometimes runs in families. The illness occurs in less than 1 percent of the general population, but it occurs in 10 percent of people who have a first-degree relative with the disorder, such as a parent, brother, or sister. People who have second-degree relatives (aunts, uncles, grandparents, or cousins) with the disease also develop schizophrenia more often than the general population. The risk is highest for an identical twin of a person with schizophrenia. He or she has a 40 to 65 percent chance of developing the disorder. Although these genetic relationships are strong, there are many people who have schizophrenia who don't have a family member with the disorder and, conversely, many people with one or more family members with the disorder who do not develop it themselves.

Scientists believe that many different genes contribute to an increased risk of schizophrenia, but that no single gene causes the disorder by itself. In fact, recent research has found that people with schizophrenia tend to have higher rates of rare genetic mutations. These genetic differences involve hundreds of different genes and probably disrupt brain development in diverse and subtle ways.

Research into various genes that are related to schizophrenia is ongoing, so it is not yet possible to use genetic information to predict who will develop the disease. Despite this, tests that scan a person's genes can be bought without a prescription or a health professional's advice. Ads for the tests suggest that with a saliva sample, a company can determine if a client is at risk for developing specific diseases, including schizophrenia. However, scientists don't yet know all of the gene variations that contribute to schizophrenia and those that are known raise the risk only by very small amounts. Therefore, these "genome scans" are unlikely to provide a complete picture of a person's risk for developing a mental disorder like schizophrenia.

In addition, it certainly takes more than genes to cause the disorder. Scientists think that interactions between genes and aspects of the individual's environment are necessary for schizophrenia to develop. Many environmental factors may be involved, such as exposure to viruses or malnutrition before birth, problems during birth, and other, not yet known, psychosocial factors.

Different Brain Chemistry and Structure

Scientists think that an imbalance in the complex, interrelated chemical reactions of the brain involving the neurotransmitters dopamine and glutamate, and possibly others, plays a role in schizophrenia. Neurotransmitters are substances that brain cells use to communicate with each other. Scientists are learning more about how brain chemistry is related to schizophrenia.

Also, the brain structures of some people with schizophrenia are slightly different than those of healthy people. For example, fluid-filled cavities at the center of the brain, called ventricles, are larger in some people with schizophrenia. The brains of people with the illness also tend to have less gray matter, and some areas of the brain may have less or more activity.

These differences are observed when brain scans from a group of people with schizophrenia are compared with those from a group of people without schizophrenia. However, the differences are not large enough to identify individuals with the disorder and are not currently used to diagnose schizophrenia.

Studies of brain tissue after death also have revealed differences in the brains of people with schizophrenia. Scientists have found small changes in the location or structure of brain cells that are formed before birth. Some experts think problems during brain development before birth may lead to faulty connections. The problem may not show up in a person until puberty. The brain undergoes major changes during puberty, and these changes could trigger psychotic symptoms in people who are vulnerable due to genetics or brain differences. Scientists have learned a lot about schizophrenia, but more research is needed to help explain how it develops.

How Can You Help a Person with Schizophrenia?

Family and friends can help their loved one with schizophrenia by supporting their engagement in treatment and pursuit of their recovery goals. Positive communication approaches will be most helpful. It can be difficult to know how to respond to someone with schizophrenia who makes strange or clearly false statements. Remember that these beliefs or hallucinations seem very real to the person. It is not helpful to say they are wrong or imaginary. But going along with the delusions is not helpful, either. Instead, calmly say that you see things differently. Tell them that you acknowledge that everyone has the right to see things his or her own way. In addition, it is important to understand that schizophrenia is a biological illness. Being respectful, supportive, and kind without tolerating dangerous or inappropriate behavior is the best way to approach people with this disorder.

Chapter 13

Seasonal Affective Disorder (SAD)

What Is Seasonal Affective Disorder (SAD)?

Seasonal affective disorder (SAD) is a type of depression that comes and goes with the seasons, typically starting in the late fall and early winter and going away during the spring and summer. Depressive episodes linked to the summer can occur, but are much less common than winter episodes of SAD.

Signs and Symptoms

Seasonal affective disorder (SAD) is not considered as a separate disorder. It is a type of depression displaying a recurring seasonal pattern. To be diagnosed with SAD, people must meet full criteria for major depression coinciding with specific seasons (appearing in the winter or summer months) for at least 2 years. Seasonal depressions must be much more frequent than any non-seasonal depressions.

Symptoms of major depression include:

- Feeling depressed most of the day, nearly every day

- Feeling hopeless or worthless

This chapter includes text excerpted from "Seasonal Affective Disorder," National Institute of Mental Health (NIMH), March 2016.

- Having low energy
- Losing interest in activities you once enjoyed
- Having problems with sleep
- Experiencing changes in your appetite or weight
- Feeling sluggish or agitated
- Having difficulty concentrating
- Having frequent thoughts of death or suicide

Symptoms of the winter pattern of SAD include:

- Having low energy
- Hypersomnia
- Overeating
- Weight gain
- Craving for carbohydrates
- Social withdrawal (feel like "hibernating")

Symptoms of the less frequently occurring summer seasonal affective disorder include:

- Poor appetite with associated weight loss
- Insomnia
- Agitation
- Restlessness
- Anxiety
- Episodes of violent behavior

Risk Factors

Attributes that may increase your risk of SAD include:

- **Being female.** SAD is diagnosed four times more often in women than men.
- **Living far from the equator.** SAD is more frequent in people who live far north or south of the equator. For example, 1 percent of those who live in Florida and 9 percent of those who live in New England or Alaska suffer from SAD.

- **Family history.** People with a family history of other types of depression are more likely to develop SAD than people who do not have a family history of depression.

- **Having depression or bipolar disorder.** The symptoms of depression may worsen with the seasons if you have one of these conditions (but SAD is diagnosed only if seasonal depressions are the most common).

- **Younger Age.** Younger adults have a higher risk of SAD than older adults. SAD has been reported even in children and teens.

The causes of SAD are unknown, but research has found some biological clues:

- People with SAD may have trouble regulating one of the key neurotransmitters involved in mood, serotonin. One study found that people with SAD have 5 percent more serotonin transporter protein in winter months than summer months. Higher serotonin transporter protein leaves less serotonin available at the synapse because the function of the transporter is to recycle neurotransmitter back into the pre-synaptic neuron.

- People with SAD may overproduce the hormone melatonin. Darkness increases production of melatonin, which regulates sleep. As winter days become shorter, melatonin production increases, leaving people with SAD to feel sleepier and more lethargic, often with delayed circadian rhythms.

- People with SAD also may produce less Vitamin D. Vitamin D is believed to play a role in serotonin activity. Vitamin D insufficiency may be associated with clinically significant depression symptoms.

Part Three

Who Develops Depression?

Chapter 14

How Depression Affects People in Different Ways

Not everyone who is depressed experiences every symptom. Some people experience only a few symptoms. Some people have many. The severity and frequency of symptoms, and how long they last, will vary depending on the individual and his or her particular illness. Symptoms may also vary depending on the stage of the illness.

Women

Women with depression do not all experience the same symptoms. However, women with depression typically have symptoms of sadness, worthlessness, and guilt. Depression is more common among women than among men. Biological, lifecycle, hormonal, and psychosocial factors that are unique to women may be linked to their higher depression rate. For example, women are especially vulnerable to developing postpartum depression after giving birth, when hormonal and physical changes and the new responsibility of caring for a newborn can be overwhelming.

This chapter contains text excerpted from the following sources: Text in this chapter begins with excerpts from "Depression: What You Need to Know," National Institute of Mental Health (NIMH), December 13, 2015; Text under the heading "Racial and Ethnic Minority Populations" is excerpted from "Racial and Ethnic Minority Populations," Substance Abuse and Mental Health Services Administration (SAMHSA), February 18, 2016; Text under the heading "LGBT Population" is excerpted from "Stigma and Discrimination," Centers for Disease Control and Prevention (CDC), February 29, 2016.

Men

Men often experience depression differently than women. While women with depression are more likely to have feelings of sadness, worthlessness, and excessive guilt, men are more likely to be very tired, irritable, lose interest in once-pleasurable activities, and have difficulty sleeping.

Men may turn to alcohol or drugs when they are depressed. They also may become frustrated, discouraged, irritable, angry, and sometimes abusive. Some men may throw themselves into their work to avoid talking about their depression with family or friends, or behave recklessly. And although more women attempt suicide, many more men die by suicide in the United States.

Children

Before puberty, girls and boys are equally likely to develop depression. A child with depression may pretend to be sick, refuse to go to school, cling to a parent, or worry that a parent may die. Because normal behaviors vary from one childhood stage to another, it can be difficult to tell whether a child is just going through a temporary "phase" or is suffering from depression. Sometimes the parents become worried about how the child's behavior has changed, or a teacher mentions that "your child doesn't seem to be himself." In such a case, if a visit to the child's pediatrician rules out physical symptoms, the doctor will probably suggest that the child be evaluated, preferably by a mental health professional who specializes in the treatment of children. Most chronic mood disorders, such as depression, begin as high levels of anxiety in children.

Teens

The teen years can be tough. Teens are forming an identity apart from their parents, grappling with gender issues and emerging sexuality, and making independent decisions for the first time in their lives. Occasional bad moods are to be expected, but depression is different.

Older children and teens with depression may sulk, get into trouble at school, be negative and irritable, and feel misunderstood. If you're unsure if an adolescent in your life is depressed or just "being a teenager," consider how long the symptoms have been present, how severe they are, and how different the teen is acting from his or her usual self. Teens with depression may also have other disorders such as anxiety, eating disorders, or substance abuse. They may also be at higher risk for suicide.

Children and teenagers usually rely on parents, teachers, or other caregivers to recognize their suffering and get them the treatment they need. Many teens don't know where to go for mental health treatment or believe that treatment won't help. Others don't get help because they think depression symptoms may be just part of the typical stress of school or being a teen. Some teens worry what other people will think if they seek mental healthcare.

Depression often persists, recurs, and continues into adulthood, especially if left untreated. If you suspect a child or teenager in your life is suffering from depression, speak up right away.

Older People

Having depression for a long period of time is not a normal part of growing older. Most older adults feel satisfied with their lives, despite having more illnesses or physical problems. But depression in older adults may be difficult to recognize because they may show different, less obvious symptoms.

Sometimes older people who are depressed appear to feel tired, have trouble sleeping, or seem grumpy and irritable. Confusion or attention problems caused by depression can sometimes look like Alzheimer disease or other brain disorders. Older adults also may have more medical conditions such as heart disease, stroke, or cancer, which may cause depressive symptoms. Or they may be taking medications with side effects that contribute to depression.

Some older adults may experience what doctors call vascular depression, also called arteriosclerotic depression or subcortical ischemic depression. Vascular depression may result when blood vessels become less flexible and harden over time, becoming constricted. The hardening of vessels prevents normal blood flow to the body's organs, including the brain. Those with vascular depression may have or be at risk for heart disease or stroke.

Sometimes it can be difficult to distinguish grief from major depression. Grief after loss of a loved one is a normal reaction and generally does not require professional mental health treatment. However, grief that is complicated and lasts for a very long time following a loss may require treatment.

Older adults who had depression when they were younger are more at risk for developing depression in late life than those who did not have the illness earlier in life.

Racial and Ethnic Minority Populations

Racial and ethnic minorities currently make up about a third of the population of the nation and are expected to become a majority by 2050. These diverse communities have unique behavioral health needs and experience different rates of mental and/or substance use disorders and treatment access.

Communities of color tend to experience greater burden of mental and substance use disorders often due to poorer access to care; inappropriate care; and higher social, environmental, and economic risk factors.

LGBT Population

Homophobia, stigma (negative and usually unfair beliefs), and discrimination (unfairly treating a person or group of people) against gay, bisexual, and other men who have sex with men still exist in the United States and can negatively affect the health and well-being of this community.

These negative beliefs and actions can affect the physical and mental health of gay, bisexual, and other men who have sex with men, whether they seek and are able to get health services, and the quality of the services they may receive. Such barriers to health must be addressed at different levels of society, such as health care settings, work places, and schools to improve the health of gay and bisexual men throughout their lives.

Chapter 15

Women and Depression

Do you feel very tired, helpless, and hopeless? Are you sad most of the time, and take no pleasure in your family, friends, or hobbies? Are you having trouble working, sleeping, eating, and functioning? Have you felt this way for a long time? If so, you may have depression.

What Is Depression?

Everyone feels low sometimes, but these feelings usually pass after a few days. When you have depression, the low feelings persist and they can be intense. These low feelings hurt your ability to do the things that make up daily life for weeks at a time. Depression is a serious illness that needs treatment.

What Are the Different Forms of Depression?

The types of depression that affect women include:

- **Major depression**: Severe symptoms that interfere with a woman's ability to work, sleep, study, eat, and enjoy life. An episode of major depression may occur only once in a person's lifetime. But more often, a person can have several episodes.

If the symptoms of depression began either during pregnancy or in the month after giving birth, a woman is said to have postpartum (or peripartum) depression. Women who have had episodes of depression

---

This chapter includes text excerpted from "Depression in Women," National Institute of Mental Health (NIMH), April 1, 2014.

109

before they became pregnant are at increased risk of postpartum depression.

- **Persistent depressive disorder**: Depressed mood that lasts for at least 2 years. A person diagnosed with persistent depressive disorder may have episodes of major depression along with periods of less severe symptoms, but symptoms must last for 2 years.

- **Premenstrual dysphoric disorder**: Symptoms include severe mood swings, depressed mood, and anxiety that appear consistently in the week before a woman's menstrual period and lift within a few days. Symptoms are severe enough to interfere with daily activities and relationships.

What Causes Depression in Women?

Different kinds of factors play a role in the risk of depression. Depression tends to run in families. One of the reasons for this has to do with genes. Some genes increase the risk of depression. Others increase resilience—the ability to recover from hardship—and protect against depression. Experiences such as trauma or abuse during childhood and stress during adulthood can raise risk. However, the same stresses or losses may trigger depression in one person and not another. Factors such as a warm family and healthy social connections can increase resilience.

Research has shown that in people with depression, there can be subtle changes in the brain systems involved in mood, energy, and thinking and how the brain responds to stress. The changes may differ from person to person, so that a treatment that works for one person may not work for another.

During childhood, girls and boys experience depression at about equal rates. By the teen years, however, girls become more likely to experience depression than boys. Researchers continue to explore the reasons for this difference and how changes in hormone levels may be involved in depression risk during a woman's lifetime.

How Is Depression Treated?

The first step to getting the right treatment is to visit a doctor or mental health professional. She can do an exam or lab tests to rule out other conditions that may have the same symptoms as depression. She can also tell if certain medications you are taking may be affecting your mood.

The doctor should get a complete history of symptoms, including when they started, how long they have lasted, and how bad they are. She should also know whether they have occurred before, and if so, how they were treated. She should also ask if there is a history of depression in your family.

Medication

Medications called antidepressants can work well to treat depression. They can take several weeks to work. Antidepressants can have side effects including:

- Headache
- Nausea, feeling sick to your stomach
- Difficulty sleeping and nervousness
- Agitation or restlessness
- Sexual problems

Most side effects lessen over time. Talk to your doctor about any side effects you may have.

It's important to know that although antidepressants can be safe and effective for many people, they may present serious risks to some, especially children, teens, and young adults.

A "black box"—the most serious type of warning that a prescription drug can have—has been added to the labels of antidepressant medications. These labels warn people that antidepressants may cause some people, especially those who become agitated when they first start taking the medication and before it begins to work, to have suicidal thoughts or make suicide attempts. Anyone taking antidepressants should be monitored closely, especially when they first start taking them. For most people, though, the risks of untreated depression far outweigh those of antidepressant medications when they are used under a doctor's careful supervision.

Therapy

Several types of therapy can help treat depression. Therapy helps by teaching new ways of thinking and behaving, and changing habits that may be contributing to the depression. Therapy can also help women understand and work through difficult relationships that may be causing their depression or making it worse. Researchers are developing new ways to treat depression more quickly and effectively.

- **If you are pregnant:**

Before taking an antidepressant during pregnancy, talk to your doctor about the risks and benefits to you and your baby. There may be a very small chance that taking the medication during certain times of your pregnancy may affect your growing baby. But not taking your medication also may be risky to you and your baby. Experts generally agree that each woman's individual situation should determine whether she can safely take an antidepressant while pregnant.

How Can I Help a Loved One Who Is Depressed?

If you know someone who has depression, first help her see a doctor or mental health professional.

- Offer her support, understanding, patience, and encouragement.

- Talk to her, and listen carefully.

- Never ignore comments about suicide, and report them to her therapist or doctor.

- Invite her out for walks, outings, and other activities. If she says no, keep trying, but don't push her to take on too much too soon.

- Remind her that with time and treatment, the depression will lift.

How Can I Help Myself If I Am Depressed?

As you continue treatment, gradually you will start to feel better. Remember that if you are taking an antidepressant, it may take several weeks for it to start working. Try to do things that you used to enjoy before you had depression. Go easy on yourself. Other things that may help include:

- Breaking up large tasks into small ones, and doing what you can as you can. Try not to do too many things at once.

- Spending time with other people and talking to a friend or relative about your feelings.

- Postponing important decisions until you feel better. Discuss decisions with others who know you well.

Where Can I Go for Help?

If you are unsure where to go for help, ask your family doctor. You can also check the phone book for mental health professionals. Hospital doctors can help in an emergency.

Women are more likely than men to attempt suicide. If you or someone you know is in crisis, get help quickly.

- Call your doctor.

- Call 911 for emergency services.

- Go to the nearest hospital emergency room.

- Call the toll-free, 24-hour hotline of the National Suicide Prevention Lifeline at 1-800-273-TALK (1-800-273-8255); TTY: 1-800-799-4TTY (4889).

Chapter 16

Men and Depression

Are you tired and irritable all the time? Have you lost interest in your work, family, or hobbies? Are you having trouble sleeping and feeling angry or aggressive, sad, or worthless? Have you been feeling like this for weeks or months?

If so, you may have depression.

What Is Depression?

Everyone feels sad or irritable sometimes, or has trouble sleeping occasionally. But these feelings and troubles usually pass after a couple of days. When a man has depression, he has trouble with daily life and loses interest in anything for weeks at a time.

Both men and women get depression. But men can experience it differently than women. Men may be more likely to feel very tired and irritable, and lose interest in their work, family, or hobbies. They may be more likely to have difficulty sleeping than women who have depression. And although women with depression are more likely to attempt suicide, men are more likely to die by suicide.

Many men do not recognize, acknowledge, or seek help for their depression. They may be reluctant to talk about how they are feeling. But depression is a real and treatable illness. It can affect any man at any age. With the right treatment, most men with depression can get better and gain back their interest in work, family, and hobbies.

This chapter includes text excerpted from "Men and Depression," National Institute of Mental Health (NIMH), 2013. Reviewed November 2016.

What Are the Different Forms of Depression?

The most common types of depression in men are:

- **Major depression**: Severe symptoms that interfere with a man's ability to work, sleep, study, eat, and enjoy most aspects of life. An episode of major depression may occur only once in a person's lifetime. But more often, a person can have several episodes.

- **Dysthymic disorder, or dysthymia**: Depressive symptoms that last a long time (2 years or longer) but are less severe than those of major depression.

- **Minor depression**: Similar to major depression and dysthymia, but symptoms are less severe and may not last as long.

What Causes Depression in Men?

Several factors may contribute to depression in men.

- **Genes**: Men with a family history of depression may be more likely to develop it than those whose family members do not have the illness.

- **Brain chemistry and hormones**: The brains of people with depression look different on scans than those of people without the illness. Also, the hormones that control emotions and mood can affect brain chemistry.

- **Stress**: Loss of a loved one, a difficult relationship or any stressful situation may trigger depression in some men.

- Most of the time, it is likely a combination of these factors.

How Is Depression Treated?

- The first step to getting the right treatment is to visit a doctor or mental health professional. He can do an exam or lab tests to rule out other conditions that may have the same symptoms as depression. He can also tell if certain medications you are taking may be affecting your mood.

The doctor needs to get a complete history of symptoms. Tell the doctor when the symptoms started, how long they have lasted, how bad they are, whether they have occurred before, and if so, how they were treated. Tell the doctor if there is a history of depression in your family.

Medication

Medications called antidepressants can work well to treat depression. But they can take several weeks to work. Antidepressants can have side effects including:

- Headache
- Nausea, feeling sick to your stomach
- Difficulty sleeping and nervousness
- Agitation or restlessness
- Sexual problems.

Most side effects lessen over time. Talk to your doctor about any side effects you may have.

It's important to know that although antidepressants can be safe and effective for many people, they may present serious risks to some, especially children, teens, and young adults. A "black box"—the most serious type of warning that a prescription drug can have—has been added to the labels of antidepressant medications. These labels warn people that antidepressants may cause some people to have suicidal thoughts or make suicide attempts, especially those who become agitated when they first start taking the medication and before it begins to work. Anyone taking antidepressants should be monitored closely, especially when they first start taking them.

For most people, though, the risks of untreated depression far outweigh those of antidepressant medications when they are used under a doctor's supervision. Careful monitoring by a professional will also minimize any potential risks.

Therapy

Several types of therapy can help treat depression. Some therapies are just as effective as medications for certain types of depression. Therapy helps by teaching new ways of thinking and behaving, and changing habits that may be contributing to the depression. Therapy can also help men understand and work through difficult situations or relationships that may be causing their depression or making it worse.

How Can I Help a Loved One Who Is Depressed?

If you know someone who has depression, first help him find a doctor or mental health professional and make an appointment.

- Offer him support, understanding, patience, and encouragement.

- Talk to him, and listen carefully.

- Never ignore comments about suicide, and report them to his therapist or doctor.

- Invite him out for walks, outings and other activities. If he says no, keep trying, but don't push him to take on too much too soon.

- Encourage him to report any concerns about medications to his healthcare provider.

- Ensure that he gets to his doctor's appointments.

- Remind him that with time and treatment, the depression will lift.

How Can I Help Myself If I Am Depressed?

As you continue treatment, gradually you will start to feel better. Remember that if you are taking an antidepressant, it may take several weeks for it to start working. Try to do things that you used to enjoy before you had depression. Go easy on yourself. Other things that may help include:

- See a professional as soon as possible. Research shows that getting treatment sooner rather than later can relieve symptoms quicker and reduce the length of time treatment is needed.

- Break up large tasks into small ones, and do what you can as you can. Don't try to do too many things at once.

- Spend time with other people and talk to a friend or relative about your feelings.

- Do not make important decisions until you feel better. Discuss decisions with others who know you well.

Where Can I Go for Help?

If you are unsure where to go for help, ask your family doctor. You can also check the phone book for mental health professionals or check with your insurance carrier to find someone who participates in your plan. Hospital doctors can help in an emergency.

What If I or Someone I Know Is in Crisis?

Men with depression are at risk for suicide. If you or someone you know is in crisis, get help quickly.

- Call your doctor.

- Call 911 for emergency services.

- Go to the nearest hospital emergency room.

- Call the toll-free, 24-hour hotline of the National Suicide Prevention Lifeline at 1-800-273-TALK (1-800-273-8255); TTY: 1-800-799-4TTY (1-800-799-4889).

Chapter 17

Depression in Children and Adolescents

Chapter Contents

Section 17.1

Understanding Depression in Children

Text in this section is excerpted from "Depression,"
© 1995–2016. The Nemours Foundation/KidsHealth®.
Reprinted with permission.

About Depression

It's normal for kids to feel sad, down, or irritated, or to be in bad moods from time to time. But when negative feelings and thoughts linger for a long time and limit a child's ability to function normally, it might be depression.

Depression is a type of mood disorder. The main sign is when kids are sad, discouraged, or irritable for weeks, months, or even longer. Another sign a kid might have depression is negative thinking. This includes focusing on problems and faults, being mostly critical and self-critical, and complaining a lot.

Depression can interfere with energy, concentration, sleep, and appetite. Kids with depression may lose interest in activities and schoolwork, seem tired, give up easily, or withdraw from friends or family.

When kids have depression, it's hard for them to make an effort, even when doing things they used to enjoy. Depression can make kids feel worthless, rejected, or unlovable. It can make everyday problems seem more difficult than they actually are. When depression is severe, it can lead kids to think about self-harm or suicide.

Recognizing Depression

- It can be hard for parents and other adults to know when a child is depressed. An irritable or angry mood might seem like a bad attitude or disrespect. Low energy and lack of interest might look like not trying. Parents (and kids and teens themselves) may not realize that these can be signs of depression. Because depression can show up in different ways and might be hard to see, it helps to let a doctor know if feelings of sadness or bad moods seem to go on for a few weeks.

Diagnosing Depression and Other Mood Disorders

When diagnosing depression and similar mood disorders, doctors, and mental health professionals use different categories. They all have depressed mood as a main symptom, but they develop in different ways. For example:

- **Major depression** is an intense episode of depression that has developed recently and has lasted for at least 2 weeks.

- **Chronic depression** (also called dysthymia) is a milder depression that has developed more gradually, and has lasted for 2 years or longer.

- **Adjustment disorder with depressed mood** is depression that has developed after an upsetting event—anything from a natural disaster to a death in the family.

- **Seasonal affective disorder** is a kind of depression that is related to light exposure. It develops when hours of daylight are shorter; for example, during winter months.

- **Bipolar disorder** (also called manic depression or bipolar depression) is a condition that includes episodes of major depression and, at other times, episodes of mania (emotional highs).

- **Disruptive mood dysregulation disorder** is a pattern of intense, frequent temper tantrums; outbursts of aggression and anger; and a usual mood of irritability that has lasted for at least a year in a child older than 6.

Getting Help

Depression and other mood disorders can get better with the right attention and care. But problems also can continue or get worse if they're not treated.

If you think your child might be depressed or has a problem with moods:

Talk with your child about depression and moods. Kids might ignore, hide, or deny how they feel. Or they might not realize that they're depressed. Older kids and teens might act like they don't want help, but talk with them anyway. Listen, offer your support, and show love.

Schedule a visit to your child's pediatrician. The doctor will probably do a complete physical exam. A full exam lets the doctor check your child for other health conditions that could cause depression-like symptoms. If the doctor thinks your child has depression, or a similar mood disorder, he or she may refer you to a specialist for evaluation and treatment.

Contact a mental health specialist. Depression can get better. But without help, it can last or get worse. A child or adolescent psychiatrist or psychologist can evaluate your child and recommend treatment.

Therapists treat depression and other mood disorders with talk therapy, sometimes medicine, or both. Parent counseling is often part of the treatment, too. It focuses on ways parents can best support and respond to a kid or teen going through depression.

More Ways to Help

Treatment with a therapist is important. But you play an important role, too. At home, these simple but powerful things can help your child deal with depression.

Be sure your child eats nutritious foods, gets enough sleep, and gets daily physical activity. These have positive effects on mood.

Enjoy time together. Spend time with your child doing things you both can enjoy. Go for a walk, play a game, cook, make a craft, watch a funny movie. Gently encouraging positive emotions and moods (such as enjoyment, relaxation, amusement, and pleasure) can slowly help to overcome the depressed moods that are part of depression.

Be patient and kind. When depression causes kids and teens to act grumpy and irritable, it's easy for parents to become frustrated or angry. Remind yourself that these moods are part of depression, not intentional disrespect. Avoid arguing back or using harsh words. Try to stay patient and understanding. A positive relationship with a parent helps strengthen a child's resilience against depression.

Section 17.2

Depression among Teens

This section includes text excerpted from "Teen Depression,"
National Institute of Mental Health (NIMH), June 11, 2015.

If you have been feeling sad, hopeless, or irritable for what seems like a long time, you might have depression.

- Depression is a real, treatable brain illness, or health problem.

- Depression can be caused by big transitions in life, stress, or changes in your body's chemicals that affect your thoughts and moods.

- Even if you feel hopeless, depression gets better with treatment.

- There are lots of people who understand and want to help you.

- Ask for help as early as you can so you can get back to being yourself.

Regular Sadness and Depression Are Not the Same

Regular Sadness

Feeling moody, sad, or grouchy? Who doesn't once in a while? It's easy to have a couple of bad days. Your schoolwork, activities, and family and friend drama, all mixed with not enough sleep, can leave you feeling overwhelmed. On top of that, teen hormones can be all over the place and also make you moody or cry about the smallest thing. Regular moodiness and sadness usually go away quickly though, within a couple of days.

Depression

Untreated depression is a more intense feeling of sadness, hopelessness, and anger or frustration that lasts much longer, such as for weeks, months, or longer. These feelings make it hard for you to function as you normally would or participate in your usual activities. You may also have trouble focusing and feel like you have little to no motivation or energy. You may not even feel like seeing your best friends. Depression can make you feel like it is hard to enjoy life or even get through the day.

Know the Signs and Symptoms of Depression

Most of the day or nearly every day you may feel one or all of the following:

- Sad
- Empty
- Hopeless
- Angry, cranky, or frustrated, even at minor things

You also may:

- Not care about things or activities you used to enjoy.
- Have weight loss when you are not dieting or weight gain from eating too much.
- Have trouble falling asleep or staying asleep, or sleep much more than usual.
- Move or talk more slowly.
- Feel restless or have trouble sitting still.
- Feel very tired or like you have no energy.
- Feel worthless or very guilty.
- Have trouble concentrating, remembering information, or making decisions.
- Think about dying or suicide or try suicide.

Not everyone experiences depression the same way. And depression can occur at the same time as other mental health problems, such as anxiety, an eating disorder, or substance abuse.

If You Think You Are Depressed, Ask for Help as Early as You Can

1. Talk to:
   - Your parents or guardian

- Your teacher or counselor

- Your doctor

- A helpline, such as 1-800-273-TALK (8255), free 24-hour help

- Or call 911 if you are in a crisis or want to hurt yourself.

2. Ask your parent or guardian to make an appointment with your doctor for a checkup. Your doctor can make sure that you do not have another health problem that is causing your depression. If your doctor finds that you do not have another health problem, he or she can treat your depression or refer you to a mental health professional. A mental health professional can give you a thorough evaluation and also treat your depression.

3. Talk to a mental health professional, such as a psychiatrist, counselor, psychologist, or other therapist. These mental health professionals can diagnose and treat depression and other mental health problems.

There Are Ways You Can Feel Better

Effective treatments for depression include talk therapy or a combination of talk therapy and medicine.

Talk Therapy

A therapist, such as a psychiatrist, a psychologist, a social worker, or counselor can help you understand and manage your moods and feelings. You can talk out your emotions to someone who understands and supports you. You can also learn how to stop thinking negatively and start to look at the positives in life. This will help you build confidence and feel better about yourself. Research has shown that certain types of talk therapy or psychotherapy can help teens deal with depression. These include cognitive behavioral therapy, which focuses on thoughts, behaviors, and feelings related to depression, and interpersonal psychotherapy, which focuses on working on relationships.

Medicines

If your doctor thinks you need medicine to help your depression, he or she can prescribe an antidepressant. There are a few antidepressants that have been widely studied and proven to help teens. If your doctor recommends medicine, it is important to see your doctor regularly and tell your parents or guardian about your feelings, especially if you start feeling worse or have thoughts of hurting yourself.

Be Good to Yourself

Besides seeing a doctor and a counselor, you can also help your depression by being patient with yourself and good to yourself. Don't expect to get better immediately, but you will feel yourself improving gradually over time.

- Daily exercise, getting enough sleep, spending time outside in nature and in the sun, or eating healthy foods can also help you feel better.

- Your counselor may teach you how to be aware of your feelings and teach you relaxation techniques. Use these when you start feeling down or upset.

- Try to spend time with supportive family members. Talking with your parents, guardian, or other family members who listen and care about you gives you support and they can make you laugh.

- Try to get out with friends and try fun things that help you express yourself.

Depression Can Affect Relationships

It's understandable that you don't want to tell other people that you have been struggling with depression. But know that depression can affect your relationships with family and friends, and how you perform at school. Maybe your grades have dropped because you find it hard to concentrate and stay on top of school. Teachers may think that you aren't trying in class. Maybe because you're feeling hopeless, peers think you are too negative and start giving you a hard time.

Know that their misunderstanding won't last forever because you are getting better with treatment. Think about talking with people you trust to help them understand what you are going through.

Depression Is Not Your Fault or Caused by Something You Did Wrong

Depression is a real, treatable brain illness, or health problem. Depression can be caused by big transitions in life, stress, or changes in your body's chemicals that affect your thoughts and moods. Depression can run in families. Maybe you haven't realized that you have depression and have been blaming yourself for being negative. Remember that depression is not your fault!

Chapter 18

Depression in College Students

Feeling moody, sad, or grouchy? Who doesn't once in a while? College is an exciting time, but it can also be very challenging. As a college student, you might be leaving home for the first time, learning to live independently, taking tough classes, meeting new people, and getting a lot less sleep. Small or large setbacks can seem like the end of the world, but these feelings usually pass with a little time.

But if you have been feeling sad, hopeless, or irritable for at least 2 weeks, you might have depression. You're not alone. Depression is the most common health problem for college students. You should know:

- Depression is a medical illness.

- Depression can be treated.

- Early treatment is best.

- Most colleges offer free or low-cost mental health services to students.

What Is Depression?

Depression is a medical illness with many symptoms, including physical ones. Sadness is only a small part of depression. Some people

---

This chapter includes text excerpted from "Depression and College Students," National Institute of Mental Health (NIMH), November 11, 2015.

with depression may not feel sadness at all, but be more irritable, or just lose interest in things they usually like to do. Depression interferes with your daily life and normal function. Don't ignore or try to hide the symptoms. It is not a character flaw, and you can't will it away.

Are There Different Types of Depression?

Yes. The most common depressive disorders include major depression (a discrete episode, clearly different from a person's usual feeling and functioning), persistent depressive disorder (a chronic, low-grade depression that can get better or worse over time), and psychotic depression (the most severe, with delusions or hallucinations). Some people are vulnerable to depression in the winter ("seasonal affective disorder"), and some women report depression in the week or two prior to their menstrual period ("premenstrual dysphoric disorder").

What Are the Signs and Symptoms of Depression?

If you have been experiencing any of the following signs and symptoms nearly every day for at least 2 weeks, you may have major (sometimes called "clinical") depression:

- Persistent sad, anxious, or "empty" mood
- Feelings of hopelessness, pessimism
- Feelings of guilt, worthlessness, helplessness
- Loss of interest or pleasure in hobbies and activities
- Decreased energy, fatigue, being "slowed down"
- Difficulty concentrating, remembering, making decisions
- Difficulty sleeping, early-morning awakening, or oversleeping
- Appetite and/or unwanted weight changes
- Thoughts of death or suicide; suicide attempts
- Restlessness, irritability
- Persistent physical symptoms, such as muscle pain or headaches

Not everyone who is depressed experiences every symptom. Some people experience only a few symptoms. Some people have many. If any of these symptoms is interfering with your functioning—or if you are having thoughts that life is not worth living or ideas of harming yourself—you should seek help immediately; it is not necessary to wait 2 weeks.

What Are "Co-Occurring" Disorders?

Depression can occur at the same time as other health problems, such as anxiety, an eating disorder, or substance abuse. It can also co-occur with other medical conditions, such as diabetes or thyroid imbalance. Certain medications—for example, those for the treatment of severe acne—may cause side effects that contribute to depression; although some women are very sensitive to hormonal changes, modern birth control pills are not associated with depression for most users.

If I Think I May Have Depression, Where Can I Get Help?

If you have symptoms of depression that are getting in the way of your ability to function with your studies and your social life, ask for help. Depression can get better with care and treatment. Don't wait for depression to go away by itself or think you can manage it all on your own, and don't ignore how you're feeling just because you think you can "explain" it. As a college student, you're busy—but you need to make time to get help. If you don't ask for help, depression may get worse and contribute to other health problems, while robbing you of the academic and social enjoyment and success that brought you to college in the first place. It can also lead to "self-medication" with high-risk behaviors with their own serious consequences, such as binge drinking and other substance abuse and having unsafe sex.

Most colleges provide mental health services through counseling centers, student health centers, or both. Check out your college website for information. If you think you might have depression, start by making an appointment with a doctor or healthcare provider for a checkup. This can be a doctor or healthcare provider at your college's student health services center, a doctor who is off-campus in your college town, or a doctor in your hometown. Your doctor can make sure that you do not have another health problem that is causing your depression.

If your doctor finds that you do not have another health problem, he or she can discuss treatment options or refer you to a mental health professional, such as a psychiatrist, counselor, or psychologist. A mental health professional can give you a thorough evaluation and also treat your depression.

If you have thoughts of wishing you were dead or of suicide, call a helpline, such as 1-800-273-TALK (8255), for free 24-hour help, call campus security or 911, or go to the nearest emergency room.

How Is Depression Treated?

Effective treatments for depression include talk therapy (also called psychotherapy), personalized for your situation, or a combination of talk therapy and medication. Early treatment is best.

What Is Talk Therapy?

A therapist, such as a psychiatrist, a psychologist, a social worker, or counselor, can help you understand and manage your moods and feelings. You can talk out your emotions to someone who understands and supports you. You can also learn how to stop thinking negatively and start to look at the positives in life. This will help you build confidence and feel better about yourself as you begin to work with your therapist to find solutions to problems that may have seemed insurmountable when you were feeling depressed and maybe even hopeless. Research has shown that certain types of talk therapy or psychotherapy can help young adults deal with depression.

These include:

- **Cognitive behavioral therapy**, or CBT, which focuses on thoughts, behaviors, and feelings related to depression

- **Interpersonal psychotherapy**, or IPT, which focuses on working on relationships

- **Dialectical behavior therapy**, or DBT, which is especially useful when depression is accompanied by self-destructive or self-harming behavior

All therapies can be adapted to each person's issues, for example, if depression is associated with an anxiety or eating disorder. Your college counseling center may offer both individual and group counseling. Many also offer workshops and outreach programs to support you.

What Medications Treat Depression?

If your doctor thinks you need medication to help your depression, he or she may prescribe an antidepressant. There are a number of antidepressants that have been widely studied and proven to help.

If your doctor recommends medication, it is important to see your doctor regularly and tell him or her about any side effects and how you are feeling, especially if you start feeling worse or have thoughts of hurting yourself. Although the doctor will attempt to "match" the best medication for your depression, sometimes it takes a little "trial and error" to find the best choice. If you or a close family member has done well on a particular medication in the past, that can be a good predictor of success again.

Always follow the directions of the doctor or healthcare provider when taking medication. You will need to take one or more regular doses of an antidepressant every day, and it may not take full effect for a few weeks. To avoid having depression return, most people continue taking medication for some months after they are feeling better. If your depression is long-lasting or comes back repeatedly, you may need to take antidepressants longer.

Although all antidepressants can cause side effects, some are more likely to cause certain side effects than others. Tell your doctor if you are often "sensitive" to medication; starting with a low dose and increasing it slowly to a full therapeutic level is the best way to minimize adverse effects. You may need to try more than one antidepressant medicine before finding the one that improves your symptoms without causing side effects that are difficult to live with.

What Else Can I Do?

- Besides seeing a doctor and a counselor, you can also help your depression by being patient with yourself and good to yourself. Don't expect to get better immediately, but you will feel yourself improving gradually over time.

- Daily exercise, spending time outside in nature and in the sun, and eating healthy foods can also help you feel better.

- Get enough sleep. Try to have consistent sleep habits and avoid all-night study sessions.

- Your counselor may teach you how to be aware of your feelings and teach you relaxation techniques. Use these when you start feeling down or upset.

- Avoid using drugs and at least minimize, if not totally avoid, alcohol.

- Break up large tasks into small ones, and do what you can as you can; try not to do too many things at once.

- Try to spend time with supportive family members or friends, and take advantage of campus resources, such as student support groups. Talking with your parents, guardian, or other students who listen and care about you gives you support.

- Try to get out with friends and try fun things that help you express yourself. As you recover from depression, you may find that even if you don't feel like going out with friends, if you push yourself to do so, you'll be able to enjoy yourself more than you thought.

Remember that, by treating your depression, you are helping yourself succeed in college and after graduation.

What Are the Warning Signs for Suicide?

Depression is also a major risk factor for suicide. The following are some of the signs you might notice in yourself or a friend that may be reason for concern.

- Talking about wanting to die or to kill oneself
- Looking for a way to kill oneself, such as searching online or buying a gun
- Talking about feeling hopeless or having no reason to live
- Talking about feeling trapped or in unbearable pain
- Talking about being a burden to others and that others would be better off if one was gone
- Increasing the use of alcohol or drugs
- Acting anxious or agitated; behaving recklessly
- Giving away prized possessions
- Sleeping too little or too much
- Withdrawing or feeling isolated
- Showing rage or talking about seeking revenge
- Displaying extreme mood swings

Where Can I Learn More about Depression and Other Mental Health Issues?

The National Institute of Mental Health (NIMH) website (www. nimh.nih.gov) provides information about various mental health disorders and mental health issues. On the website, you can also learn about the latest mental health research and news. The website is mobile-friendly. This means you can access the NIMH website anywhere, anytime, and on any device—from desktop computers to tablets and mobile phones.

Chapter 19

Depression in Older Adults

Depression Is Not a Normal Part of Growing Older

Depression is a true and treatable medical condition, not a normal part of aging. However older adults are at an increased risk for experiencing depression. If you are concerned about a loved one, offer to go with him or her to see a healthcare provider to be diagnosed and treated. Depression is not just having "the blues" or the emotions we feel when grieving the loss of a loved one. It is a true medical condition that is treatable, like diabetes or hypertension.

How Do I Know If It's Depression?

Someone who is depressed has feelings of sadness or anxiety that last for weeks at a time. He or she may also experience:

- Feelings of hopelessness and/or pessimism
- Feelings of guilt, worthlessness and/or helplessness
- Irritability, restlessness
- Loss of interest in activities or hobbies once pleasurable
- Fatigue and decreased energy
- Difficulty concentrating, remembering details and making decisions

This chapter includes text excerpted from "Depression Is Not a Normal Part of Growing Older," Centers for Disease Control and Prevention (CDC), March 5, 2015.

- Insomnia, early-morning wakefulness, or excessive sleeping

- Overeating or appetite loss

- Thoughts of suicide, suicide attempts

- Persistent aches or pains, headaches, cramps, or digestive problems that do not get better, even with treatment

How Is Depression Different for Older Adults?

- **Older adults are at increased risk.** We know that about 80% of older adults have at least one chronic health condition, and 50% have two or more. Depression is more common in people who also have other illnesses (such as heart disease or cancer) or whose function becomes limited.

- **Older adults are often misdiagnosed and undertreated.** Healthcare providers may mistake an older adult's symptoms of depression as just a natural reaction to illness or the life changes that may occur as we age, and therefore not see the depression as something to be treated. Older adults themselves often share this belief and do not seek help because they don't understand that they could feel better with appropriate treatment.

How Many Older Adults Are Depressed?

The good news is that the majority of older adults are not depressed. Some estimates of major depression in older people living in the community range from less than 1% to about 5% but rise to 13.5% in those who require home healthcare and to 11.5% in older hospital patients.

How Do I Find Help?

Most older adults see an improvement in their symptoms when treated with antidepression drugs, psychotherapy, or a combination of both. If you are concerned about a loved one being depressed, offer to go with him or her to see a healthcare provider to be diagnosed and treated.

If you or someone you care about is in crisis, please seek help immediately.

- Call 911

- Visit a nearby emergency department or your healthcare provider's office

Chapter 20

Depression in Minority Populations

Mental Health and African Americans

- Poverty level affects mental health status. African Americans living below the poverty level, as compared to those over twice the poverty level, are 3 times more likely to report psychological distress.

- African Americans are 10% more likely to report having serious psychological distress than Non-Hispanic whites.

- The death rate from suicide for African American men was more than four times greater than for African American women, in 2014.

This chapter contains text excerpted from the following sources: Text under the heading "Mental Health and African Americans" is excerpted from "Mental Health and African Americans," Office of Minority Health (OMH), U.S. Department of Health and Human Services (HHS), May 16, 2016; Text under the heading "Mental Health and American Indians/Alaska Natives" is excerpted from "Mental Health and American Indians/Alaska Natives," Office of Minority Health (OMH), U.S. Department of Health and Human Services (HHS), May 16, 2016; Text under the heading "Mental Health and Asian Americans" is excerpted from "Mental Health and Asian Americans," Office of Minority Health (OMH), U.S. Department of Health and Human Services (HHS), May 16, 2016; Text under the heading "Mental Health and Hispanics" is excerpted from "Mental Health and Hispanics," Office of Minority Health (OMH), U.S. Department of Health and Human Services (HHS), May 16, 2016.

- However, the suicide rate for African Americans is 70% lower than that of the non-Hispanic white population.

- A report from the U.S. Surgeon General found that from 1980–1995, the suicide rate among African Americans ages 10 to 14 increased 233%, as compared to 120% of non-Hispanic whites.

Table 20.1. Adults Age 18 and over with past Year Major Depressive Episode Who Received Treatment for the Depression, 2012

Non-Hispanic Black	Non-Hispanic White	Non-Hispanic Black/ Non-Hispanic White Ratio
62.1	72	0.9

Mental Health and American Indians/Alaska Natives

- In 2014, suicide was the second leading cause of death for American Indian/Alaska Natives between the ages of 10 and 34.

- In 2014, suicide was the leading cause of death for American Indian/Alaska Native girls between the ages of 10 and 14.

- American Indian/Alaska Natives are 50% more likely to experience feelings of nervousness or restlessness as compared to non-Hispanic whites.

- Violent deaths–unintentional injuries, homicide, and suicide– account for 75% of all mortality in the second decade of life for American Indian/Alaska Natives.

- While the overall death rate from suicide for American Indian/ Alaska Natives is comparable to the White population, adolescent American Indian/Alaska Native females have death rates at almost four times the rate for White females in the same age groups.

Table 20.2. Serious Psychological Distress among Adults 18 Years of Age and over, Percent, 2013-2014

American Indian/Alaska Native	Non-Hispanic White	American Indian/Alaska Native/Non-Hispanic White Ratio
5.4	3.2	1.7

Mental Health and Asian Americans

- Suicide was the 9th leading cause of death for Asian Americans, and the 10th leading cause of death for White Americans, in 2014.

- Southeast Asian refugees are at risk for posttraumatic stress disorder (PTSD) associated with trauma experienced before and after immigration to the United States. One study found that 70% of Southeast Asian refugees receiving mental healthcare were diagnosed with PTSD.

- For Asian Americans, the rate of serious psychological distress increases with lower levels of income, as it does in most other ethnic populations.

- The overall suicide rate for Asian Americans is half that of the White population.

Table 20.3. Serious Psychological Distress among Adults 18 Years of Age and over, Percent, 2009-2010

Asian American	Non-Hispanic White	Asian American/Non-Hispanic White Ratio
1.9	3.2	0.6

Mental Health and Hispanics

- Poverty level affects mental health status. Hispanics living below the poverty level, as compared to Hispanics over twice the poverty level, are over twice as likely to report psychological distress.

- The death rate from suicide for Hispanic men was four times the rate for Hispanic women, in 2014.

- However, the suicide rate for Hispanics is half that of the non-Hispanic white population.

- Suicide attempts for Hispanic girls, grades 9–12, were 50% higher than for White girls in the same age group, in 2015.

- Non-Hispanic whites received mental health treatment 2 times more often than Hispanics, in 2014.

Table 20.4. Adults Age 18 and over with past Year Major Depressive Episode Who Received Treatment for Depression, 2012

Hispanic	Non-Hispanic White	Hispanic/Non-Hispanic White Ratio
55.6	72	0.8

Chapter 21

Depression and Violence in LGBT Population

Most lesbian, gay, bisexual, transgender, and questioning (LGBTQ) youth are happy and thrive during their adolescent years. Going to a school that creates a safe and supportive learning environment for all students and having caring and accepting parents are especially important. This helps all youth achieve good grades and maintain good mental and physical health.

However, some LGBTQ youth are more likely than their heterosexual peers to experience difficulties in their lives and school environments, such as violence.

Experiences with Violence and Depression

Negative attitudes toward lesbian, gay, and bisexual (LGB) people put these youth at increased risk for experiences with violence, compared with other students. Violence can include behaviors such as bullying, teasing, harassment, physical assault, and suicide-related behaviors.

According to data from Youth Risk Behavior Surveys (YRBS) conducted during 2001–2009 in seven states and six large urban school districts, the percentage of LGB students (across the sites) who were threatened or injured with a weapon on school property in the prior year ranged from 12% to 28%. In addition, across the sites:

This chapter includes text excerpted from "LGBT Youth," Centers for Disease Control and Prevention (CDC), November 12, 2014.

- 19% to 29% of gay and lesbian students and 18% to 28% of bisexual students experienced dating violence in the prior year.

- 14% to 31% of gay and lesbian students and 17% to 32% of bisexual students had been forced to have sexual intercourse at some point in their lives.

LGBTQ youth are also at increased risk for suicidal thoughts and behaviors, suicide attempts, and suicide. A nationally representative study of adolescents in grades 7–12 found that lesbian, gay, and bisexual youth were more than twice as likely to have attempted suicide as their heterosexual peers. More studies are needed to better understand the risks for suicide among transgender youth. However, one study with 55 transgender youth found that about 25% reported suicide attempts.

Another survey of more than 7,000 seventh- and eighth-grade students from a large Midwestern county examined the effects of school [social] climate and homophobic bullying on lesbian, gay, bisexual, and questioning (LGBQ) youth and found that:

- LGBQ youth were more likely than heterosexual youth to report high levels of bullying and substance use;

- Students who were questioning their sexual orientation reported more bullying, homophobic victimization, unexcused absences from school, drug use, feelings of depression, and suicidal behaviors than either heterosexual or LGB students;

- LGB students who did not experience homophobic teasing reported the lowest levels of depression and suicidal feelings of all student groups (heterosexual, LGB, and questioning students); and

- All students, regardless of sexual orientation, reported the lowest levels of depression, suicidal feelings, alcohol and marijuana use, and unexcused absences from school when they were:

  - In a positive school climate and

  - Not experiencing homophobic teasing.

Effects on Education and Health

Exposure to violence can have negative effects on the education and health of any young person. However, for LGBT youth, a national study of middle and high school students shows that LGBT students

(61.1%) were more likely than their non-LGBT peers to feel unsafe or uncomfortable as a result of their sexual orientation.

According to data from Centers for Disease Control and Prevention's (CDC) YRBS, the percentage of gay, lesbian, and bisexual students (across sites) who did not go to school at least one day during the 30 days before the survey because of safety concerns ranged from 11% to 30% of gay and lesbian students and 12% to 25% of bisexual students. The stresses experienced by LGBT youth also put them at greater risk for depression, substance use, and sexual behaviors that place them at risk for HIV and other sexually transmitted diseases (STDs). For example, HIV infection among young men who have sex with men aged 13–24 years increased by 26% over 2008–2011.

What Schools Can Do

For youth to thrive in their schools and communities, they need to feel socially, emotionally, and physically safe and supported. A positive school climate has been associated with decreased depression, suicidal feelings, substance use, and unexcused school absences among LGBQ students.

Schools can implement clear policies, procedures, and activities designed to promote a healthy environment for all youth. For example, research has shown that in schools with LGB support groups (such as gay-straight alliances), LGB students were less likely to experience threats of violence, miss school because they felt unsafe, or attempt suicide than those students in schools without LGB support groups. A recent study found that LGB students had fewer suicidal thoughts and attempts when schools had gay-straight alliances and policies prohibiting expression of homophobia in place for 3 or more years.

To help promote health and safety among LGBTQ youth, schools can implement the following policies and practices:

- Encourage respect for all students and prohibit bullying, harassment, and violence against all students.

- Identify "safe spaces," such as counselors' offices, designated classrooms, or student organizations, where LGBTQ youth can receive support from administrators, teachers, or other school staff.

- Encourage student-led and student-organized school clubs that promote a safe, welcoming, and accepting school environment (e.g., gay-straight alliances, which are school clubs open to youth of all sexual orientations).

- Ensure that health curricula or educational materials include human immunodeficiency virus (HIV), other sexually transmitted diseases (STD), or pregnancy prevention information that is relevant to LGBTQ youth (such as, ensuring that curricula or materials use inclusive language or terminology).

- Encourage school district and school staff to develop and publicize trainings on how to create safe and supportive school environments for all students, regardless of sexual orientation or gender identity, and encourage staff to attend these trainings.

- Facilitate access to community-based providers who have experience providing health services, including HIV/STD testing and counseling, to LGBTQ youth.

- Facilitate access to community-based providers who have experience in providing social and psychological services to LGBTQ youth.

What Parents Can Do

How parents respond to their LGB teen can have a tremendous impact on their adolescent's current and future mental and physical health. Supportive reactions can help youth cope with the challenges of being an LGBTQ teen. However, some parents react negatively to learning that they may have an LGBTQ daughter or son. In some cases, parents no longer allow their teens to remain in the home. In other situations, stress and conflict at home can cause some youth to run away. As a result, LGB youth are at greater risk for homelessness than their heterosexual peers.

To be supportive, parents should talk openly with their teen about any problems or concerns and be watchful of behaviors that might indicate their child is a victim of bullying or violence?or that their child may be victimizing others. If bullying, violence, or depression is suspected, parents should take immediate action, working with school personnel and other adults in the community.

Chapter 22

Occupation-Related Depression

Leading Causes of Worry for Employers in United States

Among the leading physical and mental health conditions in terms of direct medical costs and lost productivity to United States employers are several chronic disease (e.g., heart disease), depression, and musculoskeletal disorders (e.g., back pain). With workers in America today spending more than one-third of their day on the job, employers are in a unique position to promote the health and safety of their employees. The use of effective workplace health programs and policies can reduce health risks and improve the quality of life for 138 million workers in the United States.

The workplace provides many opportunities for promoting health and preventing disease and injury. Workplace health programs can:

- Influence social norms.

- Establish health-promoting policies.

This chapter contains text excerpted from the following sources: Text under the heading "Leading Causes of Worry for Employers in United States" is excerpted from "Workplace Health Strategies," Centers for Disease Control and Prevention (CDC), November 3, 2015; Text under the heading "Workplace Health Strategies for Controlling Depression" is excerpted from "Depression," Centers for Disease Control and Prevention (CDC), March 1, 2016.

- Increase healthy behaviors such as dietary and physical activity changes.

- Improve employees' health knowledge and skills.

- Help employees get necessary health screenings, immunizations, and follow-up care.

- Reduce employees' on-the-job exposure to substances and hazards that can cause diseases and injury.

Workplace Health Strategies for Controlling Depression

The mental health of workers is an area of increasing concern to organizations. Depression is a major cause of disability, absenteeism, presenteeism, and productivity loss among working-age adults. The ability to identify major depression in the workplace is complicated by a number of issues such as employees' concerns about confidentiality or the impact it may have on their job that cause some people to avoid screening.

- In a given year, 18.8 million American adults (9.5% of the adult population) will suffer from a depressive illness

- It is estimated that 20% of people aged 55 years or older experience some type of mental health issue. Depression is the most prevalent mental health problem among older adults

- Approximately 80% of persons with depression reported some level of functional impairment because of their depression, and 27% reported serious difficulties in work and home life

- Only 29% of all persons with depression reported contacting a mental health professional in the past year, and among the subset with severe depression, only 39% reported contact

- In a 3-month period, patients with depression miss an average of 4.8 workdays and suffer 11.5 days of reduced productivity

- In 2003, national health expenditures for mental health services were estimated to be over $100 million

- Depression is estimated to cause 200 million lost workdays each year at a cost to employers of $17 to $44 billion

- Research shows that rates of depression vary by occupation and industry type. Among full-time workers aged 18 to 64 years, the highest rates of workers experiencing a major depressive episode in the past year were found in the personal care and service occupations (10.8%) and the food preparation and serving related occupations (10.3%)

- Occupations with the lowest rates of workers experiencing a major depressive episode in the past year were engineering, architecture, and surveying (4.3%); life, physical, and social science (4.4%); and installation, maintenance, and repair (4.4%)

Depression is a complex condition characterized by changes in thinking, mood, or behavior that can affect anyone. Depression is influenced by a number of factors such as genetics; physiology (e.g., neurotransmitters), psychology (e.g., personality and temperament), gender, and the environment (e.g., physical environment and social support). Depression in working populations is equally complex and the causes are not well understood. However, there is recognition that both work and non-work related risk factors play a role such as the effects of worksites that produce excessive job stress on employees and employees' depression effect on the worksite.

Evidence linking work organization with depression and other mental health problems, and with increased productivity losses, is beginning to accumulate. A number of studies of a diverse group of occupations have identified several job stressors (e.g., high job demands; low job control; lack of social support in the workplace) that may be associated with depression. Although the evidence is mounting of the links between job stress and depression, there is less evidence of effective interventions to prevent depression in the workplace. There is a need to better understand organizational practices to reduce job stress, and aspects of job design that contribute to poor mental health, so that interventions can be developed to interventions that effectively target these risk factors in the workplace.

However, there are a number of strategies employers can pursue to support employees' mental health such as holding depression recognition screenings; placing confidential self-rating sheets in cafeterias, break rooms, or bulletin boards; promoting greater awareness through employee assistance programs (EAP); training supervisors in depression recognition; and ensuring workers' access to needed psychiatric services through health insurance benefits and benefit structures.

In addition to its direct medical and workplace costs, depression also increases healthcare costs and lost productivity indirectly by contributing to the severity of other costly conditions such as heart disease, diabetes, and stroke. However, routine, systematic clinical screening can successfully identify patients who are depressed, allowing them to access care earlier in the course of their illnesses. Research suggests that 80% of patients with depression will improve with treatment.

Chapter 23

Depression Related to Pregnancy

How Do I Know If I Have Depression?

When you are pregnant or after you have a baby, you may be depressed and not know it. Some normal changes during and after pregnancy can cause symptoms similar to those of depression. But if you have any of the following symptoms of depression for more than 2 weeks, call your doctor:

- Feeling restless or moody
- Feeling sad, hopeless, and overwhelmed
- Crying a lot
- Having no energy or motivation
- Eating too little or too much
- Sleeping too little or too much
- Having trouble focusing or making decisions
- Having memory problems
- Feeling worthless and guilty
- Losing interest or pleasure in activities you used to enjoy

This chapter includes text excerpted from "Depression during and after Pregnancy Fact Sheet," Office on Women's Health (OWH), U.S. Department of Health and Human Services (HHS), February 12, 2016.

- Withdrawing from friends and family

- Having headaches, aches and pains, or stomach problems that don't go away

Your doctor can figure out if your symptoms are caused by depression or something else.

What Causes Depression? What about Postpartum Depression?

There is no single cause. Rather, depression likely results from a combination of factors:

- Depression is a mental illness that tends to run in families. Women with a family history of depression are more likely to have depression.

- Changes in brain chemistry or structure are believed to play a big role in depression.

- Stressful life events, such as death of a loved one, caring for an aging family member, abuse, and poverty, can trigger depression.

- Hormonal factors unique to women may contribute to depression in some women. We know that hormones directly affect the brain chemistry that controls emotions and mood. We also know that women are at greater risk of depression at certain times in their lives, such as puberty, during and after pregnancy, and during perimenopause. Some women also have depressive symptoms right before their period.

Depression after childbirth is called postpartum depression. Hormonal changes may trigger symptoms of postpartum depression. When you are pregnant, levels of the female hormones estrogen and progesterone increase greatly. In the first 24 hours after childbirth, hormone levels quickly return to normal. Researchers think the big change in hormone levels may lead to depression. This is much like the way smaller hormone changes can affect a woman's moods before she gets her period.

Levels of thyroid hormones may also drop after giving birth. The thyroid is a small gland in the neck that helps regulate how your body uses and stores energy from food. Low levels of thyroid hormones can cause symptoms of depression. A simple blood test can tell if this condition is causing your symptoms. If so, your doctor can prescribe thyroid medicine.

Other factors may play a role in postpartum depression. You may feel:

- tired after delivery
- tired from a lack of sleep or broken sleep
- overwhelmed with a new baby
- doubts about your ability to be a good mother
- stress from changes in work and home routines
- an unrealistic need to be a perfect mom
- loss of who you were before having the baby
- less attractive
- a lack of free time

Are Some Women More at Risk for Depression during and after Pregnancy?

Certain factors may increase your risk of depression during and after pregnancy:

- a personal history of depression or another mental illness
- a family history of depression or another mental illness
- a lack of support from family and friends
- anxiety or negative feelings about the pregnancy
- problems with a previous pregnancy or birth
- marriage or money problems
- stressful life events
- young age
- substance abuse

Women who are depressed during pregnancy have a greater risk of depression after giving birth. The U.S. Preventive Services Task Force (USPSTF) recommends screening for depression during and after pregnancy, regardless of a woman's risk factors for depression.

What Is the Difference between "Baby Blues," Postpartum Depression, and Postpartum Psychosis?

Many women have the baby blues in the days after childbirth. If you have the baby blues, you may:

- have mood swings

- feel sad, anxious, or overwhelmed
- have crying spells
- lose your appetite
- have trouble sleeping

The baby blues most often go away within a few days or a week. The symptoms are not severe and do not need treatment.

The symptoms of postpartum depression last longer and are more severe. Postpartum depression can begin anytime within the first year after childbirth. If you have postpartum depression, you may have any of the symptoms of depression listed above. Symptoms may also include:

- Thoughts of hurting the baby
- Thoughts of hurting yourself
- Not having any interest in the baby
- Postpartum depression needs to be treated by a doctor

Postpartum psychosis is rare. It occurs in about 1 to 4 out of every 1,000 births. It usually begins in the first 2 weeks after childbirth. Women who have bipolar disorder or another mental health problem called schizoaffective disorder have a higher risk for postpartum psychosis. Symptoms may include:

- seeing things that aren't there
- feeling confused
- having rapid mood swings
- trying to hurt yourself or your baby

What Should I Do If I Have Symptoms of Depression during or after Pregnancy?

Call your doctor if:

- Your baby blues don't go away after 2 weeks
- Symptoms of depression get more and more intense
- Symptoms of depression begin any time after delivery, even many months later
- It is hard for you to perform tasks at work or at home

- You cannot care for yourself or your baby

- You have thoughts of harming yourself or your baby

Your doctor can ask questions to you to test for depression. Your doctor can also refer you to a mental health professional who specializes in treating depression.

Some women don't tell anyone about their symptoms. They feel embarrassed, ashamed, or guilty about feeling depressed when they are supposed to be happy. They worry they will be viewed as unfit parents.

Any woman may become depressed during pregnancy or after having a baby. It doesn't mean you are a bad or "not together" mom. You and your baby don't have to suffer. There is help.

Here are some other helpful tips:

- Rest as much as you can. Sleep when the baby is sleeping.

- Don't try to do too much or try to be perfect.

- Ask your partner, family, and friends for help.

- Make time to go out, visit friends, or spend time alone with your partner.

- Discuss your feelings with your partner, family, and friends.

- Talk with other mothers so you can learn from their experiences.

- Join a support group. Ask your doctor about groups in your area.

- Don't make any major life changes during pregnancy or right after giving birth. Major changes can cause unneeded stress. Sometimes big changes can't be avoided. When that happens, try to arrange support and help in your new situation ahead of time.

What Can Happen If Depression Is Not Treated?

Untreated depression can hurt you and your baby. Some women with depression have a hard time caring for themselves during pregnancy. They may:

- eat poorly

- not gain enough weight

- have trouble sleeping

- miss prenatal visits

- not follow medical instructions

157

- use harmful substances, like tobacco, alcohol, or illegal drugs

Depression during pregnancy can raise the risk of:

- problems during pregnancy or delivery
- having a low-birth-weight baby
- premature birth

Untreated postpartum depression can affect your ability to parent. You may:

- Lack energy
- Have trouble focusing
- Feel moody
- Not be able to meet your child's needs

As a result, you may feel guilty and lose confidence in yourself as a mother. These feelings can make your depression worse.

Researchers believe postpartum depression in a mother can affect her baby. It can cause the baby to have:

- Delays in language development
- Problems with mother-child bonding
- Behavior problems
- Increased crying

It helps if your partner or another caregiver can help meet the baby's needs while you are depressed. All children deserve the chance to have a healthy mom. And all moms deserve the chance to enjoy their life and their children. If you are feeling depressed during pregnancy or after having a baby, don't suffer alone. Please tell a loved one and call your doctor right away.

How Common Is Depression during and after Pregnancy?

Depression is a common problem during and after pregnancy. About 13 percent of pregnant women and new mothers have depression.

Chapter 24

Depression in Prison Inmates

Prison Inmates and Depression

Inmates often view depression as a personal weakness, and they can be reluctant to discuss their feelings because of the stigma associated with a mental health problem. Clinicians, nursing staff, and social work staff can help alleviate the stress felt by inmates diagnosed with depression by emphasizing that depression is a common and highly treatable medical condition.

How Is Depression Diagnosed?

A doctor determines whether a person has depression by:

- Giving the inmate a physical examination

- Doing certain medical tests to rule out other conditions that can cause the same symptoms as depression

- Asking the inmate a number of health-related and other questions:

This chapter contains text excerpted from the following sources: Text beginning with the heading "Prison Inmates and Depression" is excerpted from "Management of Major Depressive Disorder," Federal Bureau of Prisons (BOP), May 2014; Text beginning with the heading "Mental Health Screens" is excerpted from "Mental Health Screens for Corrections," National Institute of Justice (NIJ), U.S. Department of Justice (DOJ), May 2007. Reviewed November 2016.

159

- When did the symptoms start? How long have they lasted? How severe are they? Have

- you had them before? If so, were the symptoms treated and how?

- Do you use alcohol or drugs?

- Do you have thoughts of death or suicide?

- Have other members of your family had a depressive illness?

How Is Depression Treated?

Treatment choices depend on the results of the doctor's evaluation. If the doctor sees signs of severe depression in the inmate, or suspects that suicide is a possibility, he or she may refer the inmate to a psychiatrist (a medical doctor who specializes in mental illness). In some cases, the doctor may even recommend that the inmate be hospitalized immediately.

Some people with milder forms of depression may only need counseling. Others who have moderate-to-severe depression often benefit from a combination of medication and counseling. They would receive an antidepressant medication to relieve the symptoms, and counseling to help them learn better ways to deal with their problems and with depression itself.

Once you begin treatment for depression:

- See your healthcare provider regularly so he or she can monitor your progress, give you support and encouragement, and adjust your medications as necessary.

- Take your medications exactly as your doctor has instructed. Many inmates do not feel better until 4–8 weeks after beginning their medications, so try to be patient.

- Don't isolate yourself. Participate in your normal activities.

- Join a depression support group if one is available.

- Take care of yourself. Eat a healthy diet and get the right amount of sleep and exercise.

- Don't abuse alcohol or illegal drugs; they will slow your recovery.

Mental Health Screens

As corrections staff across the United States struggle to keep up with the rapid influx of new inmates while maintaining a secure environment, their efforts are increasingly hampered by the presence of individuals with serious mental illnesses who are entering corrections facilities in growing numbers. Numerous studies show that jail detainees have a significantly higher rate of serious mental illness (e.g., bipolar disorder, major depression, schizophrenia, and other psychoses) than the general population. One pair of studies reported that approximately 6 percent of men and 15 percent of women who were admitted to Chicago's Cook County jail displayed severe symptoms of mental illness and required treatment.

Many serious mental illnesses are chronic and are subject to exacerbation and relapse. The stress of incarceration can worsen symptoms in persons with preexisting mental disorders, leading to acute psychiatric disturbances, including harm to self or others; inmates with histories of severe mental illness may present an even greater risk. Moreover, several studies have shown that inmates with psychiatric impairment may exhibit more serious and more numerous adjustment and disciplinary problems (such as refusal to leave one's cell or destruction of property) during incarceration than unimpaired inmates.

Prisons and jails have a substantial legal obligation to provide health and mental healthcare for inmates. Case law and statutes have not provided a clear definition of what constitutes adequate mental healthcare. The American Psychiatric Association (APA) has, however, recommended that all corrections facilities provide at minimum mental health screening, referral, and evaluation; crisis intervention and short-erm treatment (most often medication); and discharge and prerelease planning. A national survey of 1,706 United States jails reported that 83 percent of them provide some form of initial screening for mental health treatment needs. Still, screening procedures are highly variable; they may consist of anything from one or two questions about previous treatment to a detailed, structured mental status examination. One result of this variability is apparent in data that showed fully 63 percent of inmates who were found to have acute mental symptoms through independently administered testing were missed by routine screening performed by jail staff and remained untreated.

Clearly, there is a pressing need to develop valid and reliable procedures to screen incoming detainees for signs and symptoms of acute psychiatric disturbance and disorder.

Researchers funded by the National Institute of Justice have created and tested two brief mental health screening tools and found that they are likely to work well in correctional settings. These tools are the Correctional Mental Health Screen (CMHS) and the Brief Jail Mental Health Screen (BJMHS).

161

CMHS: The CMHS uses separate questionnaires for men and women. The version for women (CMHS–W) consists of 8 yes/no questions, and the version for men (CMHS–M) contains 12 yes/no questions about current and lifetime indications of serious mental disorder. Six questions regarding symptoms and history of mental illness are the same on both questionnaires; the remaining questions are unique to each gender screen. Each screen takes about 3–5 minutes to administer. It is recommended that male inmates who answer six or more questions "yes" and female inmates who answer five or more questions "yes" be referred for further evaluation.

BJMHS: The BJMHS has 8 yes/no questions, takes about 2–3 minutes, and requires minimal training to administer. It asks six questions about current mental disorders plus two questions about history of hospitalization and medication for mental or emotional problems. Inmates who answer "yes" to two or more questions about current symptoms or answer "yes" to either of the other two questions are referred for further evaluation. Instructions for administering the screen appear on the back of the form. Corrections classification officers, intake staff, or nursing staff can administer the screen without specialized mental health training, but may receive brief informal training before administration.

Criteria for Detecting Mental Illness in Jails

When inmates enter a corrections facility, the staff's first task is to separate out those who may be at significant risk for suicide, acute psychotic breakdown, or complications from recent substance abuse from those who are merely experiencing varying degrees of distress usually associated with arrest, conviction, and detention. Effective mental health triage in the corrections setting can be viewed as a three-stage process:

1. routine, systematic, and universal mental health *screening* performed by corrections staff during the intake or classification stage, to identify those inmates who may need closer monitoring and mental health assessment for a severe mental disorder;

2. a more in-depth *assessment* by trained mental health personnel conducted within 24 hours of a positive screen; and

3. a full-scale psychiatric *evaluation* when an inmate's degree of acute disturbances warrants it.

Screening is the crucial part of the process, because it is the primary means by which staff can determine which inmates require more specialized mental health assessment or evaluation, as well as treatment. Unless inmates are identified as potentially needing mental health treatment, they will not receive it.

Screening, however, is the weak link and, as already noted, varies considerably. Until now, there were no valid, standardized tools available that could be recommended for adoption nationwide. A valid standard screen needs to be brief, because corrections classification staff have only a limited amount of time to spend with any one inmate. It also needs to provide *explicit decision criteria*, because the mental health training and experience of corrections staff is likely to be relatively low. Corrections staff traditionally are confident in their ability to discern overtly psychotic symptoms, but are considerably more uncertain about identifying less obvious—though equally serious—signs and symptoms of anxiety and depression. Thus, they need a tool that can provide them with the basis for a clear decision ("refer" or "don' t refer").

A useful jail mental health screen also needs to exhibit a *low false-negative rate*—that is, it would not miss many inmates who have a serious mental disorder because the potential consequences of not treating an inmate with a serious mental illness could be grave. On the other hand, it must have a low *false-positive rate* too, because mental health resources in corrections settings are scarce and burdening trained mental health staff with the need to assess many people who do not have a serious mental illness is an inefficient use of their time. Thus, an effective mental health screening tool would have a high degree of *predictive validity*, in that most of the people who are flagged by it as being "positive" should, on further assessment, be found to have a treatable serious mental illness.

Chapter 25

Caregivers and Depression

Caregivers care for someone with an illness, injury, or disability. Caregiving can be rewarding, but it can also be challenging. Stress from caregiving is common. Women especially are at risk for the harmful health effects of caregiver stress. These health problems may include depression or anxiety. There are ways to manage caregiver stress.

What Is a Caregiver?

A caregiver is anyone who provides care for another person in need, such as a child, an aging parent, a husband or wife, a relative, friend, or neighbor. A caregiver also may be a paid professional who provides care in the home or at a place that is not the person's home.

People who are not paid to give care are called informal caregivers or family caregivers. This fact sheet focuses on family caregivers who provide care on a regular basis for a loved one with an injury, an illness such as dementia, or a disability. The family caregiver often has to manage the person's daily life. This can include helping with daily tasks like bathing, eating, or taking medicine. It can also include arranging activities and making health and financial decisions.

Who Are Caregivers?

Most Americans will be informal caregivers at some point during their lives. A 2012 survey found that 36% of Americans provided

This chapter includes text excerpted from "Caregiver Stress Fact Sheet," Office on Women's Health (OWH), U.S. Department of Health and Human Services (HHS), August 17, 2015.

unpaid care to another adult with an illness or disability in the past year. That percentage is expected to go up as the proportion of people in the United States who are elderly increases. Also, changes in healthcare mean family caregivers now provide more home-based medical care. Nearly half of family caregivers in the survey said they give injections or manage medicines daily.

Also, most caregivers are women. And nearly three in five family caregivers have paid jobs in addition to their caregiving.

What Is Caregiver Stress?

Caregiver stress is due to the emotional and physical strain of caregiving. Caregivers report much higher levels of stress than people who are not caregivers. Many caregivers are providing help or are "on call" almost all day. Sometimes, this means there is little time for work or other family members or friends. Some caregivers may feel overwhelmed by the amount of care their aging, sick or disabled family member needs.

Although caregiving can be very challenging, it also has its rewards. It feels good to be able to care for a loved one. Spending time together can give new meaning to your relationship.

Remember that you need to take care of yourself to be able to care for your loved one. Learn some ways to manage caregiver stress and find resources.

Who Gets Caregiver Stress?

Anyone can get caregiver stress, but more women caregivers say they have stress and other health problems than men caregivers. And some women have a higher risk for health problems from caregiver stress, including those who:

- Care for a loved one who needs constant medical care and supervision. Caregivers of people with Alzheimer disease or dementia are more likely to have health problems and to be depressed than caregivers of people with conditions that do not require constant care.

- Care for a spouse. Women who are caregivers of spouses are more likely to have high blood pressure, diabetes, and high cholesterol and are twice as likely to have heart disease as women who provide care for others, such as parents or children.

Women caregivers also may be less likely to get regular screenings, and they may not get enough sleep or regular physical activity.

What Are the Signs and Symptoms of Caregiver Stress?

Caregiver stress can take many forms. For instance, you may feel frustrated and angry one minute and helpless the next. You may make mistakes when giving medicines. Or you may turn to unhealthy behaviors like smoking or drinking too much alcohol.

Other signs and symptoms include:

- Feeling overwhelmed
- Feeling alone, isolated, or deserted by others
- Sleeping too much or too little
- Gaining or losing a lot of weight
- Feeling tired most of the time
- Losing interest in activities you used to enjoy
- Becoming easily irritated or angered
- Feeling worried or sad often
- Having headaches or body aches often

Talk to your doctor about your symptoms and ways to relieve stress. Also, let others give you a break. Reach out to family, friends, or a local resource.

How Does Caregiver Stress Affect My Health?

Some stress can be good for you, as it helps you cope and respond to a change or challenge. But long-term stress of any kind, including caregiver stress, can lead to serious health problems.

Some of the ways stress affects caregivers include:

- **Depression and anxiety.** Women who are caregivers are more likely than men to develop symptoms of anxiety and depression. Anxiety and depression also raise your risk for other health problems, such as heart disease and stroke.
- **Weak immune system.** Stressed caregivers may have weaker immune systems than noncaregivers and spend more days sick with the cold or flu. A weak immune system can also make vaccines such as flu shots less effective. Also, it may take longer to recover from surgery.
- **Obesity.** Stress causes weight gain in more women than men. Obesity raises your risk for other health problems, including heart disease, stroke, and diabetes.

- **Higher risk for chronic diseases.** High levels of stress, especially when combined with depression, can raise your risk for health problems, such as heart disease, cancer, diabetes, or arthritis.

- **Problems with short-term memory or paying attention.** Caregivers of spouses with Alzheimer disease are at higher risk for problems with short-term memory and focusing.

Caregivers also report symptoms of stress more often than people who are not caregivers.

Part Four

Causes and Risk Factors for Depression

Chapter 26

What Causes Depression?

Chapter Contents

Section 26.1

Overview of the Causes of Depression

This section includes text excerpted from "Depression:
Causes and Risk Factors," NIHSeniorHealth,
National Institute on Aging (NIA), May 2016.

What Is Depression?

Depression is more than just feeling sad or blue. It is a common but serious mood disorder that needs treatment. It causes severe symptoms that affect how you feel, think, and handle daily activities, such as sleeping, eating, or working. When you have depression, you have trouble with daily life for weeks at a time. Doctors call this condition "depressive disorder," or "clinical depression."

Depression is a real illness. It is not a sign of a person's weakness or a character flaw. You can't "snap out of" clinical depression. Most people who experience depression need treatment to get better.

Causes and Risk Factors of Depression

Several factors, or a combination of factors, may contribute to depression.

- **Genes**: People with a family history of depression may be more likely to develop it than those whose families do not have the illness.

- **Personal history**: Older adults who had depression when they were younger are more at risk for developing depression in late life than those who did not have the illness earlier in life.

- **Brain chemistry**: People with depression may have different brain chemistry than those without the illness.

- **Stress**: Loss of a loved one, a difficult relationship, or any stressful situation may trigger depression.

Vascular Depression

For older adults who experience depression for the first time later in life, the depression may be related to changes that occur in the brain and body as a person ages. For example, older adults may suffer from restricted blood flow, a condition called ischemia. Over time, blood vessels may stiffen and prevent blood from flowing normally to the body's organs, including the brain.

If this happens, an older adult with no family history of depression may develop what is sometimes called "vascular depression." Those with vascular depression also may be at risk for heart disease, stroke, or other vascular illness.

Depression Can Co-Occur with Other Illnesses

Depression, especially in midlife or older adults, can co-occur with other serious medical illnesses such as diabetes, cancer, heart disease, and Parkinson disease. Depression can make these conditions worse and vice versa. Sometimes medications taken for these physical illnesses may cause side effects that contribute to depression. A doctor experienced in treating these complicated illnesses can help work out the best treatment strategy. Because many older adults face these illnesses along with various social and economic difficulties, some healthcare professionals may wrongly conclude that these problems are the cause of the depression—an opinion often shared by patients themselves.

All these factors can cause depression to go undiagnosed or untreated in older people. Yet, treating the depression will help an older adult better manage other conditions he or she may have.

Section 26.2

Probing the Depression-Rumination Cycle

"Probing the Depression-Rumination Cycle,"
© 2017 Omnigraphics. Reviewed November 2016.

Rumination is a thought process in which people obsessively focus on negative experiences and replay them over and over in their minds. The word is derived from the Latin term for ruminant animals, which are species with digestive systems that require them to regurgitate and rechew food. People who ruminate tend to chew over unpleasant situations repeatedly or brood about troubling issues constantly. Although self-reflection and analysis of past experiences can be helpful in problem solving, rumination rarely offers new insights or leads to a better understanding of a situation. Instead, people who ruminate focus so intensely on negative feelings that they lose perspective and become unable to experience positive feelings, which can cause anxiety and depression.

Rumination and Depression

Research has found links between rumination and several mental health conditions, including depression, anxiety, posttraumatic stress disorder (PTSD), substance abuse, and eating disorders. For instance, studies indicate that people who ruminate are four times more likely than other people to develop major depression. Rumination intensifies the negative feelings associated with depression, such as hopelessness, inadequacy, and worthlessness. In addition, rumination destroys self-confidence and creates uncertainty that makes people doubt their own judgment and avoid taking positive steps toward finding solutions to problems.

Rumination also reduces the level of social support available to help with personal problems. Research has shown that ruminators seek help more often than other people. Yet their persistently negative outlook and tendency to dwell on unpleasantness can create social friction and drive friends and relatives away. After a while, people being asked for support become frustrated and respond less compassionately, perhaps telling the ruminator to just forget about whatever they are obsessing over and move on with their life. The ruminator may interpret this response as rejection or abandonment, which then provides another negative experience for them to ruminate about. In this way, rumination and depression can become locked in a self-reinforcing cycle.

Rumination Triggers

Many of the triggers for rumination are similar to those for depression. In women, grief, sadness, and regret often serve as triggers for depressive rumination. In men, anger and resentment are the most common emotions that trigger rumination. Rumination is often associated with traumatic or stressful life events, such as losing a job, experiencing the death of a loved one, or having an illness or accident.

People who are prone to rumination often share some basic personality characteristics. Many ruminators are perfectionists who struggle to cope with less-than-perfect results. Many ruminators also tend to exhibit neuroticism and place an excessive value on interpersonal relationships. Finally, ruminators are likely to feel as if they face constant sources of pressure or stress that are beyond their control. Most do not view their rumination as part of the problem, but rather as a means of gaining necessary insight to deal with their problems.

Breaking the Rumination Cycle

Since rumination and depression can become linked in a self-perpetuating cycle, finding ways to stop ruminating can also help lighten symptoms of depression. Although depression is a medical condition that cannot be simply willed away, some people experience improvements in mood when they utilize techniques to avoid ruminating on negative thoughts and feelings. Some suggested methods of stopping or preventing rumination include the following:

- **Healthy Distraction**

   With practice, many ruminators can learn to recognize when they become focused on negative thoughts and experiences and employ various methods to distract themselves. Possible distraction techniques include doing chores such as vacuuming or mowing the lawn; watching a movie; taking a nap; or engaging in meditation or prayer. It may also be helpful to imagine a soothing image, such as a slowly rotating fan, a babbling brook, or the details of a childhood bedroom or yard. Practicing mindfulness is another valuable distraction tool. When negative thoughts about past events intrude upon enjoyment of the present, it may be helpful to redirect thoughts toward the immediate moment by carefully recognizing and considering what each sense is experiencing. Research has shown that distraction techniques can help reduce the time ruminators spend dwelling on and discussing negative events, which can also help improve the quality of their relationships.

- **Positive Thinking**

  The rumination-depression cycle works by activating neural networks in the brain that are attuned to negative thoughts and emotions. One bad memory of a negative outcome triggers additional memories of negative experiences, which leads to anxiety, self-doubt, and depression. With practice, however, many people can develop the skill of deliberately shifting their focus away from these neural networks and instead activating memories of positive experiences. Interrupting rumination and shifting to a network of positive thoughts can be difficult for people with depression. Some tips for accessing positive memories include asking family and friends for help and encouragement in remembering good times; listening to music associated with happy times and good moods; looking at photographs or videos of joyful experiences and trying to remember the sounds, smells, and other sensations; and physically going to a place connected with positive outcomes and states of mind. Accessing a positive neural network can provide a change of perspective and reveal new approaches to dealing with problems.

- **Planning**

  Depressive ruminators tend to become immobilized by negative thoughts and feel incapable of moving forward. They envision terrible outcomes and become afraid to try because they might fail. Breaking the cycle requires letting go of unattainable goals and things that are beyond one's control or ability to change. It may be helpful to break down a seemingly big problem into smaller, actionable pieces. Then, instead of focusing on the big problem, it may be possible to plan a series of small steps toward solving each part of the problem. Making a plan of action and achieving small goals can help increase self-confidence and decrease feelings of inadequacy and hopelessness. To avoid becoming paralyzed by inaction, it is important to view inevitable mistakes and failures as opportunities for learning and personal growth.

- **Containment**

  Of course, it is not possible to keep negative thoughts at bay all of the time. But there are proven techniques for containing those thoughts, reducing their power, and preventing them from turning into harmful rumination. One way to eliminate the power of negative thoughts and insecurities is to identify and confront them directly. Keeping a journal of emotions and triggers can help to clarify the source of negative thoughts. Once the underlying fear has been identified, the next step is to envision the worst-case scenario. Someone who panics at the thought of speaking in front of an audience, for instance, could picture forgetting a speech and looking foolish. In most cases, confronting the worst-case scenario helps people realize that they are resilient enough to handle it. To avoid ruminating, it may be helpful to contain negative thoughts by scheduling 15 to 30 minutes of worry time per day to dwell upon them. This method makes it easier to dismiss negative thoughts when they intrude at other times.

- **Therapy**

  Seeing a professional counselor may be helpful for people whose rumination interferes with their enjoyment of life. Mental health professionals can offer support, encouragement, and additional techniques and guidance to help people break out of the rumination-depression cycle and improve their mood, confidence, and self-esteem.

References

1. Chand, Suma. "Uplift Your Mood: Stop Ruminating," Anxiety and Depression Association of America, 2016.

2. Feiner, Lauren. "Eight Tips to Help Stop Ruminating," Psych Central, February 16, 2014.

3. Law, Bridget Murray. "Probing the Depression-Rumination Cycle," APA Monitor, November 2005, p. 38.

4. Wehrenberg, Margaret. "Rumination: A Problem in Anxiety and Depression," Psychology Today, April 20, 2016.

Chapter 27

Stress, Resilience, and the Risk of Depression

Chapter Contents

Section 27.1

Stress and Your Health

This section includes text excerpted from "Coping with Stress,"
Centers for Disease Control and Prevention (CDC), October 2, 2015.

What Is Stress?

Stress is a condition that is often characterized by symptoms of physical or emotional tension. It is a reaction to a situation where a person feels threatened or anxious. Stress can be positive (e.g., preparing for a wedding) or negative (e.g., dealing with a natural disaster).

Sometimes after experiencing a traumatic event that is especially frightening—including personal or environmental disasters, or being threatened with an assault—people have a strong and lingering stress reaction to the event. Strong emotions, jitters, sadness, or depression may all be part of this normal and temporary reaction to the stress of an overwhelming event.

Common Reactions to a Stressful Event

- Disbelief, shock, and numbness
- Feeling sad, frustrated, and helpless
- Fear and anxiety about the future
- Feeling guilty
- Anger, tension, and irritability
- Difficulty concentrating and making decisions
- Crying
- Reduced interest in usual activities
- Wanting to be alone
- Loss of appetite
- Sleeping too much or too little

- Nightmares or bad memories
- Reoccurring thoughts of the event
- Headaches, back pains, and stomach problems
- Increased heart rate, difficulty breathing
- Smoking or use of alcohol or drugs

Healthy Ways to Cope with Stress

Feeling emotional and nervous or having trouble sleeping and eating can all be normal reactions to stress. Engaging in healthy activities and getting the right care and support can put problems in perspective and help stressful feelings subside in a few days or weeks. Some tips for beginning to feel better are:

- Take care of yourself.
  - Eat healthy, well-balanced meals
  - Exercise on a regular basis
  - Get plenty of sleep
  - Give yourself a break if you feel stressed out
- Talk to others. Share your problems and how you are feeling and coping with a parent, friend, counselor, doctor, or pastor.
- Avoid drugs and alcohol. Drugs and alcohol may seem to help with the stress. In the long run, they create additional problems and increase the stress you are already feeling.
- Take a break. If your stress is caused by a national or local event, take breaks from listening to the news stories, which can increase your stress.

Recognize when you need more help. If problems continue or you are thinking about suicide, talk to a psychologist, social worker, or professional counselor.

Helping Youth Cope with Stress

Because of their level of development, children and adolescents often struggle with how to cope well with stress. Youth can be particularly overwhelmed when their stress is connected to a traumatic event—like a natural disaster (earthquakes, tornados, wildfires), family loss, school shootings, or community violence. Parents and educators can take steps to provide stability and support that help young people feel better.

Tips for Parents

It is natural for children to worry, especially when scary or stressful events happen in their lives. Talking with children about these stressful events and monitoring what children watch or hear about the events can help put frightening information into a more balanced context. Some suggestions to help children cope are:

- **Maintain a normal routine.** Helping children wake up, go to sleep, and eat meals at regular times provide them a sense of stability. Going to school and participating in typical after-school activities also provide stability and extra support.

- **Talk, listen, and encourage expression.** Create opportunities to have your children talk, but do not force them. Listen to your child's thoughts and feelings and share some of yours. After a traumatic event, it is important for children to feel like they can share their feelings and to know that their fears and worries are understandable. Keep these conversations going by asking them how they feel in a week, then in a month, and so on.

- **Watch and listen.** Be alert for any change in behavior. Are children sleeping more or less? Are they withdrawing from friends or family? Are they behaving in any way out of the ordinary? Any changes in behavior, even small changes, may be signs that the child is having trouble coming to terms with the event and may support.

- **Reassure.** Stressful events can challenge a child's sense of physical and emotional safety and security. Take opportunities to reassure your child about his or her safety and well-being and discuss ways that you, the school, and the community are taking steps to keep them safe.

- **Connect with others.** Make an on-going effort to talk to other parents and your child's teachers about concerns and ways to help your child cope. You do not have to deal with problems alone—it is often helpful for parents, schools, and health professionals to work together to support and ensuring the well-being of all children in stressful times.

Tips for Kids and Teens

After a traumatic or violent event, it is normal to feel anxious about your safety and security. Even if you were not directly involved, you may worry about whether this type of event may someday affect you. How can you deal with these fears? Start by looking at the tips below for some ideas.

- **Talk to and stay connected to others.** This connection might be your parent, another relative, a friend, neighbor, teacher, coach, school nurse, counselor, family doctor, or member of your church or temple. Talking with someone can help you make sense out of your experience and figure out ways to feel better. If you are not sure where to turn, call your local crisis intervention center or a national hotline.

- **Get active.** Go for a walk, play sports, write a play or poem, play a musical instrument, or join an after-school program. Volunteer with a community group that promotes nonviolence or another school or community activity that you care about. Trying any of these can be a positive way to handle your feelings and to see that things are going to get better.

- **Take care of yourself.** As much as possible, try to get enough sleep, eat right, exercise, and keep a normal routine. It may be hard to do, but by keeping yourself healthy you will be better able to handle a tough time.

- **Take information breaks.** Pictures and stories about a disaster can increase worry and other stressful feelings. Taking breaks from the news, Internet, and conversations about the disaster can help calm you down.

Tips for School Personnel

Kids and teens who experience a stressful event, or see it on television, may react with shock, sadness, anger, fear, and confusion. They may be reluctant to be alone or fearful of leaving secure areas such as the house or classroom. School personnel can help their students restore their sense of safety by talking with the children about their fears. Other tips for school personnel include:

- **Reach out and talk.** Create opportunities to have students talk, but do not force them. Try asking questions like, what do you think about these events, or how do you think these things happen? You can be a model by sharing some of your own thoughts as well as correct misinformation. Children talking about their feelings can help them cope and to know that different feelings are normal.

- **Watch and listen.** Be alert for any change in behavior. Are students talking more or less? Withdrawing from friends? Acting out? Are they behaving in any way out of the ordinary? These changes may be early warning signs that a student is struggling and needs extra support from the school and family.

- **Maintain normal routines.** A regular classroom and school schedule can provide reassurance and promote a sense of stability and safety. Encourage students to keep up with their schoolwork and extracurricular activities but do not push them if they seem overwhelmed.

- **Take care of yourself.** You are better able to support your students if you are healthy, coping well, and taking care of yourself first.

  - Eat healthy, well-balanced meals

  - Exercise on a regular basis

  - Get plenty of sleep

  - Give yourself a break if you feel stressed out

Section 27.2

Resilience Factors and the Risk of Developing Mental Health Problems

This section includes text excerpted from "Effects of Disasters:
Risk and Resilience Factors," U.S. Department of
Veterans Affairs (VA), September 2, 2015.

Stress Reactions to a Disaster

Every year, millions of people are affected by both human-caused and natural disasters. Disasters may be explosions, earthquakes, floods, hurricanes, tornados, or fires. In a disaster, you face the danger of death or physical injury. You may also lose your home, possessions, and community. Such stressors place you at risk for emotional and physical health problems.

Stress reactions after a disaster look very much like the common reactions seen after any type of trauma. Disasters can cause a full range of mental and physical reactions. You may also react to problems that occur after the event, as well as to triggers or reminders of the trauma.

Risk Factors

A number of factors make it more likely that someone will have more severe or longer-lasting stress reactions after disasters:

Severity of Exposure

The amount of exposure to the disaster is highly related to risk of future mental problems. At highest risk are those that go through the disaster themselves. Next are those in close contact with victims. At lower risk of lasting impact are those who only had indirect exposure, such as news of the severe damage. Injury and life threat are the factors that lead most often to mental health problems. Studies have looked at severe natural disasters, such as the Armenian earthquake, mudslides in Mexico, and Hurricane Andrew in the United States. The

185

findings show that at least half of these survivors suffer from distress or mental health problems that need clinical care.

Gender and Family

Almost always, women or girls suffer more negative effects than do men or boys. Disaster recovery is more stressful when children are present in the home. Women with spouses also experience more distress during recovery. Having a family member in the home who is extremely distressed is related to more stress for everyone. Marital stress has been found to increase after disasters. Also, conflicts between family members or lack of support in the home make it harder to recover from disasters.

Age

Adults who are in the age range of 40–60 are likely to be more distressed after disasters. The thinking is that if you are in that age range, you have more demands from job and family. Research on how children react to natural disasters is limited. In general, children show more severe distress after disasters than do adults. Higher stress in the parents is related to worse recovery in children.

Other Factors Specific to the Survivor

Several factors related to a survivor's background and resources are important for recovery from disaster. Recovery is worse if you:

- Were not functioning well before the disaster
- Have had no experience dealing with disasters
- Must deal with other stressors after the disaster
- Have poor self-esteem
- Think you are uncared for by others
- Think you have little control over what happens to you
- Lack the capacity to manage stress

Other factors have also been found to predict worse outcomes:

- Bereavement (death of someone close)
- Injury to self or another family member

- Life threat

- Panic, horror, or feelings like that during the disaster

- Being separated from family (especially among youth)

- Great loss of property

- Displacement (being forced to leave home)

Developing Countries

These risk factors can be made worse if the disaster occurs in a developing country. Disasters in developing countries have more severe mental health impact than do disasters in developed countries. This is true even with less serious disasters. For example, natural disasters are generally thought to be less serious than human-caused. In developing countries, though, natural disasters have more severe effects than do human-caused disasters in developed countries.

Low or Negative Social Support

The support of others can be both a risk and a resilience factor. Social support can weaken after disasters. This may be due to stress and the need for members of the support network to get on with their own lives. Sometimes the responses from others you rely on for support are negative. For example, someone may play down your problems, needs, or pain, or expect you to recover more quickly than is realistic. This is strongly linked to long-term distress in trauma survivors.

After a mass trauma, social conflicts, even those that have been resolved, may again be seen. Racial, religious, ethnic, social, and tribal divisions may recur as people try to gain access to much-needed resources. In families, conflicts may arise if family members went through different things in the disaster. This sets up different courses of recovery that often are not well understood among family members. Family members may also serve as distressing reminders to each other of the disaster.

Keep in mind that while millions of people have been directly affected by disasters, most of them do recover. Human nature is resilient, and most people have the ability to come back from a disaster. Plus, people sometimes report positive changes after disaster. They may re-think what is truly important and come to appreciate what they value most in life.

Resilience Factors

Human resilience dictates that a large number of survivors will naturally recover from disasters over time. They will move on without having severe, long-lasting mental health issues. Certain factors increase resilience after disasters:

Social Support

Social support is one of the keys to recovery after any trauma, including disaster. Social support increases well-being and limits distress after mass trauma. Being connected to others makes it easier to obtain knowledge needed for disaster recovery. Through social support, you can also find:

- Practical help solving problems
- A sense of being understood and accepted
- Sharing of trauma experiences
- Some comfort that what you went through and how you responded is not "abnormal."
- Shared tips about coping

Coping Confidence

Over and over, research has found that coping self-efficacy—"believing that you can do it"—is related to better mental health outcomes for disaster survivors. When you think that you can cope no matter what happens to you, you tend to do better after a disaster. It is not so much feeling like you can handle things in general. Rather, it is believing you can cope with the results of a disaster that has been found to help survivors to recover.

Hope

Better outcomes after disasters or mass trauma are likely if you have one or more of the following:

- Optimism (because you can hope for the future)
- Expecting the positive
- Confidence that you can predict your life and yourself
- Belief that it is very likely that things will work out as well as can reasonably be expected

- Belief that outside sources, such as the government, are acting on your behalf with your welfare at heart

- Belief in God

- Positive superstitious belief, such as "I'm always lucky."

- Practical resources, including housing, job, money

Summing It Up

Disasters can cause both mental and physical reactions. Being closer to the disaster and having weak social support can lead to worse recovery. On the other hand, being connected to others and being confident that you can handle the results of the disaster make mental health problems less likely. Overall, human beings are resilient, and most survivors will recover from the disaster. For those with higher risk factors, self-care and seeking help are recommended.

Chapter 28

Trauma as a Risk Factor for Depression

Chapter Contents

Section 28.1

Depression, Trauma, and Posttraumatic Stress Disorder (PTSD)

This section includes text excerpted from "Depression, Trauma, and PTSD," U.S. Department of Veterans Affairs (VA), August 13, 2015.

Depression and Trauma

Depression is a common problem that can occur following trauma. It involves feelings of sadness or low mood that last more than just a few days. Unlike a blue mood that comes and goes, depression is longer lasting. Depression can get in the way of daily life and make it hard to function. It can affect your eating and sleeping, how you think, and how you feel about yourself.

How Common Is Depression Following Trauma?

In any given year, almost 1 in 10 adult Americans has some type of depression. Depression often occurs after trauma. For example, a survey of survivors from the Oklahoma City bombing showed that 23% had depression after the bombing. This was compared to 13% who had depression before the bombing. Posttraumatic stress disorder (PTSD) and depression are often seen together. Results from a large national survey showed that depression is nearly 3 to 5 times more likely in those with PTSD than those without PTSD.

What Are the Symptoms of Depression?

Depression is more than just feeling sad. Most people with depression feel down or sad more days than not for at least 2 weeks. Or they find they no longer enjoy or have interest in things anymore. If you have depression, you may notice that you're sleeping and eating a lot more or less than you used to. You may find it hard to stay focused. You may feel down on yourself or hopeless. With more severe depression, you may think about hurting or killing yourself.

How Are Depression and Trauma Related?

Depression can sometimes seem to come from out of the blue. It can also be caused by a stressful event such as a divorce or a trauma. Trouble coping with painful experiences or losses often leads to depression. For example, Veterans returning from a war zone may have painful memories and feelings of guilt or regret about their war experiences. They may have been injured or lost friends. Disaster survivors may have lost a loved one, a home, or have been injured. Survivors of violence or abuse may feel like they can no longer trust other people. These kinds of experiences can lead to both depression and PTSD.

Many symptoms of depression overlap with the symptoms of PTSD. For example, with both depression and PTSD, you may have trouble sleeping or keeping your mind focused. You may not feel pleasure or interest in things you used to enjoy. You may not want to be with other people as much. Both PTSD and depression may involve greater irritability. It is quite possible to have both depression and PTSD at the same time.

How Is Depression Treated?

There are many treatment options for depression. You should be assessed by a healthcare professional who can decide which type of treatment is best for you. In many cases, milder forms of depression are treated by counseling or therapy. More severe depression is treated with medicines or with both therapy and medicine.

Research has shown that certain types of therapy and medicine are effective for both depression and PTSD. Since the symptoms of PTSD and depression can overlap, treatment that helps with PTSD may also result in improvement of depression. Cognitive behavioral therapy (CBT) is a type of therapy that is proven effective for both problems. CBT can help patients change negative styles of thinking and acting that can lead to both depression and PTSD. A type of medicine that is effective for both depression and PTSD is a selective serotonin reuptake inhibitor (SSRI).

What Can I Do about Feelings of Depression?

Depression can make you feel worn out, worthless, helpless, hopeless, and sad. These feelings can make you feel as though you are never going to feel better. You may even think that you should just give up. Some symptoms of depression, such as being tired or not having the desire to do anything, can also get in the way of your seeking treatment.

It is very important for you to know that these negative thoughts and feelings are part of depression. If you think you might be depressed, you should seek help in spite of these feelings. You can expect them to change as treatment begins working. In the meantime, here is a list of things you can do that may improve your mood:

- Talk with your doctor or healthcare provider.

- Talk with family and friends.

- Spend more time with others and get support from them. Don't close yourself off.

- Take part in activities that might make you feel better. Do the things you used to enjoy before you began feeling depressed. Even if you don't feel like it, try doing some of these things. Chances are you will feel better after you do.

- Engage in mild exercise.

- Set realistic goals for yourself.

- Break up goals and tasks into smaller ones that you can manage.

Depression and PTSD

Depression is common in those who have PTSD. The symptoms of depression can make it hard to function, and may also get in the way of your getting treatment. Be aware that there are effective treatments for both depression and PTSD. If you think you may be depressed, talk to your doctor.

Section 28.2

Child Abuse Leaves Epigenetic Marks

This section includes text excerpted from "Child Abuse Leaves
Epigenetic Marks," National Human Genome Research
Institute (NHGRI), July 3, 2013. Reviewed November 2016.

Child abuse is a serious national and global problem that cuts across economic, racial, and cultural lines. Each year, more than 1.25 million children are abused or neglected in the United States, with that number expanding to at least 40 million per year worldwide.

In addition to harming the immediate well being of the child, maltreatment and extreme stress during childhood can impair early brain development and metabolic and immune system function, leading to chronic health problems. As a consequence, abused children are at increased risk for a wide range of physical health conditions including obesity, heart disease, and cancer, as well as psychiatric conditions such as depression, suicide, drug and alcohol abuse, high-risk behaviors and violence.

They are also more susceptible to developing posttraumatic stress disorder (PTSD)—a severe and debilitating stress-related psychiatric disorder-after experiencing other types of trauma later in life.

Part of the explanation is that child abuse can leave marks, not only physically and emotionally, but also in the form of epigenetic marks on a child's genes. Although these epigenetic marks do not cause mutations in the DNA (Deoxyribonucleic acid) itself, the chemical modifications-including DNA methylation-change gene expression by silencing (or activating) genes. This can alter fundamental biological processes and adversely affect health outcomes throughout life.

New research, published in the May 14, 2013, issue of the *Proceedings for the National Academy of Sciences* (NAS), shows that PTSD patients who were abused as children have different patterns of DNA methylation and gene expression compared to those who were not.

Researchers from the Max Planck Institute in Germany and Emory University in the United States investigated whether the timing of trauma, specifically childhood abuse early in life, had an effect on the underlying biology of PTSD at the genome-wide level. To address this question, the authors examined a subset of 169 participants from the Grady Trauma Project-a survey of more than 5,000 individuals in Atlanta with a high lifetime exposure to multiple types of trauma, violence and abuse.

Among the 169 participants in the current study, most were African Americans in their late thirties and forties, and all had suffered from at least two types of trauma other than child abuse and seven types of trauma on average. In spite of multiple trauma exposure, the majority (108 people) did not develop PTSD. Of the 61 that did, however, 32 reported a history of childhood abuse and 29 did not.

To focus on the effect of childhood abuse in PTSD, the researchers examined genetic changes in peripheral blood cells from PTSD patients with and without previous exposure to childhood maltreatment. These were then compared to the trauma-exposed group that did not develop PTSD to rule out changes associated with trauma exposure alone.

Despite sharing a few common biological pathways, 98 percent of the changes in gene expression patterns in PTSD patients with childhood abuse did not overlap with those found in PTSD patients without childhood abuse. Interestingly, PTSD patients who experienced significant abuse as children exhibited more changes in genes associated with central nervous system development and immune system regulation, whereas those without a history of childhood abuse displayed more changes in genes associated with cell death and growth rate regulation.

Furthermore, the researchers found that epigenetic marks associated with gene expression changes were up to 12-fold higher in PTSD patients with a history of childhood abuse. This suggests that although all patients with PTSD may show similar symptoms, abused children who subsequently develop PTSD may experience a systematically and biologically different form of the disorder compared to those without childhood abuse.

What this means is that we may need to rethink our classification of PTSD and the notion of providing the same treatment for all PTSD patients, said Dr. Divya Mehta, corresponding author at the Max Planck Institute of Psychiatry.

"At the biological level, these individuals may be very distinct, as we see with the epigenetics," Dr. Mehta explained. "As we move forward with more personalized medicine, we will need to delve a bit further into the environment and history of each individual to understand the biology of their PTSD and to determine the best treatment for their disorder."

Although, it is currently unclear whether the epigenetic marks left by child abuse can be removed or the damage reversed, this discovery is important in the search for biomarkers with clinical indications that can be used to identify different forms of PTSD. This will help to direct more precise avenues for therapy and guide treatments tailored specifically to the biological process of individual patients.

By starting to distinguish subtypes of PTSD, this study highlights the multi-factorial nature of psychiatric disorders triggered by a combination of environmental and genetic factors. As the next step, Dr. Mehta and her team plan to study whether the age at which abuse occurs or the type of abuse affects the biology of PTSD.

Since even small changes in DNA methylation signatures in child abuse can have long-term implications for fundamental biological processes and health, Dr. Mehta hopes their research will also increase public awareness and strengthen efforts to protect children from the consequences of childhood abuse and neglect.

Section 28.3

Adverse Childhood Experiences

This section contains text excerpted from the following sources: Text in this section begins with excerpts from "Adverse Childhood Experiences," Substance Abuse and Mental Health Services Administration (SAMHSA), March 7, 2016; Text under the heading "Psychological Consequences" is excerpted from "Long-Term Consequences of Child Abuse and Neglect," Child Welfare Information Gateway, U.S. Department of Health and Human Services (HHS), July 2013. Reviewed November 2016.

Adverse childhood experiences (ACEs) are stressful or traumatic events, including abuse and neglect. They may also include household dysfunction such as witnessing domestic violence or growing up with family members who have substance use disorders. ACEs are strongly related to the development and prevalence of a wide range of health problems throughout a person's lifespan, including those associated with substance misuse.

ACEs include:

• Physical abuse

- Sexual abuse

- Emotional abuse

- Physical neglect

- Emotional neglect

- Mother treated violently

- Substance misuse within household

- Household mental illness

- Parental separation or divorce

- Incarcerated household member

ACEs Research and Behavioral Health

Research has demonstrated a strong relationship between ACEs, substance use disorders, and behavioral problems. When children are exposed to chronic stressful events, their neurodevelopment can be disrupted. As a result, the child's cognitive functioning or ability to cope with negative or disruptive emotions may be impaired. Over time, and often during adolescence, the child may adopt negative coping mechanisms, such as substance use or self-harm. Eventually, these unhealthy coping mechanisms can contribute to disease, disability, and social problems, as well as premature mortality.

Psychological Consequences

The immediate emotional effects of abuse and neglect—isolation, fear, and an inability to trust—can translate into lifelong psychological consequences, including low self-esteem, depression, and relationship difficulties. Researchers have identified links between child abuse and neglect and the following:

Difficulties during infancy. Of children entering foster care in 2010, 16 percent were younger than 1 year. When infants and young children enter out-of-home care due to abuse or neglect, the trauma of a primary caregiver change negatively affects their attachments. Nearly half of infants in foster care who have experienced maltreatment exhibit some form of cognitive delay and have lower intelligence quotient (IQ) scores, language difficulties, and neonatal challenges compared to children who have not been abused or neglected.

Poor mental and emotional health. Experiencing childhood trauma and adversity, such as physical or sexual abuse, is a risk factor for borderline personality disorder, depression, anxiety, and other psychiatric disorders. One study using ACE data found that roughly 54 percent of cases of depression and 58 percent of suicide attempts in women were connected to adverse childhood experiences. Child maltreatment also negatively impacts the development of emotion regulation, which often persists into adolescence or adulthood.

Cognitive difficulties. National Survey of Child and Adolescent Well-Being (NSCAW) researchers found that children with substantiated reports of maltreatment were at risk for severe developmental and cognitive problems, including grade repetition. In its final report on the second NSCAW study (NSCAW II), more than 10 percent of school-aged children and youth showed some risk of cognitive problems or low academic achievement, 43 percent had emotional or behavioral problems, and 13 percent had both.

Social difficulties. Children who experience neglect are more likely to develop antisocial traits as they grow up. Parental neglect is associated with borderline personality disorders, attachment issues or affectionate behaviors with unknown/little-known people, inappropriate modeling of adult behavior, and aggression.

Chapter 29

Unemployment, Poverty, and Depression

Unemployed Adults with Mental Illness

Mental illness can make it difficult to get or maintain employment, and the strain of unemployment can make mental illness worse. According to combined data from the 2008 to 2012 National Surveys on Drug Use and Health (NSDUHs), 12.8 million adults aged 18 to 64 were unemployed in the past week, and 36.8 million persons had any mental illness (AMI) in the past year. Approximately 3.1 million adults aged 18 to 64 (1.6 percent) both were unemployed and had AMI.

NSDUH data also show that the percentages of adults aged 18 to 64 who both were unemployed and had AMI varied across States and metropolitan areas. Two States (Michigan and Ohio) had higher percentages of persons aged 18 to 64 who both were unemployed and had

---

This chapter contains text excerpted from the following sources: Text under the heading "Unemployed Adults with Mental Illness" is excerpted from "3.1 Million Adults with Mental Illness Were Unemployed," Substance Abuse and Mental Health Services Administration (SAMHSA), March 25, 2015; Text under the heading "Unemployment and Depression Among Emerging Adults" is excerpted from "Unemployment and Depression Among Emerging Adults in 12 States, Behavioral Risk Factor Surveillance System, 2010," Centers for Disease Control and Prevention (CDC), March 19, 2015; Text under the heading "Depression in the U.S. Household Population" is excerpted from "Depression in the U.S. Household Population, 2009-2012," Centers for Disease Control and Prevention (CDC), November 6, 2015.

AMI than did the nation as a whole. Nine States (Alaska, Connecticut, Georgia, Massachusetts, Minnesota, New Hampshire, North Dakota, Vermont, and Wisconsin) had significantly lower percentages than the nation as a whole. No metropolitan areas had higher percentages of persons who both were unemployed and had AMI than the nation, but six metropolitan areas (Atlanta, Houston, Kansas City, Miami, Minneapolis, and Pittsburgh) had lower percentages than did the nation as a whole.

Policymakers, communities, and treatment providers should consider the increased need for mental health services in geographic areas with high levels of unemployment. Improving mental health screening and treatment could help reduce the effects of mental illness on unemployment. This in turn could reduce the chances of unemployment, increase the chances of reemployment, and reduce the length of unemployment for those with mental illness.

Unemployment and Depression among Emerging Adults

Depressive disorders are among the most common mental health problems. As a leading cause of disability, depression is related to reduced quality of life and increased risk for physical health problems. Although depression has substantial consequences throughout the lifespan, depression during emerging adulthood, the period of transition from adolescence to adulthood, influences long-term consequences through recurrent depressive episodes and worse socioeconomic outcomes. Annually, 8.3% of adults aged 18 to 25 report having had at least 1 major depressive episode.

Although many factors contribute to depression, unemployment is consistently associated with high rates of depression among adults. Unemployment may contribute to depression because of losses in social contact and status or stress related to income loss. For emerging adults, long experiences of unemployment increase the likelihood of experiencing depression throughout the transition.

The high unemployment rate among emerging adults, around 20% in 2010, is a substantial public health problem. The potential situational stressor of being unemployed and the developmental stressor of transitioning to young adulthood may combine to increase experiences of depression. However, few studies relating unemployment and depression focus on emerging adults. For example, Brown et al excluded those aged 18 to 25 in their study examining frequent mental distress and unemployment, and Galambos et al did not measure clinically significant depression in their examination of depressive symptoms among recent graduates.

Depression in the U.S. Household Population

Depression is a serious medical illness with mood, cognitive, and physical symptoms. Depression is associated with higher rates of chronic disease, increased healthcare utilization, and impaired functioning. Rates of treatment remain low, and the treatment received is often inadequate. This data brief examines both depression and depressive symptom severity in the past 2 weeks from a symptom-based questionnaire, by demographic characteristics, functioning difficulties, and recent contact with a mental health professional. Severity is categorized as severe, moderate, mild, or no depressive symptoms. Current depression is defined as severe or moderate symptoms; no depression is defined as mild or no symptoms.

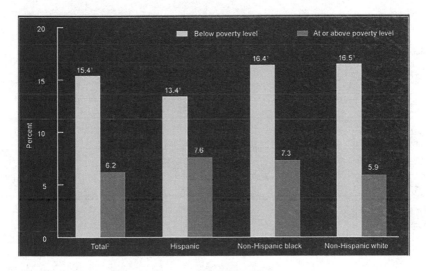

Figure 29.1. *Percentage of persons aged 12 and over with depression, by poverty status and race and Hispanic origin: United States, 2009–2012*

[1] *Significantly higher than "at or above poverty level."*
[2] *Includes race and ethnicity groups not shown separately.*
Depression is defined as moderate to severe depressive symptoms. The poverty level is set by the U.S. Department of Health and Human Services (HHS) and is based on family income and family size

Poor persons were more than twice as likely to have depression as persons living at or above the poverty level.

- More than 15% of persons living below the federal poverty level had depression compared with 6.2% of persons living at or above the poverty level.

- No significant differences were observed in rates of depression by race and Hispanic origin among persons living below the poverty level or among those living at or above the poverty level.

Chapter 30

Other Mental Health Disorders and the Relationship to Depression

Chapter Contents

Section 30.1

Anxiety Disorders and Depression among Children and Women

This section contains text excerpted from the following sources:
Text beginning with the heading "Internalizing Disorders and Children" is excerpted from "Anxiety and Depression," Centers for Disease Control and Prevention (CDC), August 8, 2016; Text under the heading "Depression and Anxiety among Women" is excerpted from "Depression and Anxiety," Office on Women's Health (OWH), U.S. Department of Health and Human Services (HHS), September 20, 2013. Reviewed November 2016.

Internalizing Disorders and Children

Many children have fears and worries, and will feel sad and hopeless from time to time. Strong fears will appear at different times in development. For example, toddlers are often very distressed about being away from their parents, even if they are safe and cared for. Persistent or extreme forms of fear and sadness feelings could be due to anxiety or depression. Because the symptoms primarily involve thoughts and feelings, they are called internalizing disorders.

Anxiety in Children

When children do not outgrow the fears and worries that are typical in young children, or when there are so many fears and worries that they interfere with school, home, or play activities, the child may be diagnosed with an anxiety disorder. Examples of different types of anxiety disorders include:

- Being very afraid when away from parents (separation anxiety)

- Having extreme fear about a specific thing or situation, such as dogs, insects, or going to the doctor (phobias)

- Being very afraid of school and other places where there are people (social anxiety)

- Being very worried about the future and about bad things happening (general anxiety)

- Having repeated episodes of sudden, unexpected, intense fear that come with symptoms like heart pounding, having trouble breathing, or feeling dizzy, shaky, or sweaty (panic disorder)

Anxiety may present as fear or worry, but can also make children irritable and angry. Anxiety symptoms can also include trouble sleeping, as well as physical symptoms like fatigue, headaches, or stomachaches. Some anxious children keep their worries to themselves and, thus, the symptoms can be missed.

Depression in Children

Occasionally being sad or feeling hopeless is a part of every child's life. However, some children feel sad or uninterested in things that they used to enjoy, or feel helpless or hopeless in situations where they could do something to address the situations. When children feel persistent sadness and hopelessness, they may be diagnosed with depression.

Examples of behaviors often seen when children are depressed include:

- Feeling sad, hopeless, or irritable a lot of the time

- Not wanting to do or enjoy doing fun things

- Changes in eating patterns—eating a lot more or a lot less than usual

- Changes in sleep patterns—sleeping a lot more or a lot less than normal

- Changes in energy—being tired and sluggish or tense and restless a lot of the time

- Having a hard time paying attention

- Feeling worthless, useless, or guilty

- Self-injury and self-destructive behavior

Extreme depression can lead a child to think about suicide or plan for suicide. For youth ages 10–24 years, suicide is the leading form of death.

Some children may not talk about helpless and hopeless thoughts, and they may not appear sad. Depression might also cause a child to make trouble or act unmotivated, so others might not notice that the child is depressed or may incorrectly label the child as a trouble-maker or lazy.

Treatment for Anxiety and Depression

The first step to treatment is to talk with a healthcare provider to get an evaluation. The American Academy of Child and Adolescent Psychiatry (AACAP) recommends that healthcare providers routinely screen children for behavioral and mental health concerns. Some of the signs and symptoms of anxiety or depression are shared with other conditions, such as trauma. Specific symptoms like having a hard time focusing could be a sign of attention-deficit hyperactivity disorder (ADHD).

It is important to get a careful evaluation to get the best diagnosis and treatment. Consultation with a health provider can help determine if medication should be part of the treatment. A mental health professional can develop a therapy plan that works best for the child and family. Behavior therapy includes child therapy, family therapy, or a combination of both. The school can also be included in the treatment plan. For very young children, involving parents in treatment is key. Cognitive-behavioral therapy (CBT) is one form of therapy that is used to treat anxiety or depression, particularly in older children. It helps the child change negative thoughts into more positive, effective ways of thinking, leading to more effective behavior. Behavior therapy for anxiety may involve helping children cope with and manage anxiety symptoms while gradually exposing them to their fears so as to help them learn that bad things do not occur.

Treatments can also include a variety of ways to help the child feel less stressed and be healthier like nutritious food, physical activity, sufficient sleep, predictable routines, and social support.

Get Help Finding Treatment

Here are tools to find a healthcare provider familiar with treatment options:

- Psychologist Locator, a service of the American Psychological Association (APA) Practice Organization.

- Child and Adolescent Psychiatrist Finder, a research tool by the American Academy of Child and Adolescent Psychiatry (AACAP).

- Find a cognitive behavioral therapist, a search tool by the Association for Behavioral and Cognitive Therapies (ABCT).

- If you need help finding treatment facilities, use the "Treatment Locator" widget.

Prevention of Anxiety and Depression

It is not known exactly why some children develop anxiety or depression. Many factors may play a role, including biology and temperament. But it is also known that some children are more likely to develop anxiety or depression when they experience trauma or stress, when they are maltreated, when they are bullied or rejected by other children, or when their own parents have anxiety or depression.

Although these factors appear to increase the risk for anxiety or depression, there are ways to decrease the chance that children experience them. Learn about public health approaches to prevent these risks:

- Bullying prevention

- Child maltreatment prevention

- Youth violence prevention

- Depression after birth

- Caring for children in a disaster

Depression and Anxiety among Women

Money worries, health problems, and the loss of loved ones become more common as we age. So it might seem "normal" for an older adult to feel depressed or anxious a lot of the time. It's not. Just like at any other age, constant worrying could be due to an anxiety disorder. And, ongoing feelings of sadness or numbness could be signs of depression.

In recent years, you have probably heard more and more about depression, anxiety, and other mental health problems. You may know how common they are and that they are real illnesses and not signs of personal weakness. Yet, many women still don't seek treatment for mental health problems because they play down or dismiss their symptoms or are embarrassed or unwilling to talk about them.

It may be hard to accept that you need help. But it's important to get it. Untreated mental health problems can reduce your quality of life. The damage can be both emotional and physical. In fact, depression may be a symptom of a physical problem. People with diabetes, heart disease, and some other health problems have a higher risk of depression. Depression and other mental health problems can make it more difficult, and more costly, to treat these and other conditions. That makes it even more important to see your doctor.

Also, untreated depression is a primary risk factor for suicide. In fact, older adults commit suicide at a higher rate than any other age group. That's why you need to get help right away if you or a loved one is having mental health problems.

Before you say, "I'm fine"...

Ask yourself if you feel:

- Nervous or "empty"
- Guilty or worthless
- Very tired and slowed down
- You don't enjoy things the way you used to
- Restless and irritable
- Like no one loves you
- Like life is not worth living

Or if you are:

- Sleeping more or less than usual
- Eating more or less than usual
- Having persistent headaches, stomach aches, or chronic pain

If these symptoms keep occurring and are interfering with your daily life, see your doctor. They may be signs of depression or an anxiety disorder, treatable medical illnesses. But your doctor can only treat you if you say how you are really feeling. Depression is not a normal part of aging. Talk to your doctor.

Reach out. It's important that you talk to someone—anyone. It could be a friend, family member, a religious leader, or your doctor. Talking to them may help you feel better, and they can help make sure you get treatment.

Section 30.2

Eating Disorders, Anxiety, and Depression

"Eating Disorders, Anxiety, and Depression,"
© 2017 Omnigraphics. Reviewed March 2016.

Depression

Depression is a mood disorder that comprises acute feelings of distress, helplessness, anxiety, and/or guilt. It is one of the most common mental-health problems, and it can seriously affect the overall well-being and productivity of the individual. Symptoms may include:

- Increased frustration

- Insomnia

- Reckless behavior

- Loss of interest in activities that were previously enjoyed

- Irritability

- Feelings of insignificance or self-hatred

- Tendency to abuse alcohol or drugs

- Frequent feelings of fatigue or pain

- Low energy level

- Fluctuations in eating habits and body weight

- Social withdrawal

- Delusions

- Suicidal thoughts

Depression can be caused by a number of factors, including hormonal imbalance, traumatic experiences, previous history of substance abuse, and side-effects of certain medication. It can either co-occur with, or lead to the development of other mental illnesses, such as anxiety, phobias, panic disorders, and eating disorders.

It is not clear whether eating disorders take root in an individual due to existing depression, or whether eating disorders cause depression. Since no two eating disorders are the same, and each is a complex condition on its own, both arguments are considered valid in different cases. For instance, feelings of worthlessness and moodiness are often identified as a sign of an eating disorder, which, on the other hand, may also be symptoms of depression. Likewise, a depressed person can indulge in emotional eating, which can subsequently lead to an eating disorder.

Anxiety

It is quite normal for people to feel anxious in stressful situations, but when an individual experiences an extreme and unreasonable level of anxiety, it is characterized as a disorder. Anxiety disorder is generally identified as a combination of psychological states, such as nervousness, fear, worry, and mistrust, that extends over a long period of time and considerably affects daily activities. Anxiety may be caused by a combination of environmental, social, psychological, genetic, and physiological factors. Some examples include:

- Hormonal imbalance

- Substance abuse, or withdrawal from an illicit drug

- History of mental illness in the family

- Traumatic episodes

- Current physical ailment

Types of anxiety disorders include generalized anxiety disorder (GAD), obsessive-compulsive disorder (OCD), phobias, social anxiety disorder, panic disorder, and posttraumatic stress disorder (PTSD).

Each of them has its own unique symptoms, which are further categorized as physical, behavioral, emotional, and cognitive. These symptoms include sweating, irregular heartbeat, difficulty in breathing, headache, irregular sleeping patterns, nervous habits, irritability, restlessness, obsessive and unwanted thoughts, and irrational fear.

Like depression, anxiety disorder can co-occur with eating disorders. And similarly, an individual suffering from an anxiety disorder can develop an eating disorder as a means of coping with anxiety. In most cases, anxiety precedes the onset of an eating disorder, such as when an individual briefly soothes symptoms of anxiety by trying to gain a sense of control over other aspects of life, like food, exercise, and weight. This, in the long run, can lead to the development of eating disorders.

Due to the complex nature of eating disorders in conjunction with depression or anxiety, there is the need for an intense treatment plan that analyzes the factors underlying these conditions. Since a number of similar factors can lead to the development of each of these illnesses, successful treatment requires an inclusive strategy that addresses the root cause of all the conditions and helps the individual learn to manage the co-occurring disorder separately and not associate it with food. In addition to medication and nutritional support, the treatment plan may also include various forms of therapy, such as group therapy, cognitive behavioral therapy (CBT), and music and art therapy.

References

1. "Eating Disorders and Other Health Problems," Eating Disorders Victoria, June 19, 2015.

2. Ekern, Jacquelyn. "Dual Diagnosis and Co-Occurring Disorders," Eating Disorder Hope, April 25, 2012.

Chapter 31

Depression, Substance Use, and Addiction

Chapter Contents

Section 31.1

Addiction Can Lead to Depression and Other Mental Disorders

This section includes text excerpted from "DrugFacts—Comorbidity: Addiction and Other Mental Disorders," National Institute on Drug Abuse (NIDA), March 2011. Reviewed November 2016.

What Is Comorbidity?

The term "comorbidity" describes two or more disorders or illnesses occurring in the same person. They can occur at the same time or one after the other. Comorbidity also implies interactions between the illnesses that can worsen the course of both.

Is Drug Addiction a Mental Illness?

Yes. Addiction changes the brain in fundamental ways, disturbing a person's normal hierarchy of needs and desires and substituting new priorities connected with procuring and using the drug. The resulting compulsive behaviors that weaken the ability to control impulses, despite the negative consequences, are similar to hallmarks of other mental illnesses.

How Common Are Comorbid Drug Addiction and Other Mental Illnesses?

Many people who are addicted to drugs are also diagnosed with other mental disorders and vice versa. For example, compared with the general population, people addicted to drugs are roughly twice as likely to suffer from mood and anxiety disorders, with the reverse also true.

Why Do These Disorders Often Co-Occur?

Although drug use disorders commonly occur with other mental illnesses, this does not mean that one caused the other, even if one appeared first. In fact, establishing which came first or why can be difficult. However, research suggests the following possibilities for this common co-occurrence:

- Drug abuse may bring about symptoms of another mental illness. Increased risk of psychosis in vulnerable marijuana users suggests this possibility.

- Mental disorders can lead to drug abuse, possibly as a means of "self-medication." Patients suffering from anxiety or depression may rely on alcohol, tobacco, and other drugs to temporarily alleviate their symptoms.

These disorders could also be caused by shared risk factors, such as:

- **Overlapping genetic vulnerabilities**: Predisposing genetic factors may make a person susceptible to both addiction and other mental disorders or to having a greater risk of a second disorder once the first appears.

- **Overlapping environmental triggers**: Stress, trauma (such as physical or sexual abuse), and early exposure to drugs are common environmental factors that can lead to addiction and other mental illnesses.

- **Involvement of similar brain regions**: Brain systems that respond to reward and stress, for example, are affected by drugs of abuse and may show abnormalities in patients with certain mental disorders.

- **Drug use disorders and other mental illnesses are developmental disorders**: That means they often begin in the teen years or even younger—periods when the brain experiences dramatic developmental changes. Early exposure to drugs of abuse may change the brain in ways that increase the risk for mental disorders. Also, early symptoms of a mental disorder may indicate an increased risk for later drug use.

How Are These Comorbid Conditions Diagnosed and Treated?

The high rate of comorbidity between drug use disorders and other mental illnesses calls for a comprehensive approach that identifies and evaluates both. Accordingly, anyone seeking help for either drug abuse/addiction or another mental disorder should be checked for both and treated accordingly.

Several behavioral therapies have shown promise for treating comorbid conditions. These approaches can be tailored to patients according to age, specific drug abused, and other factors. Some therapies have proven more effective for adolescents, while others have shown greater effectiveness for adults; some are designed for families and groups, others for individuals.

Effective medications exist for treating opioid, alcohol, and nicotine addiction and for alleviating the symptoms of many other mental disorders, yet most have not been well studied in comorbid populations. Some medications may benefit multiple problems. For example, evidence suggests that bupropion (trade names: Wellbutrin, Zyban), approved for treating depression and nicotine dependence, might also help reduce craving and use of the drug methamphetamine. More research is needed, however, to better understand how these medications work, particularly when combined in patients with comorbidities.

Section 31.2

Can Smoking Cause Depression?

This section includes text excerpted from "Depression," Centers for Disease Control and Prevention (CDC), March 15, 2015.

Who Gets Depression?

In general' about 1 out of every 6 adults will have depression at some time in their life. Depression affects about 15 million American adults every year. Anyone can get depressed. Depression can happen at any age and to any type of person. Your race, ethnicity, or how much money you make doesn't change your chance of getting depression. But some types of people seem more likely to get depressed than others. For example,

- Smokers

- People with medical problems

- People who are stressed

Why Is Depression More Common in Smokers?

Nobody knows why smokers are more likely to have depression than non–smokers, but there are a number of guesses. People who have depression might smoke to feel better. Or smokers might get depression more easily because they smoke. Other ideas are also possible. More research is needed to find out for sure. No matter what the cause, there are treatments that work for both depression and smoking.

If I Get Depressed after Quitting Smoking, Should I Start Smoking Again?

No! Look for ways to get help with your depression. Smoking does not treat depression. Remember that smoking is linked to many serious health problems for both smokers and the people around them. Finding ways to help your depression and quit smoking are the best way to go.

How Long Does It Last?

Everyone is different. For some people, it will only last a few weeks, some for many months if not treated. For many people, depression is only a problem during really stressful times (like a divorce or the death of a loved one). For other people, depression happens off and on through their life.

But, for both groups of people, there are treatments for depression that can help reduce the symptoms and shorten how long the feelings last.

Is It worth Getting Treatment for Depression?

Yes! Treatment almost always helps to reduce symptoms and shorten how long the depression lasts. A common problem is that too few people get help. Many people think that depression is not a real problem, can't be all that serious, or is a sign that they are simply not tough enough to deal with life. None of these are true.

You do not need to feel shy or embarrassed about talking openly and honestly about your feelings and worries. This is an important part of getting better. Many people benefit from treatment for depression, even if the symptoms are not serious. So you don't need to have a lot of symptoms of depression before talking to your doctor or a qualified mental health professional about getting treatment.

If you find that you have 5 or more signs from the list above, you should talk with your doctor or a qualified mental health professional. This is especially true if the feelings have lasted 2 weeks or more, are making you worried, or are getting in the way of your daily life.

What Are the Treatments for Depression?

There are many good treatments for depression, and most people who use them to get better. Treatment usually means getting psychotherapy/counseling, taking medications, or doing both. Your doctor or a qualified mental health professional can help you figure out what treatment is best for you.

What Is Therapy (Counseling, Talk Therapy, Psychotherapy)?

Therapy has shown to be quite helpful and is often an important part of treatment for depression.

Getting therapy does not mean you will be in treatment forever. Most talk therapy is for a short time. Depending on how serious your feelings are, it can mean meeting only a few times with a therapist. Most talk therapy focuses on thoughts, feelings, and issues that are happening in your life now. In some cases, understanding your past can help, but finding ways to address what is happening in your life now can help you cope and be ready for challenges in the future.

Therapy is more than just telling your therapist about your problems. It means working with your therapist to improve coping with the things happening in your life, change behaviors that are causing problems, and find solutions. Your therapist may give you some things for you to think about and work on in between meetings. Some common goals of therapy:

- Get healthier

- Get over fears or insecurities

- Cope with stress

- Make sense of past painful events

- Identify things that make your depression worse

- Have better relationships with family and friends

- Make a plan for dealing with a crisis

- Understand why something bothers you and what you can do about it

What Can I Expect from Depression Medication?

Many people with depression find that taking medication is a useful tool in improving their mood and coping. Medications for depression are called antidepressants. Antidepressants cannot solve all your problems, but they can help you to even out your mood and be more able to handle events in your life that are making your mood worse.

Antidepressants are prescription medications, so talking to your doctor about taking them might be useful to you. If your doctor writes you a prescription for an antidepressant, ask exactly how you should take the medication. There are many medications, so you and your doctor have options to choose from. Sometimes it takes trying a couple different medications to find the best one for you; be patient.

When taking these medications, it is important to stick with them for a while. Many people start feeling better a few days after starting the medication, but it often takes 1 to 2 weeks of taking it to feel a big difference, and 4 weeks to feel the most benefit. It's also common to have to change the dose, so you will want to work closely with your doctor.

How long a person takes antidepressants is very different from person to person. Many people are on them for 6 to 12 months, and some people take them for longer. Again, you and your doctor will want to talk about what is best for you.

Antidepressants are safe and work well for most people, but it is still important to talk with your doctor about side effects you may get. Side effects usually do not get in the way of daily life, and they go away as your body gets used to the medication.

If you notice that your mood is getting worse, especially if you have thoughts about hurting yourself, it is important to call your doctor right away.

How Else Can I Take Care of Myself?

There are many things you can do to help lift your mood and improve feelings of depression.

- Exercise. This can be something as simple as taking a fast walk or as involved as going to the gym or joining a team sport. The type of exercise depends on how fit you are, but any kind of activity can help. Start small and build over time. This can be hard to do when you're depressed because feeling down saps all your energy. But making the effort will pay off! It will help you feel better.

- Structure your day. Create a plan to stay busy. It is especially important to get out of the house whenever you can.

- Talk and do things with other people. Many people who are feeling depressed are cut off from other people. Having daily contact with other people will help your mood.

- Build rewards into your life. For many who are depressed, rewards and fun activities are missing from life. It is helpful to find ways to reward yourself. Even small things add up and can help your mood.

- Do what used to be fun, even if does not seem fun right now. One of the common signs of depression is not wanting to do activities that used to be fun. It may take a little time, but doing fun activities again will help improve your mood. Some people like to make a list of fun events and then do at least one a day.

- Talk with friends and loved ones. Their support is a key to you feeling better. Having a chance to tell them your concerns can help things seem less scary.

Section 31.3

Alcohol Use and Depression among Older Adults

This section includes text excerpted from "Alcohol Use and Older Adults: Alcohol and Aging," NIHSeniorHealth, National Institute on Aging (NIA), August 2015.

What Is Alcohol?

Alcohol, also known as ethanol, is a chemical found in beverages like beer, wine, and distilled spirits such as whiskey, vodka, and rum.

Through a process called fermentation, yeast converts the sugars naturally found in grains and grapes into the alcohol that is in beer and wine. Another process, called distillation, concentrates alcohol in the drink making it stronger, producing what are known as distilled spirits.

The 2012–2013 National Epidemiologic Survey on Alcohol and Related Conditions III (NESARC III) found that 55.2 percent of adults age 65 and over drink alcohol. Most of them don't have a drinking problem, but some of them drink above the recommended daily limits. Sometimes people don't know they have a drinking problem. Men are more likely than women to have problems with alcohol.

Alcohol and Aging

Adults of any age can have problems with alcohol. In general, older adults don't drink as much as younger people, but they can still have trouble with drinking. As people get older, their bodies change. They can develop health problems or chronic diseases. They may take more medications than they used to. All of these changes can make alcohol use a problem for older adults.

Older Adults Are Sensitive to Alcohol's Effects

Limited research suggests that sensitivity to alcohol's health effects may increase with age. As people age, there is a decrease in the amount of water in the body, so when older adults drink, there is less water in their bodies to dilute the alcohol that is consumed. This causes older adults to have a higher blood alcohol concentration (BAC) than younger people after consuming an equal amount of alcohol.

This means that older adults may experience the effects of alcohol, such as slurred speech and lack of coordination, more readily than when they were younger. An older person can develop problems with alcohol even though his or her drinking habits have not changed.

Excessive Drinking Can Cause/Worsen Physical and Mental Health Problems

Drinking too much alcohol can cause health problems. Heavy drinking over time can damage the liver, the heart, and the brain. It can increase the risk of developing certain cancers and immune system disorders as well as damage muscles and bones. Drinking too much alcohol can make some health conditions worse. These conditions include diabetes, high blood pressure, congestive heart failure, liver problems, and memory problems.

Other health issues include mood disorders such as depression and anxiety. Adults with major depression are more likely than adults without major depression to have alcohol problems.

Alcohol and Medicines

Many older adults take medicines, including prescription drugs, over-the-counter (non-prescription) drugs, and herbal remedies. Drinking alcohol can cause certain medicines not to work properly and other medicines to become more dangerous or even deadly. Mixing alcohol and some medicines, particularly sedative-hypnotics, can cause sleepiness, confusion, or lack of coordination, which may lead to accidents and injuries. Mixing medicines also may cause nausea, vomiting, headaches, and other more serious health problems.

Some Medicines and Alcohol Don't Mix

- Dozens of medicines interact with alcohol and those interactions can be harmful. Here are some examples.
- Taking aspirin or arthritis medications and drinking alcohol can increase the risk of bleeding in the stomach.
- Taking the painkiller acetaminophen and drinking alcohol can increase the chances of liver damage.
- Taking cold and allergy medicines that contain antihistamines often causes drowsiness. Drinking alcohol can make this drowsiness worse and impair coordination.
- Drinking alcohol and taking some medicines that aid sleep, reduce pain, or relieve anxiety or depression can cause a range of problems, including sleepiness and poor coordination as well as difficulty breathing, rapid heartbeat and memory problems.
- Drinking alcohol and taking medications for high blood pressure, diabetes, ulcers, gout, and heart failure can make those conditions worse.

Medications stay in the body for at least several hours. So, you can still experience a problem if you drink alcohol hours after taking a pill. Read the labels on all medications and follow the directions. Some medication labels warn people not to drink alcohol when taking the medicine. Ask a doctor, pharmacist, or other healthcare provider whether it's okay to drink alcohol while taking a certain medicine.

Chapter 32

Genetics and Depression

The largest genome-wide study of its kind has determined how much five major mental illnesses are traceable to the same common inherited genetic variations. Researchers funded in part by the National Institutes of Health (NIH) found that the overlap was highest between schizophrenia and bipolar disorder; moderate for bipolar disorder and depression and for Attention deficit hyperactivity disorder (ADHD) and depression; and low between schizophrenia and autism. Overall, common genetic variation accounted for 17–28 percent of risk for the illnesses.

"Since our study only looked at common gene variants, the total genetic overlap between the disorders is likely higher," explained Naomi Wray, Ph.D., University of Queensland, Brisbane, Australia, who co-led the multi-site study by the Cross Disorders Group of the Psychiatric Genomics Consortium (PGC), which is supported by the National Institutes of Health (NIH)'s National Institute of Mental Health (NIMH). "Shared variants with smaller effects, rare variants, mutations, duplications, deletions, and gene-environment interactions also contribute to these illnesses."

- Dr. Wray, Kenneth Kendler, M.D., of Virginia Commonwealth University, Richmond, Jordan Smoller, M.D., of Massachusetts General Hospital, Boston, and other members of the PGC group report on their findings in the journal Nature Genetics.

This chapter includes text excerpted from "New Data Reveal Extent of Genetic Overlap between Major Mental Disorders," National Institute of Mental Health (NIMH), August 12, 2013. Reviewed November 2016.

- "Such evidence quantifying shared genetic risk factors among traditional psychiatric diagnoses will help us move toward classification that will be more faithful to nature," said Bruce Cuthbert, Ph.D., director of the NIMH Division of Adult Translational Research and Treatment Development and coordinator of the Institute's Research Domain Criteria (RDoC) project, which is developing a mental disorders classification system for research based more on underlying causes.

- Earlier this year, PGC researchers—more than 300 scientists at 80 research centers in 20 countries—reported the first evidence of overlap between all five disorders. People with the disorders were more likely to have suspect variation at the same four chromosomal sites. But the extent of the overlap remained unclear. In the study, they used the same genome-wide information and the largest data sets currently available to estimate the risk for the illnesses attributable to any of hundreds of thousands of sites of common variability in the genetic code across chromosomes. They looked for similarities in such genetic variation among several thousand people with each illness and compared them to controls—calculating the extent to which pairs of disorders are linked to the same genetic variants.

- The overlap in heritability attributable to common genetic variation was about 15 percent between schizophrenia and bipolar disorder, about 10 percent between bipolar disorder and depression, about 9 percent between schizophrenia and depression, and about 3 percent between schizophrenia and autism.

- The newfound molecular genetic evidence linking schizophrenia and depression, if replicated, could have important implications for diagnostics and research, say the researchers. They expected to see more overlap between ADHD and autism, but the modest schizophrenia-autism connection is consistent with other emerging evidence.

- The study results also attach numbers to molecular evidence documenting the importance of heritability traceable to common genetic variation in causing these five major mental illnesses. Yet this still leaves much of the likely inherited genetic contribution to the disorders unexplained—not to mention non-inherited genetic factors. For example, common genetic variation accounted for 23 percent of schizophrenia, but evidence from twin and family studies estimate its total heritability at 81 percent. Similarly, the gaps are 25 percent vs. 75 percent for bipolar disorder, 28 percent vs. 75 percent for ADHD, 14 percent vs. 80 percent for autism, and 21 percent vs. 37 percent for depression.

Among other types of genetic inheritance known to affect risk and not detected in this study are contributions from rare variants not associated with common sites of genetic variation. However, the researchers say that their results show clearly that more illness-linked common variants with small effects will be discovered with the greater statistical power that comes with larger sample sizes.

"It is encouraging that the estimates of genetic contributions to mental disorders trace those from more traditional family and twin studies. The study points to a future of active gene discovery for mental disorders" said Thomas Lehner, Ph.D., chief of the NIMH Genomics Research Branch, which funds the project.

Part Five

Depression and Chronic Illness

Chapter 33

Chronic Illness, Pain, and Depression

Chapter Contents

Section 33.1

Chronic Illness Related to Increased Symptoms of Depression

This section includes text excerpted from "Chronic Illness and Mental Health," National Institute of Mental Health (NIMH), December 18, 2015.

Chronic Illness and Mental Health

Depression is a real illness. Treatment can help you live to the fullest extent possible, even when you have another illness.

It is common to feel sad or discouraged after a heart attack, a cancer diagnosis, or if you are trying to manage a chronic condition like pain. You may be facing new limits on what you can do and feel anxious about treatment outcomes and the future. It may be hard to adapt to a new reality and to cope with the changes and ongoing treatment that come with the diagnosis. Your favorite activities, like hiking or gardening, may be harder to do.

Temporary feelings of sadness are expected, but if these and other symptoms last longer than a couple of weeks, you may have depression. Depression affects your ability to carry on with daily life and to enjoy work, leisure, friends, and family. The health effects of depression go beyond mood—depression is a serious medical illness with many symptoms, including physical ones. Some symptoms of depression are:

- Feeling sad, irritable, or anxious

- Feeling empty, hopeless, guilty, or worthless

- Loss of pleasure in usually-enjoyed hobbies or activities, including sex

- Fatigue and decreased energy, feeling listless

- Trouble concentrating, remembering details, and making decisions

- Not being able to sleep, or sleeping too much. Waking too early

- Eating too much or not wanting to eat at all, possibly with unplanned weight gain or loss

- Thoughts of death, suicide or suicide attempts

- Aches or pains, headaches, cramps, or digestive problems without a clear physical cause and/or that do not ease even with treatment

People with Other Chronic Medical Conditions Have a Higher Risk of Depression

The same factors that increase risk of depression in otherwise healthy people also raise the risk in people with other medical illnesses. These risk factors include a personal or family history of depression or loss of family members to suicide.

However, there are some risk factors directly related to having another illness. For example, conditions such as Parkinson disease and stroke cause changes in the brain. In some cases, these changes may have a direct role in depression. Illness-related anxiety and stress can also trigger symptoms of depression.

Depression is common among people who have chronic illnesses such as the following:

- Cancer

- Coronary heart disease

- Diabetes

- Epilepsy

- Multiple sclerosis

- Stroke

- Alzheimer disease

- human immunodeficiency virus/acquired immune deficiency syndrome (HIV/AIDS)

- Parkinson disease

- Systemic lupus erythematosus

- Rheumatoid arthritis

Sometimes, symptoms of depression may follow a recent medical diagnosis but lift as you adjust or as the other condition is treated. In other cases, certain medications used to treat the illness may trigger depression. Depression may persist, even as physical health improves.

Research suggests that people who have depression and another medical illness tend to have more severe symptoms of both illnesses. They may have more difficulty adapting to their co-occurring illness and more medical costs than those who do not also have depression.

It is not yet clear whether treatment of depression when another illness is present can improve physical health. However, it is still important to seek treatment. It can make a difference in day-to-day life if you are coping with a chronic or long-term illness.

People with Depression Are at Higher Risk for Other Medical Conditions

It may have come as no surprise that people with a medical illness or condition are more likely to suffer from depression. The reverse is also true: the risk of developing some physical illnesses is higher in people with depression.

People with depression have an increased risk of cardiovascular disease, diabetes, stroke, and Alzheimer disease, for example. Research also suggests that people with depression are at higher risk for osteoporosis relative to others. The reasons are not yet clear. One factor with some of these illnesses is that many people with depression may have less access to good medical care. They may have a harder time caring for their health, for example, seeking care, taking prescribed medication, eating well, and exercising.

Ongoing research is also exploring whether physiological changes seen in depression may play a role in increasing the risk of physical illness. In people with depression, scientists have found changes in the way several different systems in the body function, all of which can have an impact on physical health:

- Signs of increased inflammation

- Changes in the control of heart rate and blood circulation

- Abnormalities in stress hormones

- Metabolic changes typical of those seen in people at risk for diabetes

It is not yet clear whether these changes, seen in depression, raise the risk of other medical illness. However, the negative impact of depression on mental health and everyday life is clear.

Depression Is Treatable Even When Other Illness Is Present

Do not dismiss depression as a normal part of having a chronic illness. Effective treatment for depression is available and can help even if you have another medical illness or condition. If you or a loved one think you have depression, it is important to tell your healthcare provider and explore treatment options.

You should also inform the healthcare provider about all treatments or medications you are already receiving, including treatment for depression (prescribed medications and dietary supplements). Sharing information can help avoid problems with multiple medications interfering with each other. It also helps the provider stay informed about your overall health and treatment issues.

Recovery from depression takes time, but treatment can improve the quality of life even if you have a medical illness. Treatments for depression include:

- Cognitive behavioral therapy (CBT), or talk therapy, that helps people change negative thinking styles and behaviors that may contribute to their depression. Interpersonal and other types of time-limited psychotherapy have also been proven effective, in some cases combined with antidepressant medication.

- Antidepressant medications, including, but not limited to, selective serotonin reuptake inhibitors (SSRIs) and serotonin and norepinephrine reuptake inhibitors (SNRIs).

- While electroconvulsive therapy (ECT) is generally reserved for the most severe cases of depression, newer brain stimulation approaches, including transcranial magnetic stimulation (TMS), can help some people with depression without the need for general anesthesia and with few side effects.

Section 33.2

Chronic Pain and PTSD

This section includes text excerpted from "Chronic Pain and PTSD: A Guide for Patients," U.S. Department of Veterans Affairs (VA), August 13, 2015.

What Is Chronic Pain?

Chronic pain is when a person suffers from pain in a particular area of the body (for example, in the back or the neck) for at least three to six months. It may be as bad as, or even worse than, short-term pain, but it can feel like more of a problem because it lasts a longer time. Chronic pain lasts beyond the normal amount of time that an injury takes to heal.

Chronic pain can come from many things. Some people get chronic pain from normal wear and tear of the body or from aging. Others have chronic pain from various types of cancer, or other chronic medical illnesses. In some cases, the chronic pain may be from an injury that happened during an accident or an assault. Some chronic pain has no explanation.

How Common Is Chronic Pain?

Approximately one in three Americans suffer from some kind of chronic pain in their lifetimes, and about one quarter of them are not able to do day to day activities because of their chronic pain. Between 80% and 90% of Americans experience chronic problems in the neck or lower back.

How Do Healthcare Providers Evaluate Pain?

Care providers generally assess chronic pain during a physical exam, but how much pain someone is in is hard to determine. Every person is different and perceives and experiences pain in different ways. There is often very little consistency when different doctors try to measure a patient's pain. Sometimes the care provider may not believe the patient, or might minimize the amount of pain. All of these things can be frustrating for the person in pain. Additionally, this kind of experience often makes patients feel helplessness and hopeless, which in turn increases tension and pain and makes the person more upset. Conversation between the doctor and patient is important, including sharing information about treatment options. If no progress is made, get a second opinion.

What Is the Experience of Chronic Pain Like Physically?

There are many forms of chronic pain, including pain felt in: the low back (most common); the neck; the mouth, face, and jaw; the pelvis; or the head (e.g., tension and migraine headaches). Of course, each type of condition results in different experiences of pain.

People with chronic pain are less able to function well in daily life than those who do not suffer from chronic pain. They may have trouble with things such as walking, standing, sitting, lifting light objects, doing paperwork, standing in line at a grocery store, going shopping, or working. Many patients with chronic pain cannot work because of their pain or physical limitations.

What Is the Experience of Chronic Pain Like Psychologically?

Research has shown that many patients who experience chronic pain (up to 100% of these patients) tend to also be diagnosed with depression. Because the pain and disability are always there and that may even become worse over time, many of them think suicide is the only way to end their pain and frustration. They think they have no control over their life. This frustration may also lead the person to use drugs or have unneeded surgery.

Chronic Pain and Posttraumatic Stress Disorder (PTSD)

Some people's chronic pain stems from a traumatic event, such as a physical or sexual assault, a motor vehicle accident, or some type of disaster. Under these circumstances the person may experience both chronic pain and PTSD. The person in pain may not even realize the connection between their pain and a traumatic event. Approximately 15% to 35% of patients with chronic pain also have PTSD. Only 2% of people who do not have chronic pain have PTSD. One study found that 51% of patients with chronic low back pain had PTSD symptoms. For people with chronic pain, the pain may actually serve as a reminder of the traumatic event, which will tend to make the PTSD even worse. Survivors of physical, psychological, or sexual abuse tend to be more at risk for developing certain types of chronic pain later in their lives.

What Is Posttraumatic Stress Disorder (PTSD)?

After a trauma or life-threatening event, it is common to have reactions such as upsetting memories of the event, increased jumpiness, or trouble sleeping. If these reactions do not go away or if they get worse, you may have posttraumatic stress disorder (PTSD).

Chapter 34

Depression and Autoimmune Diseases

Chapter Contents

Section 34.1

Depression Often Coexists with Fibromyalgia

This section contains text excerpted from the following sources: Text beginning with the heading "What Is Fibromyalgia?" is excerpted from "Questions and Answers about Fibromyalgia," National Institute of Arthritis and Musculoskeletal and Skin Diseases (NIAMS), July 2014; Text beginning with the heading "Approved Drugs" is excerpted from "Living with Fibromyalgia, Drugs Approved to Manage Pain," U.S. Food and Drug Administration (FDA), July 25, 2015.

What Is Fibromyalgia?

Fibromyalgia syndrome is a common and chronic disorder characterized by widespread pain, diffuse tenderness, and a number of other symptoms. The word "fibromyalgia" comes from the Latin term for fibrous tissue (fibro) and the Greek ones for muscle (myo) and pain (algia).

Although fibromyalgia is often considered an arthritis-related condition, it is not truly a form of arthritis (a disease of the joints) because it does not cause inflammation or damage to the joints, muscles, or other tissues. Like arthritis, however, fibromyalgia can cause significant pain and fatigue, and it can interfere with a person's ability to carry on daily activities. Also like arthritis, fibromyalgia is considered a rheumatic condition, a medical condition that impairs the joints and/or soft tissues and causes chronic pain.

In addition to pain and fatigue, people who have fibromyalgia may experience a variety of other symptoms including:

- cognitive and memory problems (sometimes referred to as "fibro fog")
- sleep disturbances
- morning stiffness
- headaches
- irritable bowel syndrome

240

- painful menstrual periods
- numbness or tingling of the extremities
- restless legs syndrome
- temperature sensitivity
- sensitivity to loud noises or bright lights

A person may have two or more coexisting chronic pain conditions. Such conditions can include chronic fatigue syndrome, endometriosis, fibromyalgia, inflammatory bowel disease, interstitial cystitis, temporomandibular joint dysfunction, and vulvodynia. It is not known whether these disorders share a common cause.

Who Gets Fibromyalgia?

Scientists estimate that fibromyalgia affects 5 million Americans age 18 or older. For unknown reasons, between 80 and 90 percent of those diagnosed with fibromyalgia are women; however, men and children also can be affected. Most people are diagnosed during middle age, although the symptoms often become present earlier in life.

What Causes Fibromyalgia?

The causes of fibromyalgia are unknown, but there are probably a number of factors involved. Many people associate the development of fibromyalgia with a physically or emotionally stressful or traumatic event, such as an automobile accident. Some connect it to repetitive injuries. Others link it to an illness. For others, fibromyalgia seems to occur spontaneously.

Many researchers are examining other causes, including problems with how the central nervous system (the brain and spinal cord) processes pain.

Some scientists speculate that a person's genes may regulate the way his or her body processes painful stimuli. According to this theory, people with fibromyalgia may have a gene or genes that cause them to react strongly to stimuli that most people would not perceive as painful. There have already been several genes identified that occur more commonly in fibromyalgia patients, and National Institute of Arthritis and Musculoskeletal and Skin Diseases (NIAMS)-supported researchers are currently looking at other possibilities.

Approved Drugs

People with fibromyalgia are typically treated with pain medicines, antidepressants, muscle relaxants, and sleep medicines. In June 2007, Lyrica (pregabalin) became the first U.S. Food and Drug Administration (FDA)-approved drug for specifically treating fibromyalgia; a year later, in June 2008, Cymbalta (duloxetine hydrochloride) became the second; and in January 2009, Savella (milnacipran HCI) became the third.

Lyrica, Cymbalta, and Savella reduce pain and improve function in some people with fibromyalgia. While those with fibromyalgia have been shown to experience pain differently from other people, the mechanism by which these drugs produce their effects is unknown. There is data suggesting that these drugs affect the release of neurotransmitters in the brain. Neurotransmitters are chemicals that transmit signals from one neuron to another. Treatment with Lyrica, Cymbalta, and Savella may reduce the level of pain experienced by some people with fibromyalgia.

Lyrica, marketed by Pfizer Inc., was previously approved to treat seizures, as well as pain from damaged nerves that can happen in people with diabetes (diabetic peripheral neuropathy) and in those who develop pain following the rash of shingles. Side effects of Lyrica including sleepiness, dizziness, blurry vision, weight gain, trouble concentrating, swelling of the hands and feet, and dry mouth. Allergic reactions, although rare, can occur.

Cymbalta, marketed by Eli Lilly and Co., was previously approved to treat depression, anxiety, and diabetic peripheral neuropathy. Cymbalta's side effects include nausea, dry mouth, sleepiness, constipation, decreased appetite, and increased sweating. Like some other antidepressants, Cymbalta may increase the risk of suicidal thinking and behavior in people who take the drug for depression. Some people with fibromyalgia also experience depression.

Savella, marketed by Forest Pharmaceuticals, Inc., is the first drug introduced primarily for treating fibromyalgia. Savella is not used to treat depression in the United States, but acts like medicines that are used to treat depression (antidepressants) and other mental disorders. Antidepressants may increase suicidal thoughts or actions in some people. Side effects include nausea, constipation, dizziness, insomnia, excessive sweating, vomiting, palpitations or increased heart rate, dry mouth and high blood pressure.

Studies of both drugs showed that a substantial number of people with fibromyalgia received good pain relief, but there were others who didn't benefit.

Lyrica and Cymbalta are approved for use in adults 18 years and older. The drug manufacturers have agreed to study their drugs in children with fibromyalgia and in breastfeeding women.

More than Medicine

People with fibromyalgia may find relief of symptoms with pain relievers, sleep medicines, antidepressants, muscle relaxants, and anti-seizure medications. But medication is just one part of the treatment approach.

What helped Matallana was a combination of medicines for pain and sleep, treatment for some of the overlapping conditions like migraines and irritable bowel syndrome, and a combination of water therapy, massage and yoga. Walking, jogging, biking, gently stretching muscles, and other exercises also can be helpful.

Emotional support also is essential, Matallana says. "My husband always believed me, and when you have that kind of support it makes a difference. It's really about facing chronic pain for the rest of your life. So dealing with the emotional impact and not just the physical side is very important."

Section 34.2

Depression and Lupus

This section includes text excerpted from "Lupus Fact Sheet," Office on Women's Health (OWH), U.S. Department of Health and Human Services (HHS), July 16, 2012. Reviewed November 2016.

What Is Lupus?

Lupus is a chronic, autoimmune disease. It can damage any part of the body (skin, joints, and/or organs inside the body). Chronic means that the signs and symptoms tend to last longer than six weeks and often for many years. In lupus, something goes wrong with your immune system, which is the part of the body that fights off viruses, bacteria, and other germs ("foreign invaders," like the flu). Normally your immune system produces proteins called antibodies that protect the body from these invaders. Autoimmune means your immune system cannot tell the difference between these invaders and your body's healthy tissues ("auto" means "self"). In lupus, your immune system creates autoantibodies, which sometimes attack and destroy healthy tissue. These autoantibodies contribute to inflammation, pain, and damage in various parts of the body.

When people talk about "lupus," they usually mean systemic lupus erythematosus or SLE. This is the most common type of lupus. It is hard to guess how many people in the United States have lupus, because the symptoms are so different for every person. Sometimes is not diagnosed. The Lupus Foundation of America thinks that about 16,000 new cases are reported across the country each year.

Although lupus can affect almost any organ system, the disease, for most people, affects only a few parts of the body. For example, one person with lupus may have swollen knees and fever. Another person may be tired all the time or have kidney trouble. Someone else may have rashes. Over time, more symptoms can develop.

Normally, lupus develops slowly, with symptoms that come and go. Women who get lupus most often have symptoms and are diagnosed between the ages of 15 and 45. But the disease also can happen in childhood or later in life.

For some people, lupus is a mild disease. But for others, it may cause severe problems. Even if your lupus symptoms are mild, it is a serious disease that needs constant monitoring and treatment. It can harm your organs and put your life at risk if untreated.

Although the term "lupus" commonly refers to SLE, there are several kinds of lupus:

- Systemic lupus erythematosus, or SLE
- Cutaneous lupus erythematosus
- Discoid lupus erythematosus
- Subacute cutaneous lupus erythematosus
- Drug-induced lupus
- Neonatal lupus

What Causes Lupus?

The cause of lupus is not known. It's not a disease you can catch from another person.

Researchers are looking at these factors:

- Environment (sunlight, stress, smoking, certain medications, and viruses might trigger symptoms in people who are prone to getting lupus)

- Hormones such as estrogen (lupus is more common in women during childbearing years)

- Problems with the immune system

- Genes play an important role, but are not the only reason a person will get lupus. Even someone who has one or more of the genes associated with lupus has a small chance of actually getting the disease. And only 10 percent of people with lupus have a parent or sibling who also has it.

What Are the Symptoms of Lupus?

The signs of lupus differ from person to person. Some people have just a few symptoms; others have more. Lupus symptoms also tend to come and go. Lupus is a disease of flares (the symptoms worsen and you feel ill) and remissions (the symptoms improve and you feel better).

Common signs of lupus are:

- Joint pain and stiffness, with or without swelling
- Muscle aches, pains, or weakness
- Fever with no known cause
- Feeling very tired
- Butterfly-shaped rash across the nose and cheeks
- Other skin rashes
- Unusual weight loss or weight gain
- Anemia (too few red blood cells)
- Trouble thinking, memory problems, confusion
- Kidney problems with no known cause
- Chest pain when taking a deep breath
- Sun or light sensitivity
- Hair loss
- Purple or pale fingers or toes from cold or stress

Less common symptoms include:

- Blood clots

- Seizures

- Sores in the mouth or nose (usually painless)

- Severe headache

- Dizzy spells

- "Seeing things", not able to judge reality

- Feeling sad

- Strokes

- Dry or irritated eyes

Will I Need to See a Special Doctor for My Lupus?

Depending on your symptoms and/or if your organs have been hurt by your lupus, you may need to see special kinds of doctors. Start by seeing your family doctor and a rheumatologist, a doctor who specializes in the diseases of joints and muscles such as lupus.

Your rheumatologist may ask that you also see:

- A clinical immunologist, a doctor who treats immune system disorders

- A nephrologist, a doctor who treats kidney diseases

- A hematologist, a doctor who treats blood disorders

- A dermatologist, a doctor who treats skin problems and diseases

- A neurologist, a doctor who treats problems with the nervous system

- A cardiologist, a doctor who specializes in the heart and blood vessels

- An endocrinologist, a doctor who specializes in problems with the glands and hormones

- A psychologist or psychiatrist, doctors who treat anxiety and depression

- An occupational therapist

- A social worker

Living with Lupus Can Be Hard. How Can I Cope?

Dealing with a long-lasting disease like lupus can be hard on your feelings. Concerns about your health and the effects of your lupus on your work and family life can be stressful. Changes in the way you look and other physical effects of lupus (and the medicines used to treat lupus) can have effect on your self-esteem. Your friends, family, and coworkers might not seem to understand how you feel. At times, you might feel sad or angry. Or, you may feel that you have no control over your life with lupus. But there are things you can do that will help you to cope and to keep a good outlook. Try to:

- **Pace yourself.** People with lupus have less energy and must manage it wisely. Most women with lupus feel much better when they get enough rest and avoid taking on too much at home and at work. To do this, pay attention to your body. Slow down or stop before you're too tired. Learn to pace yourself. Spread out your work and other activities.

- **Reduce stress.** Exercising with your doctor's okay, finding ways to relax, and staying involved in social activities you enjoy will reduce stress and help you to cope.

- **Get support.** Be open about your feelings and needs with family members and friends. Consider support groups or counseling. They can help you to see that you are not alone. Group members teach one another how to enjoy life with lupus.

- **Talk to your doctor.** The symptoms of lupus and some medications can bring on feelings of depression. People with lupus are more likely than others to be depressed and anxious. It is important to tell your doctor about your feelings, so that if it's needed, he or she can treat you for mental health disorders that are more common in people with lupus.

- **Learn about lupus.** People who are well-informed and involved in their own care have less pain, are more active, make fewer visits to the doctor, and feel better about themselves.

Section 34.3

Depression and Rheumatoid Arthritis

This section includes text excerpted from "Arthritis Types," Centers
for Disease Control and Prevention (CDC), July 22, 2016.

Rheumatoid Arthritis

Rheumatoid arthritis (RA) causes premature death, disability,
and lowers the quality of life in the industrialized and developing
world. RA is a systemic inflammatory disease that manifests itself
in multiple joints in the body. This inflammation usually affects the
lining of the joints (synovial membrane), but can also affect other
organs. This inflamed joint lining leads to erosions of the cartilage
and bone and sometimes causes joint deformity. Pain, swelling, and
redness are common joint symptoms. RA causes are unknown, but it
is believed to result from a faulty immune response. RA can begin at
any age and causes fatigue and prolonged stiffness after rest. There
is no cure for RA, but effective drugs are increasingly available to
treat RA and prevent deformed joints. In addition to medications
and surgery, scientifically-proven self-management (techniques that
people use to manage their condition on a daily basis and pursue the
activities important to them) approaches, such as exercise, can reduce
pain and disability.

Rheumatoid arthritis (RA), an autoimmune condition, is a chronic
inflammatory polyarthritis (arthritis that affects 5 or more joints). The
natural history of RA varies considerably with at least three possible
disease courses:

- **Monocyclic:** Have only one episode that ends within 2 to 5
  years of initial diagnosis. This may result from early diagnosis
  or aggressive treatment.

- **Polycyclic:** The levels of disease activity fluctuate over the
  course of the condition.

- **Progressive:** RA continues to increase in severity and does not
  go away.

Erosive changes in the bones around a joint (usually seen on an X-ray) typically occur fastest in the first year of disease.

One natural history study found that 75% of people with RA experienced remission within 5 years of diagnosis.

Diagnosis

RA is diagnosed using information from physical examination (signs and symptoms), blood tests, and X-rays. Ideally, RA is diagnosed early—within 6 months of symptom onset—so that treatment that slows or stops disease progression can begin. Early diagnosis is challenging because the symptoms of early RA can be non-specific (that is, they can be the same for many other diseases). While symptoms of RA include malaise, fatigue, weakness, muscle soreness, low-grade fever, and weight loss, these symptoms may actually be caused by other conditions.

Risk Factors

The etiology, or cause, of RA is unknown. Many cases are believed to result from an interaction between genetic factors and environmental exposures.

- Age and sex
- Genetics
- Modifiable
- Smoking
- Reproductive and breastfeeding history
- Oral contraceptives (OC)
- Hormone replacement therapy (HRT)
- Live birth history
- Breastfeeding
- Menstrual history
- Early life exposures
- Physical activity
- Vitamin D

Comorbidities

The four most common comorbidities among people with arthritis, in order of prevalence are the following:

1. **Cardiovascular disease (CVD)**, in particular ischemic heart disease, is more common among people with RA. It is unclear whether the risk of CVD is before the disease or results from it; a Rochester Epidemiology Project study found that people with RA were more likely to have a hospitalization because of myocardial infarction (MI) prior to diagnosis. However, two longitudinal cohort studies have found no difference in presence of MI, congestive heart failure or angina prior to diagnosis of RA. People with RA have greater evidence of subclinical atherosclerotic disease, and risk of silent MI. A 2015 study found that risk of CVD rose with increasing levels of disease activity. It is unknown whether the increase in CVD mortality is due to the disease, the risk factor profile of people with RA (e.g., presence of hypertension, more likely to be smokers), or the effects of the drugs used to treat the condition.

2. **Infections**, most commonly tuberculosis, are another important and primary cause of death among people with RA. Infections may be responsible for 25% of deaths among people with RA. It is unclear whether this increased susceptibility arising from immunosuppression is due to the intrinsic immune dysfunction in people with RA, the effects of the drugs used to treat it, or both.

3. **Mental health conditions:** High prevalence of anxiety and depression has been documented in several clinical populations of people with RA. Both conditions are associated with increased disease activity and decreased physical function and adherence to medical and non-medical interventions.

4. **Malignancies:** People with RA have an increased incidence of lymphoproliferative malignancies (such as leukemia and multiple myeloma). The cause of this increase is unknown.

Chapter 35

Depression and Brain Injury

What Is Traumatic Brain Injury (TBI)?

Traumatic brain injury (TBI) is the medical term for when your brain is injured by some force, such as:

- A direct hit to your head by an object.

- A fall to the ground or a hard surface.

- A car, motorcycle, or bike crash.

- An explosion or a blast very close to your head.

Doctors can tell whether your injury is mild, moderate, or severe based on what happened at the time of your injury (if you were knocked out, if you had trouble seeing clearly, or lost some memory) and by other tests. Around 1.5 million people who are not in the military experience some form of TBI each year in the United States. It is likely that more people are affected, because many people with mild TBI do not go to the emergency room or report their injury. Most TBI cases (75%) are mild.

Problems Caused by TBI

Any injury to your brain—even if it is mild—can cause problems such as headaches, ringing in your ears, mood changes, or trouble

This chapter includes text excerpted from "Depression after Brain Injury," Agency for Healthcare Research and Quality (AHRQ), U.S. Department of Health and Human Services (HHS), April 13, 2011. Reviewed November 2016.

remembering or thinking for long periods of time. You may have found that your sleeping habits are different or that you feel tired more often.

Even several months or years after your brain injury, you may notice other difficulties, including depression or anxiety.

Depression and TBI

Depression is more than feeling sad every now and then. It is normal for someone who has had a TBI to feel sad by the problems caused by this injury. But for some people, those feelings can extend beyond normal feelings of sadness. People with depression feel sad, lack energy or feel tired, or have difficulty enjoying routine events almost daily. Other symptoms include difficulty sleeping, loss of appetite, poor attention or concentration, feelings of guilt or worthlessness, or thoughts of suicide.

How Common Is Depression for People with TBI?

Research has found that patients with TBI are more likely to experience depression than those who have not had a brain injury. For every 10 people who do not have a brain injury, approximately one person will have depression. For every 10 people who DO have a brain injury, approximately three people will have depression.

What Increases My Risk of Depression?

The risk of depression after a TBI increases whether the injury is mild, moderate, or severe. Researchers cannot say if age, gender, the part of the brain that was injured, or the type of injury makes depression more likely.

How Soon after My Injury Might I Become Depressed?

Researchers do not know when depression is most likely to occur after TBI. Some people experience depression right after their injury, while others develop depression a year or more later. It is important to tell your doctor about any symptoms of depression you may be having even if it has been a while since your head injury. Your doctor or healthcare professional will ask you a series of questions or have you fill out a questionnaire or form to see if you have depression.

How Can I Tell If I Am Depressed?

There are ways to tell if you are depressed.

- Feeling down, depressed, or sad most of the day.
- Changes in your sleeping habits, such as sleeping poorly or sleeping more than usual.
- Losing interest in usual activities such as favorite hobbies, time with family members, or activities with friends.
- Increasing your use of alcohol, drugs, or tobacco.
- Not eating as much or eating more, whether or not you are hungry.
- Strong feelings of sadness, despair, or hopelessness.
- Thoughts of suicide.

You may not notice some of these symptoms, but people living and working around you may see them. You may want to ask the people close to you if they notice these signs in you.

What Should I Do If These Symptoms Start to Occur?

Tell your doctor or healthcare professional as soon as you or others around you notice any symptoms.

Your Healthcare Professional Can Help You Decide

Tell your healthcare professional:
It is important that you contact your healthcare professional when you experience:

1. Changes in sleeping or eating habits.
2. Frequent feelings of sadness, hopelessness, anxiety, or panic.
3. Disinterest in your favorite activities.
4. Thoughts about suicide.

Ask your healthcare professional:
Here are some questions you may want to ask your healthcare professional if you are going to be treated for depression or anxiety following your brain injury:

1. How often should we check to see if I am developing depression or an anxiety disorder?
2. How long do you think I will need psychotherapy or medications to treat these problems?

Chapter 36

Depression and Cancer

Depression Is Different from Normal Sadness

Depression is not simply feeling sad. Depression is a disorder with specific symptoms that can be diagnosed and treated. About one-fourth of cancer patients become depressed. The numbers of men and women affected are about the same.

A person diagnosed with cancer faces many stressful issues. These may include:

- Fear of death

- Changes in life plans

- Changes in body image and self-esteem

- Changes in day to day living

- Money and legal concerns

Sadness and grief are normal reactions to a cancer diagnosis. A person with cancer may also have:

- Feelings of disbelief, denial, or despair

- Trouble sleeping

- Loss of appetite

This chapter includes text excerpted from "Depression (PDQ®)—Patient Version," National Cancer Institute (NCI), March 30, 2016.

- Anxiety or worry about the future

Not everyone who is diagnosed with cancer reacts in the same way. Some cancer patients may not have depression or anxiety, while others may have high levels of both. Signs that you have adjusted to the cancer diagnosis and treatment include being able to stay active in daily life and continue in your roles such as:

- Spouse

- Parent

- Employee

This chapter is mainly about depression in adults with cancer. Some cancer patients may have a higher risk of depression. There are known risk factors for depression after a cancer diagnosis. Factors that increase the risk of depression are not always related to the cancer.

Risk Factors Related to Cancer

Risk factors related to cancer that may cause depression include the following:

- Learning you have cancer when you are already depressed for other reasons

- Having cancer pain that is not well controlled

- Having advanced cancer

- Being physically weakened by the cancer

- Being unmarried (for certain types of cancer)

- Having pancreatic cancer

- Taking certain medicines, such as:

  - Corticosteroids

  - Procarbazine

  - L-asparaginase

  - Interferon alfa

  - Interleukin-2

  - Amphotericin B

Risk Factors Not Related to Cancer

Risk factors not related to cancer that may cause depression include the following:

- A personal or family history of depression or suicide.
- A personal history of alcoholism or drug abuse.
- A personal history of mental problems.
- A weak social support system (not being married, having few family members or friends, having a job where you work alone).
- Stress caused by life events other than the cancer.
- Health problems that are known to cause depression (such as stroke or heart attack).

There Are Many Medical Conditions That Can Cause Depression

Medical conditions that may cause depression include the following:

- Pain that doesn't go away with treatment
- Anemia
- Fever
- Abnormal levels of calcium, sodium, or potassium in the blood
- Not enough vitamin B12 or folate in your diet
- Too much or too little thyroid hormone
- Too little adrenal hormone
- Side effects of certain medicines

Depression and anxiety are common in patients whose cancer is advanced and can no longer be treated. Patients whose cancer can no longer be treated often feel depressed and anxious. These feelings can lower the quality of life. Terminally ill patients who are depressed report being troubled about:

- Symptoms
- Relationships
- Beliefs about life

Depressed terminally ill patients feel they are "being a burden" even when they don't depend very much on others.

Family Members Also Have a Risk of Depression

Anxiety and depression are also common in family members caring for loved ones with cancer. Children are affected when a parent with cancer is depressed and may have emotional and behavioral problems themselves.

Good communication helps. Family members who talk about feelings and solve problems are more likely to have lower levels of anxiety and depression.

Diagnosis of Depression in Cancer Patients

Major depression has specific symptoms that last longer than two weeks. It's normal to feel sad after learning you have cancer, but a diagnosis of depression depends on more than being unhappy. Symptoms of depression include the following:

- Feeling sad most of the time

- Loss of pleasure and interest in activities you used to enjoy

- Changes in eating and sleeping habits

- Nervousness

- Slow physical and mental responses

- Unexplained tiredness

- Feeling worthless

- Feeling guilt for no reason

- Not being able to pay attention

- Frequent thoughts of death or suicide

Your Doctor Will Talk with You to Find out If You Have Symptoms of Depression

Your doctor wants to know how you are feeling and may want to discuss the following:

- The normal feelings cancer patients have. Talking with your doctor about this may help you see if your feelings are normal sadness or more serious.

- Your moods. You may be asked to rate your mood on a scale.

- How long the symptoms have lasted.

- How the symptoms affect your daily life, such as your relationships, your work, and your ability to enjoy your usual activities.

- All the medicines you are taking and other treatments you are receiving. Sometimes, side effects of medicines or the cancer can look like symptoms of depression. This is more likely during active cancer treatment or advanced cancer.

This information will help you and your doctor find out if you are feeling normal sadness or have a depressive disorder. Checking for depression may be repeated at times when stress increases, such as when cancer gets worse or comes back after treatment.

Physical Exams, Mental Exams, and Lab Tests Are Used to Diagnose Depression

In addition to talking with you, your doctor may do the following to check for depression:

- **Physical exam and history:** An exam of the body to check general signs of health, including checking for signs of disease, such as lumps or anything else that seems unusual. A history of your health habits, past illnesses including depression, and treatments will also be taken. A physical exam can help rule out a physical condition that may be causing your symptoms.

- **Laboratory tests:** Medical procedures that test samples of tissue, blood, urine, or other substances in the body. These tests help to diagnose disease, plan and check treatment, or monitor the disease over time. Lab tests are done to rule out a medical condition that may be causing symptoms of depression.

- **Mental status exam:** An exam done to get a general idea of your mental state by checking the following:

  - How you look and act

  - Your mood

  - Your speech

  - Your memory

  - How well you pay attention and understand simple concepts

Chapter 37

Depression and Diabetes

Depression and Medical Comorbidities

The importance of the interplay between depression and many medical comorbidities cannot be overstated. A long list of medical conditions has been associated with increased risk for depression; these include chronic pain, diabetes, cancer, human immunodeficiency virus (HIV), Parkinson disease, cardiovascular and cerebrovascular disease, and multiple sclerosis.

Individuals with diabetes have two to threefold higher odds of depression than those without diabetes. Additionally, depression earlier in life increases the risk of developing diabetes. Depressive symptom severity is associated with poor self-care and medication compliance in addition to higher healthcare-related costs. Patient physical and mental quality of life is also decreased.

Major depression was second only to back and neck pain for having the greatest effect on disability days, at $386.6 million per year. In a World Health Organization (WHO) study of more than 240,000 people

This chapter contains text excerpted from the following sources: Text under the heading "Depression and Medical Comorbidities" is excerpted from "Adult Depression in Primary Care: Percentage of Patients with Type 2 Diabetes with Documentation of Screening for Major Depression or Persistent Depressive Disorder Using Either PHQ-2 or PHQ-9," Agency for Healthcare Research and Quality (AHRQ), U.S. Department of Health and Human Services (HHS), March 2016; Text under the heading "People with Depression Are at Higher Risk for Other Medical Conditions" is excerpted from "Chronic Illness and Mental Health," by National Institute of Mental Health (NIMH), December 2015.

across 60 countries, depression was shown to produce the greatest decrease in quality of health compared to several other chronic diseases. Health scores worsened when depression was a comorbid condition, and the most disabling combination was depression and diabetes.

Depression in the elderly is widespread, often undiagnosed and usually untreated. It is a common misperception that it is a part of normal aging. Losses, social isolation and chronic medical problems that older patients experience can contribute to depression.

The rate of depression in adults older than 65 years of age treated in primary care settings ranges from 17% to 37% and is between 14% and 42% in patients who live in long-term care facilities. Comorbidities are more common in the elderly. The highest rates of depression are found in those with strokes (30% to 60%), coronary artery disease (up to 44%), cancer (up to 40%), Parkinson disease (40%), Alzheimer disease (20% to 40%), and dementia (17% to 31%). The recurrence rate is also extremely high at 40%.

Between 14% and 23% of pregnant women and 10% to 15% of postpartum women will experience a depressive disorder. A review by Milgrom and Gemmill (2014) cites a point prevalence of 13% at three months after delivery and an average of 9% during each trimester of pregnancy. According to a large-scale epidemiological study by Vesga-López et al., depression during the postpartum period may be more common than at other times in a woman's life.

With growing understanding of the systemic impact of perinatal stressors, there is a new body of research examining paternal depression. A recent meta-analysis shows a 10% to 14% incidence of paternal depression during the perinatal period, with a moderate positive correlation with maternal depression.

From 50% to 85% of people who suffer an episode of major depression will have a recurrence, usually within two or three years. Patients who have had three or more episodes of major depression are at 90% risk of having another episode.

Depression Is Treatable

Major depression is a treatable cause of pain, suffering, disability and death, yet primary care clinicians detect major depression in only one-third to one-half of their patients with major depression. Additionally, more than 80% of patients with depression have a medical comorbidity. Usual care for depression in the primary care setting has resulted in only about half of depressed adults getting treated and only 20% to 40% showing substantial improvement over 12 months.

Approximately 70% to 80% of antidepressants are prescribed in primary care, making it critical that clinicians know how to use them and have a system that supports best practices.

People with Depression Are at Higher Risk for Other Medical Conditions.

It may have come as no surprise that people with a medical illness or condition are more likely to suffer from depression. The reverse is also true: the risk of developing some physical illnesses is higher in people with depression.

People with depression have an increased risk of cardiovascular disease, diabetes, stroke, and Alzheimer disease, for example. Research also suggests that people with depression are at higher risk for osteoporosis relative to others. The reasons are not yet clear. One factor with some of these illnesses is that many people with depression may have less access to good medical care. They may have a harder time caring for their health, for example, seeking care, taking prescribed medication, eating well, and exercising.

Ongoing research is also exploring whether physiological changes seen in depression may play a role in increasing the risk of physical illness. In people with depression, scientists have found changes in the way several different systems in the body function, all of which can have an impact on physical health:

- Signs of increased inflammation

- Changes in the control of heart rate and blood circulation

- Abnormalities in stress hormones

- Metabolic changes typical of those seen in people at risk for diabetes

Chapter 38

Depression and Heart Disease

Life after a Heart Attack

Full recovery is possible. There are millions of people who have survived a heart attack. Many recover fully and are able to lead normal lives.

If you have already had a heart attack, your goals are to:

- recover and resume normal activities as much as possible

- prevent another heart attack, and

- prevent complications, such as heart failure or cardiac arrest

Follow-Up Care

After a heart attack, you will need to see your doctor regularly for checkups and tests to see how your heart is doing. Your doctor may recommend:

- lifestyle changes, such as quitting smoking, changing your diet, or increasing your physical activity

This chapter includes text excerpted from "Heart Attack: Life after a Heart Attack," NIHSeniorHealth, National Institute on Aging (NIA), May 2016.

- medications such as aspirin and nitroglycerin tablets for angina (chest pain)

- medications to control chest pain or discomfort, high cholesterol, high blood pressure, and your heart's workload

- participation in a cardiac rehabilitation program

Resuming Normal Activities

Most people who do not have chest pain or other complications are able to return to their normal activities within a few weeks after an uncomplicated heart attack. Most can begin walking immediately and resume sexual activity within a few weeks.

Most patients who do not have chest pain or other complications can usually begin driving within a week, if allowed by state law. Each state has rules for driving a motor vehicle following a serious illness. Patients with complications or chest pain should not drive until their symptoms have been stable for a few weeks.

If You Feel Worried or Depressed

After a heart attack, many people worry about having another heart attack. They often feel depressed and may have trouble adjusting to a new lifestyle. Discuss your feelings with your doctor. Your doctor can give you medication for anxiety or depression, and may recommend professional counseling. Spend time with family, friends, and even pets. Affection can make you feel better and less lonely. Most people stop feeling depressed after they have fully recovered.

Have an Emergency Action Plan

Having a heart attack increases your chances of having another one. Therefore, it is very important that you and your family know how and when to seek medical attention. Talk to your doctor about making an emergency action plan and discuss it with your family.

The emergency action plan should include:

- warning signs or symptoms of a heart attack

- information about how to access emergency medical services in your community, including calling 9-1-1

- steps you can take while waiting for medical help to arrive, such as taking aspirin

- important information to take along with you to the hospital, such as a list of medications that you take or that you are allergic to, and name and number of whom you should contact if you go to the hospital

- your healthcare provider's phone numbers (both during and after office hours)

If You Experience Chest Pain

Many heart attack survivors also have chest pain, also called angina. The pain usually occurs after exertion or with emotional stress and goes away in a few minutes when you rest or take your angina medication as directed. In a heart attack, the pain is usually more severe than in angina, and it does not go away when you rest or take your angina medication. If you think your chest pain could be a heart attack, call 9-1-1.

Chapter 39

Depression and Human Immunodeficiency Virus (HIV)

If you are diagnosed with human immunodeficiency virus (HIV), your physical health is not the only issue you have to deal with. Along with the physical illness are mental health conditions that may come up. Mental health refers to the overall well-being of a person, including a person's mood, emotions, and behavior.

Human immunodeficiency virus / Acquired immune deficiency syndrome (HIV/AIDS) can have a major impact on many parts of your life. People with HIV and those close to them are subject to many things that may affect their mental health.

Many people are surprised when they learn that they have been diagnosed with HIV. Some people feel overwhelmed by the changes that they will need to make in their lives. It is normal to have strong reactions when you find out you are HIV positive, including feelings such as fear, anger, and a sense of being overwhelmed. Often people feel helpless, sad, and anxious about the illness.

There are many things you can do to deal with the emotional aspects of having HIV/AIDS. What follows are some of the most common feelings associated with a diagnosis of HIV/AIDS and suggestions on how to cope with these feelings. You may experience some, all, or none of these feelings, and you may experience them at different times.

This chapter includes text excerpted from "Coping with HIV/AIDS: Mental Health," U.S. Department of Veterans Affairs (VA), July 30, 2015.

Denial

People who find out that they are HIV positive often deal with the news by denying that it is true. You may believe that the HIV test came out wrong or that there was a mix-up of test results. This is a natural and normal first reaction.

At first, this denial may even be helpful, because it can give you time to get used to the idea of infection. However, if not dealt with, denial can be dangerous—you may fail to take certain precautions or reach out for the necessary help and medical support.

Anger

Anger is another common and natural feeling related to being diagnosed with HIV. Many people are upset about how they got the virus or angry that they didn't know they had the virus.

Ways to deal with feelings of anger include the following:

- Talk about your feelings with others, such as people in a support group, or with a counselor, friend, or social worker.

- Try to get some exercise—like gardening, walking, or dancing—to relieve some of the tension and angry feelings you may be experiencing.

- Avoid situations—involving certain people, places, and events—that cause you to feel angry or stressed out.

Sadness or Depression

It is also normal to feel sad when you learn you have HIV/AIDS. If, over time, you find that the sadness doesn't go away or is getting worse, talk with your doctor or someone else you trust. You may be depressed.

Symptoms of depression can include the following, especially if they last for more than two weeks:

- Feeling sad, anxious, irritable, or hopeless

- Gaining or losing weight

- Sleeping more or less than usual

- Moving slower than usual or finding it hard to sit still

- Losing interest in the things you usually enjoy

- Feeling tired all the time

- Feeling worthless or guilty

- Having a hard time concentrating

- Thinking about death or giving up

  To deal with these symptoms, you may want to:

- Talk with your doctor about treatments for depression, such as therapy or medicines

- Get involved with a support group

- Spend time with supportive people, such as family members and friends

If your mood swings or depression get very severe, or if you ever think about suicide, call your doctor right away. Your doctor can help you.

Finding the right treatment for depression takes time—so does recovery. If you think you may be depressed, don't lose hope. Instead, talk to your healthcare provider and seek help for depression.

Fear and Anxiety

Fear and anxiety may be caused by not knowing what to expect now that you've been diagnosed with HIV, or not knowing how others will treat you after they find out you have HIV. You also may be afraid of telling people—friends, family members, and others—that you are HIV positive.

Fear can make your heart beat faster or make it hard for you to sleep. Anxiety also can make you feel nervous or agitated. Fear and anxiety might make you sweat, feel dizzy, or feel short of breath.

Ways to control your feelings of fear and anxiety include the following:

- Learn as much as you can about HIV/AIDS.

- Get your questions answered by your VA healthcare provider.

- Talk with your friends, family members, and healthcare providers.

- Join a support group.

- Help others who are in the same situation, such as by volunteering at an HIV/AIDS service organization. This may empower you and lessen your feelings of fear.

271

- Talk to your doctor about medicines for anxiety if the feelings don't lessen with time or if they get worse.

Stress

If you are HIV positive, you and your loved ones constantly have to deal with stress. Stress is unique and personal to each of us. When stress does occur, it is important to recognize and deal with it. Some ways to handle stress are discussed below. As you gain more understanding about how stress affects you, you will come up with your own ideas for coping with stress.

- **Try physical activity.** When you are nervous, angry, or upset, try exercise or some other kind of physical activity. Walking, yoga, and gardening are just some of the activities you might try to release your tension.

- **Take care of yourself.** Be sure you get enough rest and eat well. If you are irritable from lack of sleep or if you are not eating right, you will have less energy to deal with stressful situations. If stress keeps you from sleeping, you should ask your doctor for help.

- **Talk about it.** It helps to talk to someone about your concerns and worries. You can talk to a friend, family member, counselor, or VA health provider.

- **Let it out.** A good cry can bring relief to your anxiety, and it might even prevent a headache or other physical problem. Taking some deep breaths also releases tension.

AIDS Dementia

HIV/AIDS and some medications for treating HIV may affect your brain. When HIV itself infects the brain, it sometimes can cause problems with thinking, emotions, and movement HIV-Associated Neurocognitive Disorders (HAND). Symptoms can include the following:

- Forgetfulness
- Confusion
- Difficulty paying attention
- Slurred speech
- Sudden shifts in mood or behavior

- Muscle weakness

- Clumsiness

If you think you may have HAND:

- Don't be afraid to tell your healthcare provider that you think something is wrong.

- Keep a notepad with you and write down your symptoms whenever they occur. This information can help your doctor to help you.

- Build as much support as possible, including friends, family, and healthcare providers. Although it's possible to treat HAND successfully, it may take a while for some symptoms to go away.

Coping Tips

It is completely normal to have an emotional reaction upon learning that you are HIV positive, such as anxiety, anger, or depression. These feelings do not last forever. As noted above, there are many things that you can do to help take care of your emotional needs. Here are just a few ideas:

- Talk about your feelings with your doctor, friends, family members, or other supportive people.

- Try to find activities that relieve your stress, such as exercise or hobbies.

- Try to get enough sleep each night to help you feel rested.

- Learn relaxation methods like meditation, yoga, or deep breathing.

- Limit the amount of caffeine and nicotine you use.

- Eat small, healthy meals throughout the day.

- Join a support group.

There are many kinds of support groups that provide a place where you can talk about your feelings, help others, and get the latest information about HIV/AIDS.

More specific ways to care for your emotional well-being include various forms of therapy and medication. Used by themselves or in combination, these may be helpful in dealing with the feelings you are experiencing. Therapy can help you better express your feelings and find ways to cope with your emotions. Medicines that may be able to help with anxiety and depression are also available.

You should always talk with your doctor about your options. There are many ways to care for your emotional health, but treatments must be carefully chosen by your physician based on your specific circumstances and needs.

The most important thing to remember is that you are not alone; there are support systems in place to help you, including doctors, psychiatrists, family members, friends, support groups, and other services.

Chapter 40

Depression and Multiple Sclerosis

What Is Multiple Sclerosis?

Multiple sclerosis (MS) is the most common disabling neurological disease of young adults. It most often appears when people are between 20 to 40 years old. However, it can also affect children and older people.

The course of MS is unpredictable. A small number of those with MS will have a mild course with little to no disability, while another smaller group will have a steadily worsening disease that leads to increased disability over time. Most people with MS, however, will have short periods of symptoms followed by long stretches of relative relief, with partial or full recovery. There is no way to predict, at the beginning, how an individual person's disease will progress.

Researchers have spent decades trying to understand why some people get MS and others don't, and why some individuals with MS have symptoms that progress rapidly while others do not. How does the disease begin? Why is the course of MS so different from person to person? Is there anything we can do to prevent it? Can it be cured?

Multiple sclerosis (MS) is a neuro-inflammatory disease that affects myelin, a substance that makes up the membrane (called the myelin sheath) that wraps around nerve fibers (axons). Myelinated axons

This chapter includes text excerpted from "Multiple Sclerosis: Hope through Research," National Institute of Neurological Disorders and Stroke (NINDS), November 19, 2015.

are commonly called white matter. Researchers have learned that MS also damages the nerve cell bodies, which are found in the brain's gray matter, as well as the axons themselves in the brain, spinal cord, and optic nerve (the nerve that transmits visual information from the eye to the brain). As the disease progresses, the brain's cortex shrinks (cortical atrophy).

The term multiple sclerosis refers to the distinctive areas of scar tissue (sclerosis or plaques) that are visible in the white matter of people who have MS. Plaques can be as small as a pinhead or as large as the size of a golf ball. Doctors can see these areas by examining the brain and spinal cord using a type of brain scan called magnetic resonance imaging (MRI).

While MS sometimes causes severe disability, it is only rarely fatal and most people with MS have a normal life expectancy.

What Are the Signs and Symptoms of MS?

The symptoms of MS usually begin over one to several days, but in some forms, they may develop more slowly. They may be mild or severe and may go away quickly or last for months. Sometimes the initial symptoms of MS are overlooked because they disappear in a day or so and normal function returns. Because symptoms come and go in the majority of people with MS, the presence of symptoms is called an attack, or in medical terms, an exacerbation. Recovery from symptoms is referred to as remission, while a return of symptoms is called a relapse. This form of MS is therefore called relapsing-remitting MS, in contrast to a more slowly developing form called primary progressive MS. Progressive MS can also be a second stage of the illness that follows years of relapsing-remitting symptoms.

A diagnosis of MS is often delayed because MS shares symptoms with other neurological conditions and diseases.

The first symptoms of MS often include:

- vision problems such as blurred or double vision or optic neuritis, which causes pain in the eye and a rapid loss of vision

- weak, stiff muscles, often with painful muscle spasms

- tingling or numbness in the arms, legs, trunk of the body, or face

- clumsiness, particularly difficulty staying balanced when walking

- bladder control problems, either inability to control the bladder or urgency

- dizziness that doesn't go away

MS may also cause later symptoms such as:

- mental or physical fatigue which accompanies the above symptoms during an attack
- mood changes such as depression or euphoria
- changes in the ability to concentrate or to multitask effectively
- difficulty making decisions, planning, or prioritizing at work or in private life

Depression is a common feature of MS. A small number of individuals with MS may develop more severe psychiatric disorders such as bipolar disorder and paranoia, or experience inappropriate episodes of high spirits, known as euphoria.

People with MS, especially those who have had the disease for a long time, can experience difficulty with thinking, learning, memory, and judgment. The first signs of what doctors call cognitive dysfunction may be subtle. The person may have problems finding the right word to say, or trouble remembering how to do routine tasks on the job or at home. Day-to-day decisions that once came easily may now be made more slowly and show poor judgment. Changes may be so small or happen so slowly that it takes a family member or friend to point them out.

What Causes MS?

The ultimate cause of MS is damage to myelin, nerve fibers, and neurons in the brain and spinal cord, which together make up the central nervous system (CNS). But how that happens, and why, are questions that challenge researchers. Evidence appears to show that MS is a disease caused by genetic vulnerabilities combined with environmental factors.

Although there is little doubt that the immune system contributes to the brain and spinal cord tissue destruction of MS, the exact target of the immune system attacks and which immune system cells cause the destruction isn't fully understood.

Researchers have several possible explanations for what might be going on. The immune system could be:

- fighting some kind of infectious agent (for example, a virus) that has components which mimic components of the brain (molecular mimicry)

- destroying brain cells because they are unhealthy

- mistakenly identifying normal brain cells as foreign

The last possibility has been the favored explanation for many years. Research now suggests that the first two activities might also play a role in the development of MS. There is a special barrier, called the blood-brain barrier, which separates the brain and spinal cord from the immune system. If there is a break in the barrier, it exposes the brain to the immune system for the first time. When this happens, the immune system may misinterpret the brain as "foreign."

Genetic susceptibility. Susceptibility to MS may be inherited. Studies of families indicate that relatives of an individual with MS have an increased risk for developing the disease. Experts estimate that about 15 percent of individuals with MS have one or more family members or relatives who also have MS. But even identical twins, whose deoxyribonucleic acid (DNA) is exactly the same, have only a 1 in 3 chance of both having the disease. This suggests that MS is not entirely controlled by genes. Other factors must come into play.

Current research suggests that dozens of genes and possibly hundreds of variations in the genetic code (called gene variants) combine to create vulnerability to MS. Some of these genes have been identified. Most of the genes identified so far are associated with functions of the immune system. Additionally, many of the known genes are similar to those that have been identified in people with other autoimmune diseases as type 1 diabetes, rheumatoid arthritis or lupus. Researchers continue to look for additional genes and to study how they interact with each other to make an individual vulnerable to developing MS.

Sunlight and vitamin D. A number of studies have suggested that people who spend more time in the sun and those with relatively high levels of vitamin D are less likely to develop MS. Bright sunlight helps human skin produce vitamin D. Researchers believe that vitamin D may help regulate the immune system in ways that reduce the risk of MS. People from regions near the equator, where there is a great deal of bright sunlight, generally have a much lower risk of MS than people from temperate areas such as the United States and Canada. Other studies suggest that people with higher levels of vitamin D generally have less severe MS and fewer relapses.

Smoking. A number of studies have found that people who smoke are more likely to develop MS. People who smoke also tend to have more brain lesions and brain shrinkage than non-smokers. The reasons for this are currently unclear.

Infectious factors and viruses. A number of viruses have been found in people with MS, but the virus most consistently linked to the development of MS is Epstein Barr Virus (EBV), the virus that causes mononucleosis.

Only about 5 percent of the population has not been infected by EBV. These individuals are at a lower risk for developing MS than those who have been infected. People who were infected with EBV in adolescence or adulthood and who therefore develop an exaggerated immune response to EBV are at a significantly higher risk for developing MS than those who were infected in early childhood. This suggests that it may be the type of immune response to EBV that predisposes to MS, rather than EBV infection itself. However, there is still no proof that EBV causes MS.

Autoimmune and inflammatory processes. Tissue inflammation and antibodies in the blood that fight normal components of the body and tissue in people with MS are similar to those found in other autoimmune diseases. Along with overlapping evidence from genetic studies, these findings suggest that MS results from some kind of disturbed regulation of the immune system.

How Do Doctors Treat the Symptoms of MS?

MS causes a variety of symptoms that can interfere with daily activities but which can usually be treated or managed to reduce their impact. Many of these issues are best treated by neurologists who have advanced training in the treatment of MS and who can prescribe specific medications to treat the problems.

Fatigue

Fatigue is a common symptom of MS and may be both physical (for example, tiredness in the legs) and psychological (due to depression). Probably the most important measures people with MS can take to counter physical fatigue are to avoid excessive activity and to stay out of the heat, which often aggravates MS symptoms. On the other hand, daily physical activity programs of mild to moderate intensity can significantly reduce fatigue. An antidepressant such as fluoxetine may be prescribed if the fatigue is caused by depression. Other drugs that may reduce fatigue in some individuals include amantadine and modafinil.

Fatigue may be reduced if the person receives occupational therapy to simplify tasks and/or physical therapy to learn how to walk in a way that saves physical energy or that takes advantage of an assistive device. Some people benefit from stress management programs, relaxation training, membership in an MS support group, or individual psychotherapy. Treating sleep problems and MS symptoms that interfere with sleep (such as spastic muscles) may also help.

Depression

Studies indicate that clinical depression is more frequent among people with MS than it is in the general population or in persons with many other chronic, disabling conditions. MS may cause depression as part of the disease process, since it damages myelin and nerve fibers inside the brain. If the plaques are in parts of the brain that are involved in emotional expression and control, a variety of behavioral changes can result, including depression. Depression can intensify symptoms of fatigue, pain, and sexual dysfunction. It is most often treated with selective serotonin reuptake inhibitor (SSRI) antidepressant medications, which are less likely than other antidepressant medications to cause fatigue.

Inappropriate Laughing or Crying

MS is sometimes associated with a condition called pseudobulbar affect that causes inappropriate and involuntary expressions of laughter, crying, or anger. These expressions are often unrelated to mood; for example, the person may cry when they are actually very happy, or laugh when they are not especially happy. In 2010 the U.S. Food and Drug Administration (FDA) approved the first treatment specifically for pseudobulbar affect, a combination of the drugs dextromethorphan and quinidine. The condition can also be treated with other drugs such as amitriptyline or citalopram.

Chapter 41

Depression and Neurological Disorders

Chapter Contents

Section 41.1

Depression and Alzheimer Disease

This section includes text excerpted from "Assessing Risk Factors for
Cognitive Decline and Dementia," National Institute on Aging (NIA),
December 21, 2012. Reviewed November 2016.

Alzheimer Disease

Age and genetics are the best-known risk factors for Alzheimer
disease. While these factors are beyond our control, we may be able to
influence other risk factors involved in age-related cognitive decline and
dementia. Scientists are exploring whether or not exercise and diet or
other lifestyle choices, and certain medical conditions, including mental
health conditions, can influence risk for cognitive decline or dementia.

For instance, recent research has examined the possible role of
depression in the risk for age-related cognitive decline. Scientists are
also continuing to study the possibility that engagement in intellectu-
ally stimulating activities throughout the lifespan can help stave off
age-related cognitive decline. Finally, researchers are finding that in
some people, the brain can compensate for the toxic buildup of amyloid.

Depression

Many scientists suspect that depression increases the risk of age-related cognitive decline in older people. Two studies in very large populations lend further support to this idea.

A retrospective study led by researchers at the University of California, San Francisco, analyzed 45 years of medical records from more
than 13,500 people enrolled in the Kaiser Permanente Medical Care
Program in Northern California. People who had reported on Kaiser
health surveys that they felt depressed or were hospitalized for depression in midlife (40s to early 50s) and/or late life (70s) were at greater
risk of developing dementia in their 80s than people who had never
been depressed.

The age at which people became depressed also influenced their
likelihood of developing Alzheimer or vascular dementia (dementia

associated with stroke or other vascular disease). The risk of developing vascular dementia was increased threefold in people who experienced depression both in midlife and late life, but only by 50 percent in those who first became depressed in late life. In contrast, the risk of developing Alzheimer was increased twofold in both groups.

Similarly, researchers at Emory University, Atlanta, looked at the possible link between depression and cognitive decline in a group of more than 8,000 volunteers. They used data stored at the NIA-supported National Alzheimer Coordinating Center (NACC) database that had been collected at 30 Alzheimer Disease Centers between 2005 and 2011. About one-third of the participants (average age, 73) had mild cognitive impairment (MCI), and the rest were cognitively normal when first evaluated. Twenty-two percent of the participants had recent (within the past 2 years) depression, as defined by clinician judgment.

The Emory researchers found that volunteers who were recently or currently depressed at the first evaluation performed significantly worse on cognitive tests than did their non-depressed peers. In addition, cognitively normal people with recent or current depression were at significantly greater risk of developing MCI within the next 3 years; the risk was highest for those who continued to experience depression during that time. Significantly, treatment with antidepressant medications did not alter the risk of progression from normal cognition to MCI among depressed volunteers. The relationship between late-life depression and cognitive decline warrants further study.

Section 41.2

Depression and Parkinson Disease

This section includes text excerpted from "Parkinson's Disease: Hope through Research," National Institute of Neurological Disorders and Stroke (NINDS), July 21, 2016.

What Is Parkinson Disease (PD)?

Parkinson disease (PD) is a degenerative disorder of the central nervous system that belongs to a group of conditions called movement disorders. It is both chronic, meaning it persists over a long period of time, and progressive, meaning its symptoms grow worse over time. As nerve cells (neurons) in parts of the brain become impaired or die, people may begin to notice problems with movement, tremor, stiffness in the limbs or the trunk of the body, or impaired balance. As these symptoms become more pronounced, people may have difficulty walking, talking, or completing other simple tasks. Not everyone with one or more of these symptoms has PD, as the symptoms appear in other diseases as well.

The precise cause of PD is unknown, although some cases of PD are hereditary and can be traced to specific genetic mutations. Most cases are sporadic—that is, the disease does not typically run in families. It is thought that PD likely results from a combination of genetic susceptibility and exposure to one or more unknown environmental factors that trigger the disease.

PD is the most common form of parkinsonism, in which disorders of other causes produce features and symptoms that closely resemble PD. While most forms of parkinsonism have no known cause, there are cases in which the cause is known or suspected or where the symptoms result from another disorder.

No cure for PD exists today, but research is ongoing and medications or surgery can often provide substantial improvement with motor symptoms.

What Causes the Disease?

PD occurs when nerve cells, or neurons, in the brain die or become impaired. Although many brain areas are affected, the most common symptoms result from the loss of neurons in an area near the base of the brain called the substantia nigra. Normally, the neurons in this area produce an important brain chemical known as dopamine. Dopamine is a chemical messenger responsible for transmitting signals between the substantia nigra and the next "relay station" of the brain, the corpus striatum, to produce smooth, purposeful movement. Loss of dopamine results in abnormal nerve firing patterns within the brain that cause impaired movement.

Studies have shown that most people with Parkinson have lost 60 to 80 percent or more of the dopamine-producing cells in the substantia nigra by the time symptoms appear, and that people with PD also have loss of the nerve endings that produce the neurotransmitter norepinephrine. Norepinephrine, which is closely related to dopamine, is the main chemical messenger of the sympathetic nervous system, the part of the nervous system that controls many automatic functions of the body, such as pulse and blood pressure. The loss of norepinephrine might explain several of the non-motor features seen in PD, including fatigue and abnormalities of blood pressure regulation.

The affected brain cells of people with PD contain Lewy bodies— deposits of the protein alpha-synuclein. Researchers do not yet know why Lewy bodies form or what role they play in the disease. Some research suggests that the cell's protein disposal system may fail in people with PD, causing proteins to build up to harmful levels and trigger cell death. Additional studies have found evidence that clumps of protein that develop inside brain cells of people with PD may contribute to the death of neurons. Some researchers speculate that the protein buildup in Lewy bodies is part of an unsuccessful attempt to protect the cell from the toxicity of smaller aggregates, or collections, of synuclein.

Genetics. Scientists have identified several genetic mutations associated with PD, including the alpha-synuclein gene, and many more genes have been tentatively linked to the disorder. Studying the genes responsible for inherited cases of PD can help researchers understand both inherited and sporadic cases. The same genes and proteins that are altered in inherited cases may also be altered in sporadic cases by environmental toxins or other factors. Researchers also hope that discovering genes will help identify new ways of treating PD.

Environment. Exposure to certain toxins has caused parkinsonian symptoms in rare circumstances (such as exposure to 1-methyl-4-phenyl-1,2,3,6-tetrahydropyridine (MPTP), an illicit drug, or in miners exposed to the metal manganese). Other still-unidentified environmental factors may also cause PD in genetically susceptible individuals.

Mitochondria. Several lines of research suggest that mitochondria may play a role in the development of PD. Mitochondria are the energy-producing components of the cell and abnormalities in the mitochondria are major sources of free radicals—molecules that damage membranes, proteins, Deoxyribonucleic acid (DNA), and other parts of the cell. This damage is often referred to as oxidative stress. Oxidative stress-related changes, including free radical damage to DNA, proteins, and fats, have been detected in the brains of individuals with PD. Some mutations that affect mitochondrial function have been identified as causes of PD.

While mitochondrial dysfunction, oxidative stress, inflammation, toxins, and many other cellular processes may contribute to PD, the actual cause of the cell loss death in PD is still undetermined.

What Are the Symptoms of the Disease?

The four primary symptoms of PD are:

- **Tremor.** The tremor associated with PD has a characteristic appearance. Typically, the tremor takes the form of a rhythmic back-and-forth motion at a rate of 4–6 beats per second. It may involve the thumb and forefinger and appear as a "pill rolling" tremor. Tremor often begins in a hand, although sometimes a foot or the jaw is affected first. It is most obvious when the hand is at rest or when a person is under stress. Tremor usually disappears during sleep or improves with intentional movement. It is usually the first symptom that causes people to seek medical attention.

- **Rigidity.** Rigidity, or a resistance to movement, affects most people with PD. The muscles remain constantly tense and contracted so that the person aches or feels stiff. The rigidity becomes obvious when another person tries to move the individual's arm, which will move only in ratchet-like or short, jerky movements known as "cogwheel" rigidity.

- **Bradykinesia.** This slowing down of spontaneous and automatic movement is particularly frustrating because it may make simple tasks difficult. The person cannot rapidly perform routine movements. Activities once performed quickly and easily—such as washing or dressing—may take much longer. There is often a decrease in facial expressions.

- **Postural instability.** Postural instability, or impaired balance, causes affected individuals to fall easily.

A number of other symptoms may accompany PD, and some can be treated with medication or physical therapy.

- **Depression.** This common disorder may appear early in the course of the disease, even before other symptoms are noticed. Some people lose their motivation and become dependent on family members. Fortunately, depression typically can be treated successfully with antidepressant medications such as amytriptyline or fluoxetine.

- **Emotional changes.** Some people with PD become fearful and insecure, while others may become irritable or uncharacteristically pessimistic.

- **Urinary problems or constipation.** In some people with PD, bladder and bowel problems can occur due to the improper functioning of the autonomic nervous system, which is responsible for regulating smooth muscle activity. Medications can effectively treat some of these symptoms.

- **Sleep problems.** Sleep problems are common in PD and include difficulty staying asleep at night, restless sleep, nightmares and emotional dreams, and drowsiness or sudden sleep onset during the day. Another common problem is "REM behavior disorder," in which people act out their dreams, potentially resulting in injury to themselves or their bed partners. The medications used to treat PD may contribute to some of these sleep issues. Many of these problems respond to specific therapies.

- **Dementia or other cognitive problems.** Some people with PD may develop memory problems and slow thinking. Cognitive problems become more severe in late stages of PD, and a diagnosis of Parkinson disease dementia (PDD) may be given. Memory, social judgment, language, reasoning, or other mental skills may be affected. There is currently no way to halt PD dementia, but drugs such as rivastigmine, donepezil, or memantine may help. The medications used to treat the motor symptoms of PD may cause confusion and hallucinations.

- **Fatigue and loss of energy.** Many people with PD often have fatigue, especially late in the day. Fatigue may be associated with depression or sleep disorders, but it may also result from muscle stress or from overdoing activity when the person feels well. Fatigue may also result from akinesia—trouble initiating or carrying out movement. Exercise, good sleep habits, staying mentally active, and not forcing too many activities in a short time may help to alleviate fatigue.

- **Sexual dysfunction.** Because of its effects on nerve signals from the brain, PD may cause sexual dysfunction. PD-related depression or use of certain medications may also cause decreased sex drive and other problems. People should discuss these issues with their physician as they may be treatable.

Hallucinations, delusions, and other psychotic symptoms can be caused by the drugs prescribed for PD. Reducing PD medications dosages or changing medications may be necessary if hallucinations occur. If such measures are not effective, doctors sometimes prescribe drugs called atypical antipsychotics, which include clozapine and quetiapine. The typical antipsychotic drugs, which include haloperidol, worsen the motor symptoms of PD and should not be used.

How Is PD Diagnosed?

There are currently no blood or laboratory tests that diagnose sporadic PD. Therefore the diagnosis is based on medical history and a neurological examination. In some cases PD can be difficult to diagnose accurately early on in the course of the disease. Early signs and symptoms of PD may sometimes be dismissed as the effects of normal aging. Doctors may sometimes request brain scans or laboratory tests in order to rule out other disorders. However, computed tomography (CT) and magnetic resonance imaging (MRI) brain scans of people with PD usually appear normal. Since many other diseases have similar features but require different treatments, making a precise diagnosis is important so that people can receive the proper treatment.

What Is the Prognosis?

The average life expectancy of a person with PD is generally the same as for people who do not have the disease. Fortunately, there are many treatment options available for people with PD. However, in the late stages, PD may no longer respond to medications and can become associated with serious complications such as choking, pneumonia, and falls.

PD is a slowly progressive disorder. It is not possible to predict what course the disease will take for an individual person. One commonly used scale neurologists use for describing how the symptoms of PD have progressed in a patient is the Hoehn and Yahr scale.

Chapter 42

Depression and Stroke

Stroke is a leading cause of death in the United States. Many factors can raise your risk of having a stroke. Talk with your doctor about how you can control these risk factors and help prevent a stroke.

If you have a stroke, prompt treatment can reduce damage to your brain and help you avoid lasting disabilities. Prompt treatment also may help prevent another stroke.

Researchers continue to study the causes and risk factors for stroke. They're also finding new and better treatments and new ways to help the brain repair itself after a stroke.

What Is a Stroke?

A stroke occurs if the flow of oxygen-rich blood to a portion of the brain is blocked. Without oxygen, brain cells start to die after a few minutes. Sudden bleeding in the brain also can cause a stroke if it damages brain cells.

If brain cells die or are damaged because of a stroke, symptoms occur in the parts of the body that these brain cells control. Examples of stroke symptoms include sudden weakness; paralysis or numbness of the face, arms, or legs (paralysis is an inability to move); trouble speaking or understanding speech; and trouble seeing.

A stroke is a serious medical condition that requires emergency care. A stroke can cause lasting brain damage, long-term disability, or even death.

This chapter includes text excerpted from "Life after a Stroke," National Heart, Lung, and Blood Institute (NHLBI), June 22, 2016.

If you think you or someone else is having a stroke, call 9–1–1 right away. Do not drive to the hospital or let someone else drive you. Call an ambulance so that medical personnel can begin life-saving treatment on the way to the emergency room. During a stroke, every minute counts.

Who Is at Risk for a Stroke?

Certain traits, conditions, and habits can raise your risk of having a stroke or transient ischemic attack (TIA). These traits, conditions, and habits are known as risk factors.

The more risk factors you have, the more likely you are to have a stroke. You can treat or control some risk factors, such as high blood pressure and smoking. Other risk factors, such as age and gender, you can't control.

The major risk factors for stroke include:

- **High blood pressure.** High blood pressure is the main risk factor for stroke. Blood pressure is considered high if it stays at or above 140/90 millimeters of mercury (mmHg) over time. If you have diabetes or chronic kidney disease, high blood pressure is defined as 130/80 mmHg or higher.

- **Diabetes.** Diabetes is a disease in which the blood sugar level is high because the body doesn't make enough insulin or doesn't use its insulin properly. Insulin is a hormone that helps move blood sugar into cells where it's used for energy.

- **Heart diseases.** Coronary heart disease, cardiomyopathy, heart failure, and atrial fibrillation can cause blood clots that can lead to a stroke.

- **Smoking.** Smoking can damage blood vessels and raise blood pressure. Smoking also may reduce the amount of oxygen that reaches your body's tissues. Exposure to secondhand smoke also can damage the blood vessels.

- **Age and gender.** Your risk of stroke increases as you get older. At younger ages, men are more likely than women to have strokes. However, women are more likely to die from strokes. Women who take birth control pills also are at slightly higher risk of stroke.

- **Race and ethnicity.** Strokes occur more often in African American, Alaska Native, and American Indian adults than in White, Hispanic, or Asian American adults.

- **Personal or family history of stroke or TIA.** If you've had a stroke, you're at higher risk for another one. Your risk of having a repeat stroke is the highest right after a stroke. A TIA also increases your risk of having a stroke, as does having a family history of stroke.

- **Brain aneurysms or arteriovenous malformations (AVMs).** Aneurysms are balloon-like bulges in an artery that can stretch and burst. AVMs are tangles of faulty arteries and veins that can rupture (break open) within the brain. AVMs may be present at birth, but often aren't diagnosed until they rupture.

Other risk factors for stroke, many of which of you can control, include:

- Alcohol and illegal drug use, including cocaine, amphetamines, and other drugs

- Certain medical conditions, such as sickle cell disease, vasculitis (inflammation of the blood vessels), and bleeding disorders

- Lack of physical activity

- Overweight and obesity

- Stress and depression

- Unhealthy cholesterol levels

- Unhealthy diet

- Use of nonsteroidal anti-inflammatory drugs (NSAIDs), but not aspirin, may increase the risk of heart attack or stroke, particularly in patients who have had a heart attack or cardiac bypass surgery. The risk may increase the longer NSAIDs are used. Common NSAIDs include ibuprofen and naproxen.

Life after a Stroke

The time it takes to recover from a stroke varies—it can take weeks, months, or even years. Some people recover fully, while others have long-term or lifelong disabilities.

Ongoing care, rehabilitation, and emotional support can help you recover and may even help prevent another stroke.

If you've had a stroke, you're at risk of having another one. Know the warning signs and what to do if a stroke or transient ischemic attack (TIA) occurs. Call 9–1–1 as soon as symptoms start.

Do not drive to the hospital or let someone else drive you. By calling an ambulance, medical personnel can begin lifesaving treatment on the way to the emergency room. During a stroke, every minute counts.

Mental Healthcare and Support

After a stroke, you may have changes in your behavior or judgment. For example, your mood may change quickly. Because of these and other changes, you may feel scared, anxious, and depressed. Recovering from a stroke can be slow and frustrating.

Talk about how you feel with your healthcare team. Talking to a professional counselor also can help. If you're very depressed, your doctor may recommend medicines or other treatments that can improve your quality of life.

Joining a patient support group may help you adjust to life after a stroke. You can see how other people have coped with having strokes. Talk with your doctor about local support groups, or check with an area medical center.

Support from family and friends also can help relieve fear and anxiety. Let your loved ones know how you feel and what they can do to help you.

Transient Ischemic Attack and Depression

Depression is the most common psychiatric disorder affecting patients who have suffered a stroke. A study reveals that patients with stroke or transient ischemic attack (TIA), a " warning stroke" not usually associated with long-lasting functional deficit, have similar frequency of depression and newly identified depression between 3 and 12 months after hospitalization. The North Carolina researchers used a patient registry to identify depression and antidepressant medication use 3 and 12 months after hospitalization among 1,450 individuals with ischemic stroke and 397 individuals with TIA. Three months following hospitalization for stroke or TIA, 17.9 percent of stroke patients had depression compared to 14.3 percent of TIA patients; at 12 months, the percentages were 16.4 percent and 12.8 percent respectively. Persistent depression (diagnosis of depression at both 3 and 12 months) was present in 9.2 percent of those with stroke and 7.6 percent of those with TIA. A high proportion of patients with persistent depression was untreated with antidepressants (67.9 percent of those with stroke, 70 percent of those with TIA).

The risk of depression after even mild stroke or TIA was higher than the general population with a comparable age distribution. The researchers suggest that systematic evaluation for depression in patients with stroke or TIA may improve detection and treatment of this condition.

Part Six

Diagnosis and Treatment of Depression

Chapter 43

Recognizing Signs of Depression in You and Your Loved Ones

Depression

Depression is a serious medical illness. It's more than just a feeling of being "down in the dumps" or "blue" for a few days. Depression is a disorder of the brain. There are a variety of causes, including genetic, environmental, psychological, and biochemical factors. Depression can range from mild to severe, and symptoms can include many of feelings or behaviors listed below.

How Do I Know If Something Is Wrong and How Can I Find Help

Almost everyone faces mental health challenges at some point. A support network can help you cope during these tough times. But

---

This chapter contains text excerpted from the following sources: Text beginning with the heading "Depression" is excerpted from "Taking Care of Yourself: Mental Health," AIDS.gov, U.S. Department of Health and Human Services (HHS), March 7, 2014; Text under the heading "Talking about Depression to Loved Ones" is excerpted from "Depression: Conversation Starters," Office of Disease Prevention and Health Promotion (ODPHP), U.S. Department of Health and Human Services (HHS), February 8, 2016.

when your mental health symptoms begin to affect your ability to cope and carry out typical functions in your life, it's important to get help.

So how do you know when it's time to get help? Sometimes, you can notice a change in yourself—and, sometimes, the people around you are the ones who notice. Some changes that might be significant include:

- No longer finding enjoyment in activities which usually make you happy
- Withdrawing from social interaction
- Change in memory functioning
- Sleeping too much—or being unable to sleep
- Feeling "sad" or "empty" much of the time
- Feeling guilty
- Feeling tired all the time
- Experiencing sudden and repeated attacks of fear known as "panic attacks"
- Having racing thoughts
- Loss of sexual interest
- Worrying what others are thinking about you
- Hearing voices in your head
- Feelings of wanting to hurt yourself or others
- Intense anger or rage toward others

Get Help

If you feel that something might be different or "wrong," it's important to tell your doctor or other healthcare provider—including your nurse, case manager, or social worker—so that he or she can help you. Don't be embarrassed to talk about your feelings. Your feelings are important and valid and the members of your healthcare team should be concerned about you and respect you.

If what you are describing is pattern of behavior and feelings you have experienced over time, your healthcare provider may offer treatment or a referral to a mental health services provider. Mental health providers (psychologists, therapists, psychiatrists, social workers, or nurses) can use many forms of treatment, including medications and/ or "talk therapy."

Talking about Depression to Loved Ones

Depression can be hard to talk about. But if a friend or loved one is depressed, having a conversation about getting help can make a big difference. Use these tips to start talking.

Show you care:

- "Tell me how you are feeling. I'm here to support and listen to you."

- "I'm worried about you. I think you may need to talk to a doctor about depression."

- "Let me remind you of all the great things I love about you."

- "I really like to spend time with you. Let's take a walk or go to a movie together."

Offer hope:

- "You aren't alone. Many people suffer from depression, and it's nothing to be ashamed of."

- "Depression is an illness that can be treated. Getting help is the best thing you can do."

- "Most people get better with treatment—even people who have severe depression."

- "There are different ways to treat depression, including medicine and talk therapy. Getting active might also help you feel better."

Offer to help:

- "Let me help you figure out what's going on. You can start by making an appointment with your doctor—or I can help you find someone else to talk to, like a psychologist (therapist) or social worker."

- "Get help right away if you are having hopeless thoughts or are thinking about hurting yourself. You can call the National Suicide Prevention Lifeline at 1-800-273-TALK (1-800-273-8255) anytime."

- "You can call or text me anytime if you need support or you just want to talk."

Chapter 44

Diagnosing Depression

What Is Depression?

Depression is an illness that involves the brain. It can affect your thoughts, mood, and daily activities. Depression is more than feeling sad for a few days. Depression can be mild or severe. Mild depression can become more serious if it's not treated.

If you are diagnosed with depression, you aren't alone. Depression is a common illness that affects millions of adults in the United States every year. The good news is that depression can be treated. Getting help is the best thing you can do for yourself and your loved ones. You can feel better.

Common Symptoms

There are many symptoms associated with depression, and some will vary depending on the individual. However, some of the most common symptoms are listed below. If you have several of these symptoms for more than two weeks, you may have depression.

This chapter contains text excerpted from the following sources: Text under the heading "What Is Depression?" is excerpted from "Talk with Your Doctor about Depression," Office of Disease Prevention and Health Promotion (ODPHP), U.S. Department of Health and Human Services (HHS), February 25, 2016; Text beginning with the heading "Common Symptoms" is excerpted from "Depression," NIHSeniorHealth, National Institute of Aging (NIA), May 15, 2016; Text under the heading "Diagnostic Criteria" is excerpted from "Depression," Centers for Disease Control and Prevention (CDC), March 30, 2016.

- persistent sad, anxious or "empty" mood
- feelings of hopelessness, pessimism
- irritability, restlessness or having trouble sitting still
- feelings of guilt, worthlessness, helplessness
- loss of interest in once pleasurable activities, including sex
- decreased energy or fatigue
- moving or talking more slowly
- difficulty concentrating, remembering, making decisions
- difficulty sleeping, early-morning awakening, or oversleeping
- eating more or less than usual, usually with unplanned weight gain or loss
- feeling like life is not worth living
- thoughts of death or suicide, suicide attempts
- aches or pains, headaches, cramps, or digestive problems without a clear physical cause and/or that do not ease even with treatment
- frequent crying

Is It Depression or Something Else?

The first step to getting appropriate treatment is to visit a doctor. Certain medications or conditions can cause symptoms similar to depression. A doctor can rule out these factors by doing a complete physical exam, interview, and lab tests.

If these other factors can be ruled out, the doctor may refer you to a mental health professional, such as a psychologist, counselor, social worker, or psychiatrist. Some doctors called geriatric psychiatrists and clinical geropsychologists are specially trained to treat depression and other mental illnesses in older adults.

The doctor or mental health professional will ask about the history of your symptoms, such as when they started, how long they have lasted, their severity, whether they have occurred before, and if so, whether they were treated and how. He or she will then diagnose the depression and work with you to choose the most appropriate treatment.

Making an Appointment

If you need to make an appointment, here are some things you could say during the first call: "I haven't been myself lately, and I'd like to talk to the provider about it," or "I think I might have depression, and I'd like some help."

Talking to Your Doctor

How well you and your doctor talk to each other is one of the most important parts of getting good healthcare. But talking to your doctor isn't always easy. It takes time and effort on your part as well as your doctor's.

To prepare for your appointment, make a list of:

- any symptoms you've had, including any that may seem unrelated to the reason for your appointment

- key personal information, including any major stresses or recent life changes

- all medications, vitamins, or other supplements that you're taking, including how much and how often

- questions to ask your health provider.

Diagnostic Criteria

According to the American Psychiatric Association (APA)'s diagnostic criteria for major depressive disorder, a person must experience five or more symptoms below for a continuous period of at least two weeks.

- Feelings of sadness, hopelessness, depressed mood

- Loss of interest or pleasure in activities that used to be enjoyable

- Change in weight or appetite (either increase or decrease)

- Change in activity: psychomotor agitation (being more active than usual) or psychomotor retardation (being less active than usual)

- Insomnia (difficulty sleeping) or sleeping too much

- Feeling tired or not having any energy

- Feelings of guilt or worthlessness

- Difficulties concentrating and paying attention

- Thoughts of death or suicide.

Most symptoms must be present every day or nearly every day and must cause significant distress or problems in daily life functioning.

Chapter 45

Paying for Mental Healthcare

Chapter Contents

Section 45.1

Finding Low-Cost Mental Healthcare and Help Paying for Prescriptions

Text in this section is excerpted from "Finding Low-Cost Mental Healthcare," © 1995–2016. The Nemours Foundation/KidsHealth®. Reprinted with permission.

What should you do if you're under a lot of stress or dealing with a mental health issue and you don't have the money for treatment?

You're not alone if you're concerned about paying for mental healthcare. Lots of people need help and worry that they can't afford it. Even though health insurance covers mental health issues, it can still be challenging. Some insurance companies don't cover mental health services very much, and they often have expensive copays and deductibles.

Still, it is possible to find affordable—sometimes even free—mental healthcare or support.

Free or Low-Cost Counseling

When it comes to finding a counselor, start at school. School counselors and school psychologists can provide a good listening ear—for free! They can help you size up the situation you're dealing with and, if needed, refer you to more support in your county or community.

If your school counselor can't help, you'll need to do a little more research to figure out how to get help. Some of the free or low-cost mental healthcare possibilities to explore include:

- **Local mental health centers and clinics.** These groups are funded by federal and state governments so they charge less than you might pay a private therapist. Search online for "mental health services" and the name of the county or city where you live.

  One thing to keep in mind: Not every mental health clinic will fit your needs. Some might not work with people your age (for example, a clinic might specialize in veterans or kids with developmental disabilities). It's still worth a call, though. Even if a clinic can't help you, the people who work there might recommend someone who can.

- **Hospitals.** Call your local hospitals and ask what kinds of mental health services they offer—and at what price. Teaching hospitals, where doctors are trained, often provide low- or no-cost services.

- **Colleges and universities.** If a college in your area offers graduate degrees in psychology or social work, the students might run free or low-cost clinics as part of their training.

- **On-campus health services.** If you're in college or about to start, find out what kind of counseling and therapy your school offers and at what cost. Ask if they offer financial assistance for students.

- **Employee Assistance Programs (EAPs).** These free programs provide professional therapists to evaluate people for mental health conditions and offer short-term counseling. Not everyone has access to this benefit: EAPs are run through workplaces, so you (or your parents) need to work for an employer that offers this type of program.

- **Private therapists.** Ask trusted friends and adults for recommendations, then call to see if they offer a "sliding fee scale" (this means they charge based on how much you can afford to pay). Some psychologists even offer certain services for free, if necessary. To find a therapist in your area, check the websites of your state's mental health association or the American Psychological Association (APA).

To qualify for low-cost services, you may need to prove financial need. If you still live at home, that could mean getting parents or guardians involved in filling out paperwork. But your therapist will keep everything confidential.

If you're under 26, your mental healthcare should still be covered under your parent's insurance policy. It's worth a call to the insurance company to find out what services the policy covers and how much of those services it pays for.

Financial Help

Programs like Medicaid or the State Children's Health Insurance Program (SCHIP) offer free or reduced-fee medical insurance to teens who are not covered. To find out if you qualify for mental health assistance through these programs, call your doctor's office or hospital and ask to speak to a financial counselor. Your school counselor also might be able to help you figure out what kind of public medical assistance you could qualify for and guide you through the process of applying.

People under age 18 who live at home will need a parent or guardian to sign off on the paperwork for these programs. After that, though, your care will be confidential. A therapist won't tell parents what you've talked about—unless he or she thinks you may harm yourself or another person.

Getting Help in a Crisis

If you're feeling suicidal, very hopeless or depressed, or like you might harm yourself or others in any way, call a suicide or crisis hotline. These offer free help right away.

- **Suicide hotlines.** Toll-free confidential lines like 1-800-SUI-CIDE or 1-800-999-9999 are staffed 24 hours a day, 7 days a week by trained professionals who can help you without ever knowing your name or seeing your face. They can often give you a referral to a mental health professional you can follow up with in your area.

- **Crisis hotlines.** These help survivors of rape, violence, and other traumas. Some may also provide short-term counseling. To find one, do an online search for your state and "crisis hotline."

Other cost-effective ways to help you work through crisis situations are:

- **Emergency rooms (ERs).** Emergency rooms are required to evaluate and care for people who have emotional emergencies as well as physical ones. If you think you might hurt yourself or someone else, you can also call 911.

- **Local crisis centers.** Some states have walk-in crisis centers for people coping with mental health problems, abuse, or sexual assault. They're a bit like ERs for people who are having an emotional crisis.

Each county and state does things differently. A few might not have crisis centers. Others may have mobile units that come to you in an emergency. Some crisis centers operate in hospitals, others are run by non-profits or county mental health services. To see if there's a crisis center near you, search online for your city, county, or state and terms like "crisis center," "crisis counseling center," "psychiatric emergency services," or "crisis intervention."

If you need help finding any kind of services, contact your state's mental health association or the American Psychological Association (APA) to find out where you can get therapy and treatment near you.

Prescriptions

Paying for prescriptions can really drain your wallet. Here are some ways to be smart about the money you spend on medicines:

- **Find out if you can take generic or non-brand medicines.** Ask your doctor or pharmacist if there are over-the-counter versions of the same kinds of prescription medications.

- **Find out about prescription assistance programs** (also called "patient assistance programs"). The Partnership for Prescription Association gives free or low-cost prescriptions to people who qualify based on income.

- **Compare prices at local pharmacies.** Call each to ask what they're charging for your prescriptions.

- **Contact the pharmaceutical company that makes the medication.** All the big pharmaceutical companies have prescription assistance numbers you can call for help.

- **Beware of free prescription samples (or coupons and rebates).** They sound appealing, but they are often for expensive, name-brand medications. That's fine while the samples last. But since doctors don't like to change a medication if it's working, you could get stuck paying full price after the samples run out.

Before accepting a free sample, talk to your doctor about whether you can afford that medication in the long term. If it's something you'll only need for as long as the samples last, take advantage of the freebie!

If you're already taking medication, there are two things to know:

1. Never stop taking a prescribed medication or reduce your dosage because you can't afford to fill the prescription. Some medications can cause side effects if they're adjusted or stopped without a doctor's advice.

2. Never use someone else's medicine. Even if the person has the same health condition you do, medications work differently for different people.

If you can't afford to refill a prescription, call the prescribing doctor. Say you're having a hard time affording your meds and need some advice. It's not unusual these days for people to ask for this kind of help, and doctor's offices often know how to get it or put you in touch with someone who can.

Parents and Other Adults

Navigating your way through the healthcare system can be confusing (even for adults). That's why it's a good idea to have a parent, relative, doctor, school counselor, or social worker help you connect with a mental health professional.

But what if you want to get counseling without a parent (or guardian) knowing?

In many states, teens can be given mental health treatment without parental consent. When you call a clinic, hospital, or therapist, ask about your state's rules on parental consent for mental health services. And, when you see a counselor, find out about the rules when it comes to filling a prescription. Even if you can get confidential care, your parents may need to give the OK to fill prescriptions.

Whatever happens, don't let money hold you back from getting help. Affordable mental healthcare options are out there—it may just take some time and effort to find them. But don't give up. Stress and mental health problems don't usually get better on their own.

Section 45.2

Medicare and Your Mental Healthcare Benefits

This section includes text excerpted from "Medicare and Your Mental Health Benefits," Centers for Medicare and Medicaid Services (CMS), April 2016.

Mental health conditions, like depression or anxiety, can happen to anyone at any time. If you think you may have problems that affect your mental health, you can get help. Talk to your doctor or other healthcare provider if you have:

- Thoughts of ending your life (like a fixation on death or suicidal thoughts or attempts)

- Sad, empty, or hopeless feelings

- Loss of self-worth (like worries about being a burden, feelings of worthlessness, or self-loathing)

- Social withdrawal and isolation (don't want to be with friends, engage in activities, or leave home)

- Little interest in things you used to enjoy

- A lack of energy

- Trouble concentrating

- Trouble sleeping (like difficulty falling asleep or staying asleep, oversleeping, or daytime sleepiness)

- Weight loss or loss of appetite

- Increased use of alcohol or other drugs

Mental healthcare includes services and programs to help diagnose and treat mental health conditions. These services and programs may be provided in outpatient and inpatient settings. Medicare helps cover outpatient and inpatient mental healthcare, as well as prescription drugs you may need to treat a mental health condition.

Medicare Helps Cover Mental Health Services

Medicare Part A (Hospital Insurance) helps cover mental healthcare if you're a hospital inpatient. Part A covers your room, meals, nursing care, therapy or other treatment for your condition, lab tests, medications, and other related services and supplies.

Medicare Part B (Medical Insurance) helps cover mental health services that you would get from a doctor and services that you generally get outside of a hospital, like visits with a psychiatrist or other doctor, visits with a clinical psychologist or clinical social worker, and lab tests ordered by your doctor. Part B may also pay for partial hospitalization services if you need intensive coordinated outpatient care.

Medicare prescription drug coverage (Part D) helps cover drugs you may need to treat a mental health condition.

Outpatient Mental Healthcare and Professional Services

What Original Medicare Covers

Medicare Part B (Medical Insurance) helps cover mental health services and visits with these types of health professionals (deductibles and coinsurance may apply):

- Psychiatrist or other doctor
- Clinical psychologist
- Clinical social worker
- Clinical nurse specialist
- Nurse practitioner
- Physician assistant

Psychiatrists and other doctors must accept assignment if they participate in Medicare. Ask your doctor or psychiatrist if they accept assignment before you schedule an appointment. The other health professionals listed above must always accept assignment.

Part B covers outpatient mental health services, including services that are usually provided outside a hospital (like in a clinic, doctor's office, or therapist's office) and services provided in a hospital's outpatient department. Part B also covers outpatient mental health services for treatment of inappropriate alcohol and drug use. Part B helps pay for these covered outpatient services (deductibles and coinsurance may apply):

- One depression screening per year. The screening must be done in a primary care doctor's office or primary care clinic that can provide follow-up treatment and referrals. You pay nothing for your yearly depression screening if your doctor or healthcare provider accepts assignment.

- Individual and group psychotherapy with doctors or certain other licensed professionals allowed by the state where you get the services.

- Family counseling, if the main purpose is to help with your treatment.

- Testing to find out if you're getting the services you need and if your current treatment is helping you.

- Psychiatric evaluation.

- Medication management.

- Certain prescription drugs that aren't usually "self-administered" (drugs you would normally take on your own), like some injections.

- Diagnostic tests.

- Partial hospitalization.

- A one-time "Welcome to Medicare" preventive visit. This visit includes a review of your potential risk factors for depression. You pay nothing for this visit if your doctor or other healthcare provider accepts assignment. (Note: This visit is only covered if you get it within the first 12 months you have Part B.)

- A yearly "Wellness" visit. Medicare covers a yearly "Wellness" visit once every 12 months (if you've had Part B for longer than 12 months). This is a good time to talk to your doctor or other healthcare provider about changes in your mental health so they can evaluate your changes year to year. You pay nothing for your yearly "Wellness" visit if your doctor or other healthcare provider accepts assignment.

What You Pay

In general, after you pay your yearly Part B deductible for visits to a doctor or other healthcare provider to diagnose or treat your condition, you pay 20% of the Medicare-approved amount if your healthcare provider accepts assignment.

If you get your services in a hospital outpatient clinic or hospital outpatient department, you may have to pay an additional copayment or coinsurance amount to the hospital.

If you have a Medicare Supplement Insurance (Medigap) policy or other health coverage, tell your doctor or other healthcare provider so your bills get paid correctly.

Medicare May Cover Partial Hospitalization

Part B covers partial hospitalization in some cases. Partial hospitalization is a structured program of outpatient psychiatric services provided to patients as an alternative to inpatient psychiatric care. It's more intense than the care you get in a doctor's or therapist's office. This type of treatment is provided during the day and doesn't require an overnight stay. Medicare helps cover partial hospitalization services when they're provided through a hospital outpatient department or community mental health center. As part of your partial hospitalization program, Medicare may cover occupational therapy that's part of your mental health treatment and/or individual patient training and education about your condition.

For Medicare to cover a partial hospitalization program, you must meet certain requirements, and your doctor must certify that you would otherwise need inpatient treatment. Your doctor and the partial hospitalization program must accept Medicare payment.

You pay a percentage of the Medicare-approved amount for each service you get from a doctor or certain other qualified mental health professionals if your healthcare professional accepts assignment. You also pay coinsurance for each day of partial hospitalization services provided in a hospital outpatient setting or community mental health center.

What Original Medicare Doesn't Cover

- Meals

- Transportation to or from mental healthcare services

- Support groups that bring people together to talk and socialize (Note: This is different from group psychotherapy, which is covered.)

- Testing or training for job skills that isn't part of your mental health treatment.

Inpatient Mental Healthcare

What Original Medicare Covers

Medicare Part A (Hospital Insurance) helps pay for mental health services you get in a hospital that require you to be admitted as an inpatient. You can get these services either in a general hospital or in a psychiatric hospital that only cares for people with mental health conditions. No matter which type of hospital you choose, Part A will help cover mental health services.

If you're in a psychiatric hospital (instead of a general hospital), Part A only pays for up to 190 days of inpatient psychiatric hospital services during your lifetime.

What You Pay

Medicare measures your use of hospital services (including services you get in a psychiatric hospital) in benefit periods. A benefit period begins the day you're admitted as an inpatient in a general or psychiatric hospital. The benefit period ends after you haven't had any inpatient hospital care for 60 days in a row. If you go into a hospital again after 60 days, a new benefit period begins, and you must pay a new deductible for any inpatient hospital services you get.

There's no limit to the number of benefit periods you can have when you get mental healthcare in a general hospital. You can also have multiple benefit periods when you get care in a psychiatric hospital, but there's a lifetime limit of 190 days.

As a hospital inpatient, you pay these amounts in 2016:

- $1,288 deductible for each benefit period

- Days 1–60: $0 coinsurance per day of each benefit period

- Days 61–90: $322 coinsurance per day of each benefit period

- Days 91 and beyond: $644 coinsurance per each "lifetime reserve day" after day 90 for each benefit period (up to 60 days over your lifetime)

- Beyond lifetime reserve days: all costs

Part B also helps cover mental health services provided by doctors and other healthcare professionals if you're admitted as a hospital inpatient. You pay 20% of the Medicare-approved amount for these mental health services while you're a hospital inpatient.

317

If you have a Medicare Supplement Insurance (Medigap) policy or other health coverage, tell your doctor or other healthcare provider so your bills get paid correctly.

What Original Medicare Doesn't Cover

- Private duty nursing
- A phone or television in your room
- Personal items (like toothpaste, socks, or razors)
- A private room (unless medically necessary)

Medicare Prescription Drug Coverage (Part D)

To get Medicare prescription drug coverage, you must join a Medicare Prescription Drug Plan. Medicare drug plans are run by insurance companies and other private companies approved by Medicare. Each Medicare drug plan can vary in cost and in the specific drugs it covers. It's important to know your plan's coverage rules and your rights.

Medicare Drug Plans Have Special Rules

Will My Plan Cover the Drugs I Need?

Most Medicare drug plans have a list of drugs that the plan covers, called a formulary. Medicare drug plans aren't required to cover all drugs, but they're required to cover all (with limited exceptions) antidepressant, anticonvulsant, and antipsychotic medications, which may be necessary to keep you mentally healthy. Medicare reviews each plan's formulary to make sure it contains a wide range of drugs and that it doesn't discriminate against certain groups (like people with disabilities or mental health conditions).

Can My Drug Plan's Formulary Change?

A Medicare drug plan can make some changes to its formulary during the year within guidelines set by Medicare. If the change involves a drug you're currently taking, your plan must do one of these:

- Provide written notice to you at least 60 days prior to the date the change becomes effective.
- At the time you request a refill, provide written notice of the change and a 60-day supply of the drug under the same plan rules as before the change.

What If My Prescriber Thinks I Need a Certain Drug That My Plan Doesn't Cover?

If you belong to a Medicare drug plan, you have the right to request a coverage determination (including an exception). You can appoint a representative to help you. Your representative can be a family member, friend, advocate, attorney, doctor, or someone else you trust who will act on your behalf. You, your representative, or your doctor or other prescriber must contact your plan to ask for a coverage determination.

Request a Coverage Determination

You, your representative, or your doctor or other prescriber can request that your plan cover a drug you need. You can request a coverage determination in certain situations, like if your pharmacist or plan tells you:

- A drug you believe should be covered isn't covered

- A drug is covered at a higher cost sharing amount than you think you should have to pay

- You have to meet a plan coverage rule (like prior authorization) before you can get the drug you requested

- The plan won't cover a drug because the plan believes you don't need the drug

If you request a coverage determination, your doctor or other prescriber may need to give a supporting statement to your plan explaining why you need the drug you're requesting. You, your representative, or your doctor or other prescriber can request a coverage determination orally or in writing. Your plan may request additional written information from your prescriber.

Request an Exception

You, your representative, or your doctor or other prescriber can request an exception (a type of coverage determination) if:

- You think your plan should cover a drug that's not on its formulary because the other treatment options on your plan's formulary won't work for you.

- Your doctor or other prescriber believes you can't meet one of your plan's coverage rules (like prior authorization, step therapy, or quantity or dosage limits).

- You think your plan should charge a lower amount for a drug you're taking on the plan's non-preferred drug tier because the other treatment options in your plan's preferred drug tier won't work for you.

If you request an exception, your doctor or other prescriber will need to give a supporting statement to your plan explaining why you need the drug you're requesting. You, your representative, or your doctor or other prescriber can request an exception orally or in writing. Your plan may request additional written information from your prescriber.

What If I Disagree with My Plan's Coverage Determination or Exception Decision?

Once your plan has gotten your request, in most cases, it has 72 hours (or 24 hours if you request that a fast decision be made) to notify you of its decision. If you disagree with your Medicare drug plan's coverage determination or exception decision, you have the right to appeal the decision. The plan's written decision will explain how to file an appeal. Read this decision carefully.

Chapter 46

Finding and Choosing a Therapist

Chapter Contents

Section 46.1

Types of Therapist

This section includes text excerpted from "Types of Therapists," U.S. Department of Veterans Affairs (VA), August 14, 2015.

There are many types of professionals who provide evidence-based psychotherapy and medication to people who have experienced trauma. Mental health professionals can have different training, credentials, or licenses. Providers can also offer different services, based upon their expertise.

If you are looking for a particular type of treatment (like medications) or expert focus, the license and specialized training of the mental health provider is important. The information below reviews the most common types of licensed mental health providers and generally explains their education, training, and services offered. Whether or not a therapist needs a license to provide psychotherapy and the requirements to be licensed varies by state. Your health insurance provider may also allow you to see only certain types of mental health providers. Check your policy for details.

Who Is Licensed to Provide Psychotherapy for Posttraumatic Stress Disorder (PTSD)?

The mental health professionals below provide psychotherapy for PTSD, and in most states, are not licensed to prescribe medications.

Psychologists: Licensed clinical psychologists focus on mental health assessment and treatment. They have a doctoral degree (e.g., PhD, PsyD, EdD) from 4 or more years of graduate training in clinical or counseling psychology. To be licensed to practice, psychologists must have another 1 to 2 years of supervised clinical experience. Psychologists have the title of "doctor" because of their doctoral degree, but in most states they cannot prescribe medicine.

Clinical Social Workers: The purpose of social work is to enhance human well-being by helping people meet basic human needs.

Licensed social workers also focus on diagnosis and treatment, and specialize in areas such as mental health, aging, of family and children. Most licensed social workers have a master's degree from 2 years of graduate training (e.g., MSW) or a doctoral degree in social work (e.g., DSW or PhD).

Master's Level Clinicians: Master's level clinicians have a master's degree in counseling, psychology, or marriage and family therapy (e.g., MA, MFT). To be licensed to provide individual and/or group counseling, master's level clinicians must meet requirements that vary by state.

Who Is Licensed to Provide Medications for PTSD?

Working with a specialist who commonly sees patients with PTSD is ideal. However, in addition to the mental health providers listed below, primary care physicians, physician's assistants and nurse practitioners are usually qualified to prescribe medications for PTSD.

Psychiatrists: Psychiatrists have either a Doctor of Allopathic Medicine (MD) or Doctor of Osteopathic Medicine (DO) degree in addition to specialized training in the diagnosis and treatment of mental health problems. Since they are medical doctors, psychiatrists can prescribe medicine. Some may also provide psychotherapy.

Psychiatric Nurses or Nurse Practitioners: Psychiatric mental health nurses (PMHN) can have different levels of training. Most are registered nurses (RN) with additional training in psychiatry or psychology. Psychiatric mental health advanced practice registered nurses (PMH-APRN) have a graduate degree. Psychiatric nurse practitioners are registered nurse practitioners with specialized training in the diagnosis and treatment of mental health problems. In most states, psychiatric nurses and psychiatric nurse practitioners can prescribe medicine.

More Information

There are more types of therapists, counselors, and mental health providers who are qualified to treat issues related to trauma. You can learn more in the career services department of your college or university. Professional associations for mental health providers are also a good resource for gathering information.

Section 46.2

Finding a Therapist

This section includes text excerpted from "Finding a
Therapist," U.S. Department of Veterans Affairs (VA),
October 27, 2015.

Things to Consider

Here are some suggestions for finding a therapist, counselor, or
mental healthcare provider who can help your recovery.

- Make sure the provider has experience treating people who have
  experienced a trauma.

- Try to find a provider who specializes in evidence-based medications for posttraumatic stress disorder (PTSD) or effective psychotherapy for PTSD (e.g., cognitive behavioral therapy (CBT); cognitive processing therapy (CPT); prolonged exposure therapy (PE);
  or eye movement desensitization and reprocessing (EMDR)).

- Find out what type(s) of insurance the provider accepts and
  what you will have to pay (out-of-pocket costs) for care.

First Steps

- Contact your family doctor to ask for a recommendation. You
  can also ask friends and family if they can recommend someone.

- If you have health insurance, call to find out which mental
  health providers your insurance company will pay for. Your
  insurance company may require that you choose a provider from
  among a list they maintain.

Finding a Provider Using the Internet

These resources can help you locate a therapist, counselor, or mental health provider who is right for you.

- **Sidran Institute Help Desk** will help you find therapists who
  specialize in trauma treatment. Email or call the Help Desk at
  (410) 825-8888.

- **Anxiety and Depression Association of America** offers a therapist search by location and mental health disorder. Call (240) 485-1011 or email.

- **Association for Behavioral and Cognitive Therapies** offers a search of licensed therapists who offer cognitive or behavioral therapies.

- **EMDR International Association** has a locator listing professionals who provide EMDR.

- **ISTSS Clinician Directory** is a service provided by the International Society for Traumatic Stress Studies (ISTSS) that lets you consider many factors in searching for a clinician, counselor, or mental health professional.

- **American Psychological Association** has a Psychologist Locator that allows you to search by location, specialty, insurance accepted, and gender of provider.

- **Psychology Today** offers a therapist directory by location. You can also find treatment centers here.

- **Substance Abuse and Mental Health Services Administration (SAMHSA)** offers a Mental Health Services Locator by location and type of facility (inpatient, outpatient, residential). Call for assistance 24 hours a day 1-800-662-HELP (4357).

Finding a Provider by Phone

In addition to the numbers listed above. You can also find a therapist, counselor, or mental health provider in the following ways:

- Some mental health services are listed in the phone book. In the Government pages, look in the "County Government Offices" section, and find "Health Services (Dept. of)" or "Department of Health Services." "Mental Health" will be listed.

- In the yellow pages, mental health providers are listed under "counseling," "psychologists," "social workers," "psychotherapists," "social and human services," or "mental health."

- You can also call the psychology department of a local college or university.

Section 46.3

Choosing a Therapist

This section contains text excerpted from the following
sources: Text in this section begins with excerpts from "Choosing
a Therapist," U.S. Department of Veterans Affairs (VA),
August 14, 2015; Text under the heading "Things to Know When
Selecting a Complementary Health Practitioner" is excerpted
from "6 Things to Know When Selecting a Complementary Health
Practitioner," National Center for Complementary and
Integrative Health (NCCIH), October 11, 2016.

There are a many things to consider when choosing a therapist.
Some practical issues are location, cost, and what insurance the therapist accepts. Other issues include the therapist's background, training,
and the way he or she works with people.

Your therapist should explain the therapy, how long treatment is
expected to last, and how to tell if it is working. The information below
can help you choose a therapist who is right for you.

Questions to Ask before Therapy

Here is a list of questions you may want to ask a possible therapist:

- What is your education? Are you licensed? How many years have
  you been practicing?

- What are your special areas of practice?

- Have you ever worked with people who have been through
  trauma? Do you have any special training in PTSD treatment?

- What kinds of PTSD treatments do you use? Have they been
  proven effective for dealing with my kind of problem or issue?
  How much therapy would you recommend?

- Do you prescribe medications?

- What are your fees? (Fees are usually based on a 45-minute to
  50-minute session.) Do you have any discounted fees?

- What types of insurance do you accept? Do you file insurance claims? Do you contract with any managed care organizations? Do you accept Medicare or Medicaid insurance?

These questions are just guidelines. In the end, your choice of a therapist will be based on many factors. Think about your comfort with the person as well as his or her qualifications and experience treating PTSD. And keep in mind the importance of evidence-based, trauma-focused treatments like Cognitive Processing Therapy (CPT), Prolonged Exposure (PE), and Eye Movement Desensitization and Reprocessing (EMDR).

Paying for Therapy

If you have health insurance, check to see what mental health services are covered. Medicare, Medicaid, and most major health plans typically cover a certain number of mental health counseling sessions per year. Note that you may have a small additional amount you will have to pay, called a co-payment (or co-pay). Call your insurance company to see what they cover so you won't be surprised by a big bill.

If you don't have health insurance that will cover your therapy, you may still be able to get counseling, even if you can't afford to pay full price. Many community mental health centers have sliding scales that base your fee on what you are able to pay.

Making Your Therapy a Good "Fit"

In PTSD treatment, or any mental health therapy, you work together with your therapist to get better. A good "fit" between a therapist and a patient can make a difference. You will want to choose a therapist you are comfortable with so that you can get better. This means you should feel like you can ask questions that help you understand treatment and your progress in therapy.

The most effective PTSD treatments are time-limited, usually lasting 10–12 weeks. If you are not getting better or if you feel your therapist is not a good fit for you, look for someone else to work with. Sometimes it takes a few tries to find just the right therapist. This is not unusual and your therapist should be understanding.

Things to Know When Selecting a Complementary Health Practitioner

If you're looking for a complementary health practitioner to help treat a medical problem, it is important to be as careful and thorough in your search as you are when looking for conventional care. Here are some tips to help you in your search:

- If you need names of practitioners in your area, first check with your doctor or other healthcare provider. A nearby hospital or medical school, professional organizations, state regulatory agencies or licensing boards, or even your health insurance provider may be helpful. Unfortunately, the National Center for Complementary and Integrative Health (NCCIH) cannot refer you to practitioners.

- Find out as much as you can about any potential practitioner, including education, training, licensing, and certifications. The credentials required for complementary health practitioners vary tremendously from state to state and from discipline to discipline.

Once you have found a possible practitioner, here are some tips about deciding whether he or she is right for you:

- Find out whether the practitioner is willing to work together with your conventional healthcare providers. For safe, coordinated care, it's important for all of the professionals involved in your health to communicate and cooperate.

- Explain all of your health conditions to the practitioner, and find out about the practitioner's training and experience in working with people who have your conditions. Choose a practitioner who understands how to work with people with your specific needs, even if general well-being is your goal. And, remember that health conditions can affect the safety of complementary approaches; for example, if you have glaucoma, some yoga poses may not be safe for you.

- Don't assume that your health insurance will cover the practitioner's services. Contact your health insurance provider and ask. Insurance plans differ greatly in what complementary health approaches they cover, and even if they cover a particular approach, restrictions may apply.

- Tell all your healthcare providers about the complementary approaches you use and about all practitioners who are treating you. Keeping your healthcare providers fully informed helps you to stay in control and effectively manage your health.

Chapter 47

Therapy for Depression

Chapter Contents

Section 47.1

Psychotherapy (Talk Therapy)

This section includes text excerpted from "Psychotherapies," National
Institute of Mental Health (NIMH), November 2016.

What Is Psychotherapy?

Psychotherapy (sometimes called "talk therapy") is a term for a variety of treatment techniques that aim to help a person identify and change
troubling emotions, thoughts, and behavior. Most psychotherapy takes
place with a licensed and trained mental healthcare professional and
a patient meeting one on one or with other patients in a group setting.
Someone might seek out psychotherapy for different reasons:

- You might be dealing with severe or long-term stress from a job
  or family situation, the loss of a loved one, or relationship or other
  family issues. Or you may have symptoms with no physical explanation: changes in sleep or appetite, low energy, a lack of interest or
  pleasure in activities that you once enjoyed, persistent irritability,
  or a sense of discouragement or hopelessness that won't go away.

- A health professional may suspect or have diagnosed a condition
  such as depression, bipolar disorder, posttraumatic stress or
  other disorder and recommended psychotherapy as a first treatment or to go along with medication.

- You may be seeking treatment for a family member or child who
  has been diagnosed with a condition affecting mental health and
  for whom a health professional has recommended treatment.

An exam by your primary care practitioner can ensure there is
nothing in your overall health that would explain your or a loved one's
symptoms.

What to Consider When Looking for a Therapist

**Therapists have different professional backgrounds and
specialties.** There are resources at the end of this material that can

help you find out about the different credentials of therapists and resources for locating therapists.

There are many different types of psychotherapy. Different therapies are often variations on an established approach, such as cognitive behavioral therapy (CBT). There is no formal approval process for psychotherapies as there is for the use of medications in medicine. For many therapies, however, research involving large numbers of patients has provided evidence that treatment is effective for specific disorders. These "evidence-based therapies" have been shown in research to reduce symptoms of depression, anxiety, and other disorders.

The particular approach a therapist uses depends on the condition being treated and the training and experience of the therapist. Also, therapists may combine and adapt elements of different approaches.

One goal of establishing an evidence base for psychotherapies is to prevent situations in which a person receives therapy for months or years with no benefit. If you have been in therapy and feel you are not getting better, talk to your therapist, or look into other practitioners or approaches. The object of therapy is to gain relief from symptoms and improve quality of life.

Once you have identified one or more possible therapists, a preliminary conversation with a therapist can help you get an idea of how treatment will proceed and whether you feel comfortable with the therapist. Rapport and trust are important. Discussions in therapy are deeply personal and it's important that you feel comfortable and trusting with the therapist and have confidence in his or her expertise. Consider asking the following questions:

- What are the credentials and experience of the therapist? Does he or she have a specialty?

- What approach will the therapist take to help you? Does he or she practice a particular type of therapy? What can the therapist tell you about the rationale for the therapy and the evidence base?

- Does the therapist have experience in diagnosing and treating the age group (for example, a child) and the specific condition for which treatment is being sought? If a child is the patient, how will parents be involved in treatment?

- What are the goals of therapy? Does the therapist recommend a specific time frame or number of sessions? How will progress be assessed and what happens if you (or the therapist) feel you aren't starting to feel better?

- Will there be homework?

- Are medications an option? How will medications be prescribed if the therapist is not an M.D.?

- Are our meetings confidential? How can this be assured?

Psychotherapies and Other Treatment Options

Psychotherapy can be an alternative to medication or can be used along with other treatment options, such as medications. Choosing the right treatment plan should be based on a person's individual needs and medical situation and under a mental health professional's care.

Even when medications relieve symptoms, psychotherapy and other interventions can help a person address specific issues. These might include self-defeating ways of thinking, fears, problems with interactions with other people, or dealing with situations at home and at school or with employment.

Elements of Psychotherapy

A variety of different kinds of psychotherapies and interventions have been shown to be effective for specific disorders. Psychotherapists may use one primary approach, or incorporate different elements depending on their training, the condition being treated, and the needs of the person receiving treatment.

Here are examples of the elements that psychotherapies can include:

- Helping a person become aware of ways of thinking that may be automatic but are inaccurate and harmful. (An example might be someone who has a low opinion of his or her own abilities.) The therapist helps the person find ways to question these thoughts, understand how they affect emotions and behavior, and try ways to change self-defeating patterns. This approach is central to cognitive behavioral therapy (CBT).

- Identifying ways to cope with stress.

- Examining in depth a person's interactions with others and offering guidance with social and communication skills, if needed.

- Relaxation and mindfulness techniques.

- Exposure therapy for people with anxiety disorders. In exposure therapy, a person spends brief periods, in a supportive environment, learning to tolerate the distress certain items, ideas, or imagined scenes cause. Over time the fear associated with these things dissipates.

- Tracking emotions and activities and the impact of each on the other.

- Safety planning can include helping a person recognize warning signs, and thinking about coping strategies, such as contacting friends, family, or emergency personnel.

- Supportive counseling to help a person explore troubling issues and provide emotional support.

eHealth

The telephone, Internet, and mobile devices have opened up new possibilities for providing interventions that can reach people in areas where mental health professionals may be not be easily available, and can be at hand 24/7. Some of these approaches involve a therapist providing help at a distance, but others—such as web-based programs and cell phone apps—are designed to provide information and feedback in the absence of a therapist.

Taking the First Step

The symptoms of mental disorders can have a profound effect on someone's quality of life and ability to function. Treatment can address symptoms as well as assist someone experiencing severe or ongoing stress. Some of the reasons that you might consider seeking out psychotherapy include:

- Overwhelming sadness or helplessness that doesn't go away

- Serious, unusual insomnia or sleeping too much

- Difficulty focusing on work, or carrying out other everyday activities

- Constant worry and anxiety

- Drinking to excess or any behavior that harms self or others

- Dealing with a difficult transition, such as a divorce, children leaving home, job difficulties, or the death of someone close

- Children's behavior problems that interfere with school, family, or peers

Seeking help is not an admission of weakness, but a step towards understanding and obtaining relief from distressing symptoms.

Finding a Therapist

Many different professionals offer psychotherapy. Examples include psychiatrists, psychologists, social workers, counselors, and psychiatric nurses. Information on the credentials of providers is available from the National Alliance on Mental Illness (NAMI).

Your health plan may have a list of mental health practitioners who participate in the plan. Other resources on the "Help for Mental Illnesses" page can help you look for reduced cost health services. The resources listed there include links to help find reduced cost treatment. When talking with a prospective therapist, ask about treatment fees, whether the therapist participates in insurance plans, and whether there is a sliding scale for fees according to income.

Section 47.2

Cognitive Processing Therapy

This section includes text excerpted from "Cognitive Processing Therapy for PTSD," U.S. Department of Veterans Affairs (VA), September 8, 2016.

Practice guidelines have identified the treatments that have the most evidence for treating posttraumatic stress disorder (PTSD). The best treatments include different talk therapies (or psychotherapy) and medications. Cognitive processing therapy (CPT) is one of these treatments.

What Type of Treatment Is This?

CPT is one specific type of cognitive behavioral therapy. It is a 12-session psychotherapy for PTSD. CPT teaches you how to evaluate and change the upsetting thoughts you have had since your trauma. By changing your thoughts, you can change how you feel.

How Does It Work?

Trauma can change the way you think about yourself and the world. You may believe you are to blame for what happened or that the world is a dangerous place. These kinds of thoughts keep you stuck in your PTSD and cause you to miss out on things you used to enjoy. CPT teaches you a new way to handle these upsetting thoughts. In CPT, you will learn skills that can help you decide whether there are more helpful ways to think about your trauma. You will learn how to examine whether the facts support your thought or do not support your thought. And ultimately, you can decide whether or not it makes sense to take a new perspective.

What Will I Do?

Your provider will start off by giving you an overview of the treatment. Together, you will review some information about PTSD in order to help you better understand your symptoms. Your provider probably will ask about the type of trauma you experienced, but you will not need to go into great detail right away.

Your provider will also ask you to do some writing about how your trauma has affected you. Over the next several sessions, you will talk about any negative or unhelpful thoughts you have been having about the trauma, and you will work together to learn to consider other ways of thinking about the situation.

You will use worksheets in session and at home that help you learn this strategy. CPT can also include writing about the details of your trauma (although sometimes this can be skipped). This may sound difficult at first, but you may be more able to cope with emotions like anger, sadness and guilt by talking it over with your therapist. Towards the end of therapy, you and your therapist will focus on some specific areas of your life that may have been affected by the trauma, including your sense of safety, trust, control, self-esteem, and intimacy.

How Long Does Treatment Last?

CPT usually takes 12 weekly sessions, so treatment lasts about 3 months. Sessions are 60 to 90 minutes each. You may start to feel better after a few sessions. And the benefits of CPT often last long after your final session with your provider.

What Are the Risks?

The risks of doing CPT are mild to moderate discomfort when talking or writing about trauma-related memories or beliefs. These feelings are usually brief and people tend to feel better as they keep doing CPT. Most people who complete CPT find that the benefits outweigh any initial discomfort.

Group or Individual?

CPT can be done individually, where you meet one-to-one with a provider. CPT can also be done in a group with one or two providers and about 6–10 other people who also have PTSD.

Will I Talk in Detail about My Trauma?

Around your third session, you may be asked to write about the details of your trauma. This writing assignment will be done at home. You will read this written trauma account out loud in your next session. If you are in group CPT, you will read through your written trauma account with a provider—but not in front of the whole group. There is also another type of CPT that does not ask you to write about the details of your trauma.

Will I Have Homework?

Yes, you will do some writing and complete worksheets between sessions. Take home worksheets help you practice in real life the skills you learn in the therapist's office. Most people find that the more effort and energy they put into these assignments, the more they get out of CPT.

Chapter 48

Mental Health Medications

Chapter Contents

Section 48.1

Understanding Mental Health Medications

This section contains text excerpted from the following sources:
Text in this chapter begins with excerpts from "Mental Disorders,"
National Institutes of Health (NIH), April 28, 2015; Text beginning
with the heading "What Are Antidepressants?" is excerpted from
"Mental Health Medications," National Institute of
Mental Health (NIMH), October 2016.

Mental disorders include a wide range of problems, including:

- Anxiety disorders, including panic disorder, obsessive-compulsive disorder (OCD), posttraumatic stress disorder (PTSD), and phobias

- Bipolar disorder

- Depression

- Mood disorders

- Personality disorders

- Psychotic disorders, including schizophrenia

There are many causes of mental disorders. Your genes and family history may play a role. Your life experiences, such as stress or a history of abuse, may also matter. Biological factors can also be part of the cause. A traumatic brain injury can lead to a mental disorder. A mother's exposure to viruses or toxic chemicals while pregnant may play a part. Other factors may increase your risk, such as use of illegal drugs or having a serious medical condition like cancer.

What Are Antidepressants?

Antidepressants are medications commonly used to treat depression. Antidepressants are also used for other health conditions, such as anxiety, pain and insomnia. Although antidepressants are not U.S. Food and Drug Administration (FDA)-approved specifically to treat Attention deficit hyperactivity disorder (ADHD), antidepressants are sometimes used to treat ADHD in adults.

The most popular types of antidepressants are called selective serotonin reuptake inhibitors (SSRIs). Examples of SSRIs include:

- Fluoxetine

- Citalopram

- Sertraline

- Paroxetine

- Escitalopram

Other types of antidepressants are serotonin and norepinephrine reuptake inhibitors (SNRIs). SNRIs are similar to SSRIs and include venlafaxine and duloxetine.

Another antidepressant that is commonly used is bupropion. Bupropion is a third type of antidepressant which works differently than either SSRIs or SNRIs. Bupropion is also used to treat seasonal affective disorder and to help people stop smoking.

SSRIs, SNRIs, and bupropion are popular because they do not cause as many side effects as older classes of antidepressants, and seem to help a broader group of depressive and anxiety disorders. Older antidepressant medications include tricyclics, tetracyclics, and monoamine oxidase inhibitors (MAOIs). For some people, tricyclics, tetracyclics, or MAOIs may be the best medications.

How Do People Respond to Antidepressants?

According to a research review by the Agency for Healthcare Research and Quality (AHRQ), all antidepressant medications work about as well as each other to improve symptoms of depression and to keep depression symptoms from coming back. For reasons not yet well understood, some people respond better to some antidepressant medications than to others.

Therefore, it is important to know that some people may not feel better with the first medicine they try and may need to try several medicines to find the one that works for them. Others may find that a medicine helped for a while, but their symptoms came back. It is important to carefully follow your doctor's directions for taking your medicine at an adequate dose and over an extended period of time (often 4 to 6 weeks) for it to work.

Once a person begins taking antidepressants, it is important to not stop taking them without the help of a doctor. Sometimes people taking antidepressants feel better and stop taking the medication too soon, and the depression may return. When it is time to stop the medication, the doctor will help the person slowly and safely decrease the dose. It's important to give the body time to adjust to the change. People don't get addicted (or "hooked") on these medications, but stopping them abruptly may also cause withdrawal symptoms.

What Are the Possible Side Effects of Antidepressants?

Some antidepressants may cause more side effects than others. You may need to try several different antidepressant medications before finding the one that improves your symptoms and that causes side effects that you can manage.

The most common side effects listed by the U.S. Food and Drug Administration (FDA) include:

- Nausea and vomiting

- Weight gain

- Diarrhea

- Sleepiness

- Sexual problems

Call your doctor right away if you have any of the following symptoms, especially if they are new, worsening, or worry you:

- Thoughts about suicide or dying

- Attempts to commit suicide

- New or worsening depression

- New or worsening anxiety

- Feeling very agitated or restless

- Panic attacks

- Trouble sleeping (insomnia)

- New or worsening irritability

- Acting aggressively, being angry, or violent

- Acting on dangerous impulses

- An extreme increase in activity and talking (mania)

- Other unusual changes in behavior or mood

Combining the newer SSRI or SNRI antidepressants with one of the commonly-used "triptan" medications used to treat migraine headaches could cause a life-threatening illness called "serotonin syndrome." A person with serotonin syndrome may be agitated, have hallucinations (see or hear things that are not real), have a high temperature, or have unusual blood pressure changes. Serotonin syndrome is usually associated with the older antidepressants called MAOIs, but it can happen with the newer antidepressants as well, if they are mixed with the wrong medications.

What Are Anti-Anxiety Medications?

Anti-anxiety medications help reduce the symptoms of anxiety, such as panic attacks, or extreme fear and worry. The most common anti-anxiety medications are called benzodiazepines. Benzodiazepines can treat generalized anxiety disorder. In the case of panic disorder or social phobia (social anxiety disorder), benzodiazepines are usually second-line treatments, behind SSRIs or other antidepressants.

Benzodiazepines used to treat anxiety disorders include:

- Clonazepam

- Alprazolam

- Lorazepam

Short half-life (or short-acting) benzodiazepines (such as Lorazepam) and beta-blockers are used to treat the short-term symptoms of anxiety. Beta-blockers help manage physical symptoms of anxiety, such as trembling, rapid heartbeat, and sweating that people with phobias (an overwhelming and unreasonable fear of an object or situation, such as public speaking) experience in difficult situations. Taking these medications for a short period of time can help the person keep physical symptoms under control and can be used "as needed" to reduce acute anxiety.

Buspirone (which is unrelated to the benzodiazepines) is sometimes used for the long-term treatment of chronic anxiety. In contrast to the benzodiazepines, buspirone must be taken every day for a few weeks to reach its full effect. It is not useful on an "as-needed" basis.

How Do People Respond to Anti-Anxiety Medications?

Anti-anxiety medications such as benzodiazepines are effective in relieving anxiety and take effect more quickly than the antidepressant medications (or buspirone) often prescribed for anxiety. However, people can build up a tolerance to benzodiazepines if they are taken over a long period of time and may need higher and higher doses to get the same effect. Some people may even become dependent on them. To avoid these problems, doctors usually prescribe benzodiazepines for short periods, a practice that is especially helpful for older adults who have substance abuse problems and people who become dependent on medication easily. If people suddenly stop taking benzodiazepines, they may have withdrawal symptoms or their anxiety may return. Therefore, benzodiazepines should be tapered off slowly.

What Are the Possible Side Effects of Anti-Anxiety Medications?

Like other medications, anti-anxiety medications may cause side effects. Some of these side effects and risks are serious. The most common side effects for benzodiazepines are drowsiness and dizziness. Other possible side effects include:

- Nausea
- Blurred vision
- Headache
- Confusion
- Tiredness
- Nightmares

Tell your doctor if any of these symptoms are severe or do not go away:

- Drowsiness
- Dizziness
- Unsteadiness
- Problems with coordination
- Difficulty thinking or remembering
- Increased saliva
- Muscle or joint pain
- Frequent urination

- Blurred vision
- Changes in sex drive or ability

If you experience any of the symptoms below, call your doctor immediately:

- Rash
- Hives
- Swelling of the eyes, face, lips, tongue, or throat
- Difficulty breathing or swallowing
- Hoarseness
- Seizures
- Yellowing of the skin or eyes
- Depression
- Difficulty speaking
- Yellowing of the skin or eyes
- Thoughts of suicide or harming yourself
- Difficulty breathing

Common side effects of beta-blockers include:

- Fatigue
- Cold hands
- Dizziness or light-headedness
- Weakness

Beta-blockers generally are not recommended for people with asthma or diabetes because they may worsen symptoms related to both.

Possible side effects from buspirone include:

- Dizziness
- Headaches
- Nausea
- Nervousness
- Lightheadedness

- Excitement

- Trouble sleeping

Anti-anxiety medications may cause other side effects that are not included in the lists above.

What Are Stimulants?

As the name suggests, stimulants increase alertness, attention, and energy, as well as elevate blood pressure, heart rate, and respiration. Stimulant medications are often prescribed to treat children, adolescents, or adults diagnosed with ADHD.

Stimulants used to treat ADHD include:

- Methylphenidate

- Amphetamine

- Dextroamphetamine

- Lisdexamfetamine Dimesylate

Stimulants are also prescribed to treat other health conditions, including narcolepsy, and occasionally depression (especially in older or chronically medically ill people and in those who have not responded to other treatments).

How Do People Respond to Stimulants?

Prescription stimulants have a calming and "focusing" effect on individuals with ADHD. Stimulant medications are safe when given under a doctor's supervision. Some children taking them may feel slightly different or "funny."

Some parents worry that stimulant medications may lead to drug abuse or dependence, but there is little evidence of this when they are used properly as prescribed. Additionally, research shows that teens with ADHD who took stimulant medications were less likely to abuse drugs than those who did not take stimulant medications.

What Are the Possible Side Effects of Stimulants?

Stimulants may cause side effects. Most side effects are minor and disappear when dosage levels are lowered. The most common side effects include:

- Difficulty falling asleep or staying asleep

- Loss of appetite

- Stomach pain

- Headache

Less common side effects include:

- Motor tics or verbal tics (sudden, repetitive movements or sounds)

- Personality changes, such as appearing "flat" or without emotion

Call your doctor right away if you have any of these symptoms, especially if they are new, become worse, or worry you. Stimulants may cause other side effects that are not included in the list above.

What Are Antipsychotics?

Antipsychotic medicines are primarily used to manage psychosis. The word "psychosis" is used to describe conditions that affect the mind, and in which there has been some loss of contact with reality, often including delusions (false, fixed beliefs) or hallucinations (hearing or seeing things that are not really there). It can be a symptom of a physical condition such as drug abuse or a mental disorder such as schizophrenia, bipolar disorder, or very severe depression (also known as "psychotic depression").

Antipsychotic medications are often used in combination with other medications to treat delirium, dementia, and mental health conditions, including:

- Attention-Deficit Hyperactivity Disorder (ADIID)

- Severe Depression

- Eating Disorders

- Posttraumatic Stress Disorder (PTSD)

- Obsessive Compulsive Disorder (OCD)

- Generalized Anxiety Disorder

Antipsychotic medicines do not cure these conditions. They are used to help relieve symptoms and improve quality of life.

347

Older or first-generation antipsychotic medications are also called conventional "typical" antipsychotics or "neuroleptics". Some of the common typical antipsychotics include:

- Chlorpromazine

- Haloperidol

- Perphenazine

- Fluphenazine

Newer or second generation medications are also called "atypical" antipsychotics. Some of the common atypical antipsychotics include:

- Risperidone

- Olanzapine

- Quetiapine

- Ziprasidone

- Aripiprazole

- Paliperidone

- Lurasidone

According to a 2013 research review by the Agency for Healthcare Research and Quality, typical and atypical antipsychotics both work to treat symptoms of schizophrenia and the manic phase of bipolar disorder.

Several atypical antipsychotics have a "broader spectrum" of action than the older medications, and are used for treating bipolar depression or depression that has not responded to an antidepressant medication alone.

How Do People Respond to Antipsychotics?

Certain symptoms, such as feeling agitated and having hallucinations, usually go away within days of starting an antipsychotic medication. Symptoms like delusions usually go away within a few weeks, but the full effects of the medication may not be seen for up to six weeks. Every patient responds differently, so it may take several trials of different antipsychotic medications to find the one that works best.

Some people may have a relapse—meaning their symptoms come back or get worse. Usually relapses happen when people stop taking their medication, or when they only take it sometimes. Some people stop taking the medication because they feel better or they may feel that they don't need it anymore, but no one should stop taking an antipsychotic medication without talking to his or her doctor. When a doctor says it is okay to stop taking a medication, it should be gradually tapered off—never stopped suddenly. Many people must stay on an antipsychotic continuously for months or years in order to stay well; treatment should be personalized for each individual.

What Are the Possible Side Effects of Antipsychotics?

Antipsychotics have many side effects (or adverse events) and risks. The FDA lists the following side effects of antipsychotic medicines:

- Drowsiness
- Dizziness
- Restlessness
- Weight gain (the risk is higher with some atypical antipsychotic medicines)
- Dry mouth
- Constipation
- Nausea
- Vomiting
- Blurred vision
- Low blood pressure
- Uncontrollable movements, such as tics and tremors (the risk is higher with typical antipsychotic medicines)
- Seizures
- A low number of white blood cells, which fight infections

A person taking an atypical antipsychotic medication should have his or her weight, glucose levels, and lipid levels monitored regularly by a doctor.

Typical antipsychotic medications can also cause additional side effects related to physical movement, such as:

- Rigidity
- Persistent muscle spasms

- Tremors

- Restlessness

Long-term use of typical antipsychotic medications may lead to a condition called tardive dyskinesia (TD). TD causes muscle movements, commonly around the mouth, that a person can't control. TD can range from mild to severe, and in some people, the problem cannot be cured. Sometimes people with TD recover partially or fully after they stop taking typical antipsychotic medication. People who think that they might have TD should check with their doctor before stopping their medication. TD rarely occurs while taking atypical antipsychotics.

Antipsychotics may cause other side effects that are not included in this list above.

What Are Mood Stabilizers?

Mood stabilizers are used primarily to treat bipolar disorder, mood swings associated with other mental disorders, and in some cases, to augment the effect of other medications used to treat depression. Lithium, which is an effective mood stabilizer, is approved for the treatment of mania and the maintenance treatment of bipolar disorder. A number of cohort studies describe anti-suicide benefits of lithium for individuals on long-term maintenance. Mood stabilizers work by decreasing abnormal activity in the brain and are also sometimes used to treat:

- Depression (usually along with an antidepressant)

- Schizoaffective Disorder

- Disorders of impulse control

- Certain mental illnesses in children

Anticonvulsant medications are also used as mood stabilizers. They were originally developed to treat seizures, but they were found to help control unstable moods as well. One anticonvulsant commonly used as a mood stabilizer is valproic acid (also called divalproex sodium). For some people, especially those with "mixed" symptoms of mania and depression or those with rapid-cycling bipolar disorder, valproic acid may work better than lithium. Other anticonvulsants used as mood stabilizers include:

- Carbamazepine

- Lamotrigine
- Oxcarbazepine

What Are the Possible Side Effects of Mood Stabilizers?

Mood stabilizers can cause several side effects, and some of them may become serious, especially at excessively high blood levels. These side effects include:

- Itching, rash
- Excessive thirst
- Frequent urination
- Tremor (shakiness) of the hands
- Nausea and vomiting
- Slurred speech
- Fast, slow, irregular, or pounding heartbeat
- Blackouts
- Changes in vision
- Seizures
- Hallucinations (seeing things or hearing voices that do not exist)
- Loss of coordination
- Swelling of the eyes, face, lips, tongue, throat, hands, feet, ankles, or lower legs.

If a person with bipolar disorder is being treated with lithium, he or she should visit the doctor regularly to check the lithium levels his or her blood, and make sure the kidneys and the thyroid are working normally.

Lithium is eliminated from the body through the kidney, so the dose may need to be lowered in older people with reduced kidney function. Also, loss of water from the body, such as through sweating or diarrhea, can cause the lithium level to rise, requiring a temporary lowering of the daily dose. Although kidney functions are checked periodically during lithium treatment, actual damage of the kidney is uncommon in people whose blood levels of lithium have stayed within the therapeutic range.

Mood stabilizers may cause other side effects that are not included in this list.

Some possible side effects linked anticonvulsants (such as valproic acid) include:

- Drowsiness
- Dizziness
- Headache
- Diarrhea
- Constipation
- Changes in appetite
- Weight changes
- Back pain
- Agitation

- Mood swings
- Abnormal thinking
- Uncontrollable shaking of a part of the body
- Loss of coordination
- Uncontrollable movements of the eyes
- Blurred or double vision
- Ringing in the ears
- Hair loss

These medications may also:

- Cause damage to the liver or pancreas, so people taking it should see their doctors regularly

- Increase testosterone (a male hormone) levels in teenage girls and lead to a condition called polycystic ovarian syndrome (a disease that can affect fertility and make the menstrual cycle become irregular)

Medications for common adult health problems, such as diabetes, high blood pressure, anxiety, and depression may interact badly with anticonvulsants. In this case, a doctor can offer other medication options.

Section 48.2

Ketamine Lifts Depression via Metabolite

This section includes text excerpted from "Ketamine Lifts Depression via a Byproduct of Its Metabolism," National Institute of Mental Health (NIMH), May 4, 2016.

A chemical byproduct, or metabolite, created as the body breaks down ketamine likely holds the secret to its rapid antidepressant action, National Institutes of Health (NIH) scientists and grantees have discovered. This metabolite singularly reversed depression-like behaviors in mice without triggering any of the anesthetic, dissociative, or addictive side effects associated with ketamine.

"This discovery fundamentally changes our understanding of how this rapid antidepressant mechanism works and holds promise for development of more robust and safer treatments," said Carlos Zarate, M.D. of the NIH's National Institute of Mental Health (NIMH), a study co-author and a pioneer of research using ketamine to treat depression. "By using a team approach, researchers were able to reverse-engineer ketamine's workings from the clinic to the lab to pinpoint what makes it so unique."

NIMH grantee Todd Gould, M.D., of the University Of Maryland School Of Medicine, in collaboration with Zarate and other colleagues, report on their findings May 4, 2016 in the journal Nature. The team also included researchers at the NIH's National Center for Advancing Translational Sciences (NCATS) and National Institute on Aging (NIA), and the University of North Carolina.

"Now that we know that ketamine's antidepressant actions in mice are due to a metabolite, not ketamine itself, the next steps are to confirm that it works similarly in humans, and determine if it can lead to improved therapeutics for patients," explained Gould.

Clinical trials by Zarate and others have shown that ketamine can lift depression in hours, or even minutes—much faster than the most commonly used antidepressant medications now available, which often require weeks to take effect. Further, the antidepressant effects of a single dose can last for a week or longer. However, despite legitimate medical uses, ketamine also has dissociative, euphoric, and addictive properties, making it a potential drug of abuse and limiting its usefulness as a depression medication.

In hopes of finding leads to a more practical treatment, the research team sought to pinpoint the exact mechanism by which ketamine relieves depression. Ketamine belongs to a class of drugs that block cellular receptors for glutamate, the brain's chief excitatory chemical messenger. Until now, the prevailing view was that ketamine produced its antidepressant effects by blocking N-methyl-D-aspartic acid (NMDA) glutamate receptors.

However, human trials of other NMDA-receptor blockers failed to produce ketamine's robust and sustained antidepressant effects. So the team explored the effects of ketamine on antidepressant-responsive behaviors in mice. Ketamine harbors two chemical forms that are mirror images of each other, denoted (S)- and (R)-ketamine. The investigators found that while (S)-ketamine is more potent at blocking NMDA receptors, it is less effective in reducing depression-like behaviors than the (R) form.

The team then looked at the effects of the metabolites created as the body breaks down (S)- and (R)-ketamine. It was known that ketamine's antidepressant effects are greater in female mice. NIA researchers Irving Wainer, Ph.D., and Ruin Moaddel, Ph.D. identified a key metabolite (2S, 6S; 2R, 6R)-HNK (hydroxynorketamine) and showed that it is pharmacologically active. The team then discovered that levels of this metabolite were three times higher in female mice, hinting that it might be responsible for the sex difference in the antidepressant-like effect. To find out, the researchers chemically blocked the metabolism of ketamine. This prevented formation of the metabolite, which blocked the drug's antidepressant-like effects.

Like ketamine, this metabolite includes two forms that mirror each other. By testing both forms, they found that one—(2R, 6R)-HNK—had antidepressant-like effects similar to ketamine, lasting for at least three days in mice. Notably, unlike ketamine, the compound does not inhibit NMDA receptors. It instead activates, possibly indirectly, another type of glutamate receptor, α-amino-3-hydroxy-5-methyl-4-isoxazole propionic acid (AMPA). Blocking AMPA receptors prevented the antidepressant-like effects of (2R, 6R)-HNK in mice. The experiments confirmed that the rapid antidepressant-like effects require activation of AMPA receptors, not inhibition of NMDA receptors.

Ketamine also has effects in mice that mimic its dissociative, euphoric effects in humans and underlie its abuse and addictive potential; however, these effects were not observed with (2R, 6R)-HNK.

(2R, 6R)-HNK did not cause the changes in physical activity, sensory processing, and coordination in mice that occur with ketamine. In an experimental situation where mice were able to self-administer medication, they did so with ketamine but not the (2R, 6R)-HNK metabolite, indicating that (2R, 6R)-HNK is not addictive.

Section 48.3

Medications for Treating Depression in Women

This section includes text excerpted from "Depression—Medicines to Help You," U.S. Food and Drug Administration (FDA), December 18, 2014.

Depression—Medicines for Women

Women are more likely than men to feel depressed. About 1 woman in 5 has depression in the United States.

There is hope.

Depression can be treated with medicine or counseling. Sometimes both are used. Talk to your doctor to find out what will work best for you.

This section will help you talk to your doctor or pharmacist about medicines called antidepressants that can help to treat depression. Ask your doctor to tell you about all of the risks of taking the different medicines. This section only talks about some of the risks.

The Baby Blues

Having a baby can be a joyful time. However, some women cry a lot and feel sad right after they have a baby. This is called "the baby blues". This feeling usually goes away after about two weeks.

If you still feel sad after two weeks, go to your doctor or clinic. You may be depressed. This type of depression is called postpartum depression because it starts after a woman has a baby. A woman can have this kind of depression up to one year after she has a baby.

Depression and Your Children

Like adults, kids can also feel depressed. You should watch your children for signs of depression. Talk to your children if you notice changes in their behavior. Talk to your doctor or nurse if you are still concerned.

Children and teens can take medicines for depression. Prozac (Fluoxetine) is the only U.S. Department of Food and Drug Administration (FDA)-approved antidepressant for children and teens with depression. Talk to your doctor about important warnings for children and teens who take medicines for depression.

Important Warnings about Medicines for Depression

Children and teens who take antidepressants may be more likely to try to hurt or kill themselves.

Call 911 if the person:

- Tries to hurt or kill himself/herself.

- Talks about specific ways they plan to hurt or kill himself/herself.

- Talks about or tries to harm others.

Call your doctor right away if the person shows any of these signs:

- Talks about dying or suicide

- Starts acting very differently

- Is abnormally active

- Has severe problems sleeping

- Becomes violent or abnormally angry

- Becomes agitated or can't sit still

Medicines for Depression

There are many different kinds of medicine for depression.

- Selective Serotonin Reuptake Inhibitors (SSRIs)

- Monoamine Oxidase Inhibitors (MAOIs)

- Tricyclic Antidepressants

- Atypical Antidepressants

- Selective Serotonin and Norepinephrine Reuptake Inhibitors (SNRI)

Tell your doctor about any medicines that you are taking. Do not forget about cold medicines and herbs like St. John's Wort. Some medicines will make you very sick if you take them while you are taking antidepressants.

Like any drug, depression medicines may cause some side effects. Do not stop taking your medicines without first talking to your doctor. Tell your doctor about any problems you are having. Your doctor will help you find the medicine that is best for you.

Section 48.4

Medications for Treating Depression in Elders

This section includes text excerpted from "Depression: Medication," NIHSeniorHealth, National Institute on Aging (NIA), May 2016.

Antidepressants

Antidepressants are medicines that treat depression. They may help improve the way your brain uses certain chemicals that control mood or stress. You may need to try several different antidepressant medicines before finding the one that improves your symptoms and has manageable side effects. A medication that has helped you or a close family member in the past will often be considered.

Types of Antidepressants

There are several types of antidepressants.

- selective serotonin reuptake inhibitors (SSRIs)

- serotonin and norepinephrine reuptake inhibitors (SNRIs)

- tricyclic antidepressants (TCAs)

- monoamine oxidase inhibitors (MAOIs)

There are other antidepressants that don't fall into any of these categories and are considered unique, such as Mirtazapine and Bupropion.

Taking Antidepressants

Antidepressants take time usually 2–4 weeks to work, and often symptoms such as sleep, appetite, and concentration problems improve before mood lifts, so it is important to give medication a chance before reaching a conclusion about its effectiveness.

If you begin taking antidepressants, do not stop taking them without the help of a doctor. Sometimes people taking antidepressants feel better and then stop taking the medication on their own, and the depression returns. When you and your doctor have decided it is time to stop the medication, usually after a course of 6–12 months, the doctor will help you slowly and safely decrease your dose. Stopping them abruptly can cause withdrawal symptoms.

Side Effects

Although all antidepressants can cause side effects, some are more likely to cause certain side effects than others. You may need to try several different antidepressant medicines before finding the one that improves your symptoms and has side effects that you can manage.

Common side effects listed by the U.S. Food and Drug Administration (FDA) for antidepressants are:

- nausea and vomiting

- weight gain

- diarrhea

- sleepiness

- sexual problems

Other more serious but much less common side effects listed by the FDA for antidepressant medicines can include seizures, heart problems, and an imbalance of salt in your blood, liver damage, suicidal thoughts, or serotonin syndrome (a life-threatening reaction where your body makes too much serotonin). Serotonin syndrome can cause shivering, diarrhea, fever, seizures, and stiff or rigid muscles.

Most antidepressants are generally safe, but the FDA requires that all antidepressants carry black box warnings, the strictest warnings for prescriptions. The warning says that patients of all ages taking antidepressants should be watched closely, especially during the first few weeks of treatment.

For older adults who are already taking several medications for other conditions, it is important to talk with a doctor about any adverse drug interactions that may occur while taking antidepressants.

Herbal and Natural Products

You may have heard about an herbal medicine called St. John's wort. Although it is a top-selling botanical product, the FDA has not approved its use as an over-the-counter or prescription medicine for depression and there are serious concerns about its safety and effectiveness.

Do not use St. John's wort before talking to your healthcare provider. It should never be combined with a prescription antidepressant, and you should not use it to replace conventional care or to postpone seeing a healthcare provider.

Other natural products sold as dietary supplements, including omega-3 fatty acids and S-adenosylmethionine (SAMe) remain under study but have not been proven safe and effective for routine use.

Keep in mind that dietary supplements can cause medical problems if not used correctly or if used in large amounts, and some may interact with medications you take. Your healthcare provider can advise you.

Chapter 49

Combination Treatment

Depression is a complex mental illness associated with disability and reduced quality of life for the person with depression, as well as substantial societal burden. Major depressive disorder (MDD) is the second leading medical cause of long-term disability, the fourth leading cause of global burden of disease, and is predicted to become the second highest cause of disability by 2020. Depression exerts a negative impact on physical health; it reduces adherence to medical treatment, reduces participation in preventive activities, and increases the likelihood of risk factors such as obesity, smoking, and sedentary lifestyles. MDD may be associated with immune dysfunction and cardiovascular disease, endocrine and neurological diseases, and a general increase in chronic disease incidence. Mortality rates are high: approximately 4 percent of adults with a mood disorder die by their own hand, and about two-thirds of suicides are preceded by depression. In adolescents, untreated depression results in significant impairment in school performance, interpersonal relationships, risk of suicidal behavior and completion of suicide, risk of early pregnancy, occupational maladjustment, and impaired social and family functioning.

Pharmacological agents are one of several treatment modalities used for depression, and one of the most frequently utilized classes of antidepressant medications are the selective serotonin reuptake

This chapter includes text excerpted from "Treatment for Depression after Unsatisfactory Response to SSRIs," Agency for Healthcare Research and Quality (AHRQ), U.S. Department of Health and Human Services (HHS), April 2012. Reviewed November 2016.

inhibitors (SSRIs). The rate of treatment response following first-line treatment with SSRIs is moderate, varying from 40 to 60 percent; remission rates vary from 30 to 45 percent. Up to one-third of persons taking antidepressant medications will develop recurrent symptoms of depression while on therapy. The target goal for acute treatment should be remission, which is defined as a resolution of depressive symptoms (a score within the normal range of the symptom scale). Response to treatment (usually defined as at least a 50 percent reduction in symptom levels) may not be sufficient as a target outcome because residual depressive symptoms are risk factors for relapse and negative predictors of long-term outcome.

Clinicians are faced with a number of treatment options following an inadequate response to an SSRI, and these include monotherapy or combined therapy. Monotherapy options include:

1. an optimization strategy (increasing the dose or extending the duration of the SSRI)

2. switching to another SSRI

3. switching to another class of antidepressants

4. switching to a nonpharmacological intervention.

Combination or add on therapy options include:

1. combining the SSRI with an augmenting agent

2. combining antidepressants

3. combining the SSRI with a nonpharmacological therapy (such as psychological therapies, exercise, etc.)

It is also an option to switch to a new antidepressant and simultaneously combine that antidepressant with a second pharmacological or nonpharmacological treatment. This is sometimes referred to as an acceleration strategy.

The number of studies comparing single medications against each other (monotherapy compared with monotherapy) following an inadequate response to an SSRI are few and evaluate different agents. Extant studies are limited in type of agents utilized, sample sizes, and population characteristics. There is insufficient evidence to determine whether there is a difference between various single-agent therapies in the outcomes of response and remission following an inadequate response to an SSRI.

There is insufficient evidence to evaluate the benefits of ongoing monotherapy with an SSRI compared with combination treatment involving the addition of another antidepressant medication to the initial SSRI. There is low-grade evidence that comparable results are achieved following the switch to an alternate antidepressant medication (monotherapy with a new antidepressant) when compared with adding a nonantidepressant treatment to the initial SSRI (traditional augmentation approach). There is low-grade evidence that adding an atypical antipsychotic medication to ongoing SSRI treatment is associated with higher response and remission rates compared with adding a placebo to ongoing SSRI treatment (following inadequate response to the SSRI). There is insufficient evidence to confirm that there is an improvement in response and remission rates following the addition of any other augmentation agents. There is insufficient evidence to evaluate the benefits or harms of specific combinations of treatments relative to alternative combinations.

Chapter 50

Brain Stimulation Therapies for Severe Depression

Brain Stimulation Therapies

Brain stimulation therapies can play a role in treating certain mental disorders. Brain stimulation therapies involve activating or inhibiting the brain directly with electricity. The electricity can be given directly by electrodes implanted in the brain, or noninvasively through electrodes placed on the scalp. The electricity can also be induced by using magnetic fields applied to the head. While these types of therapies are less frequently used than medication and psychotherapies, they hold promise for treating certain mental disorders that do not respond to other treatments.

Electroconvulsive therapy is the best studied brain stimulation therapy and has the longest history of use. Other stimulation therapies discussed here are newer, and in some cases still experimental methods. These include:

- vagus nerve stimulation (VNS)

- repetitive transcranial magnetic stimulation (rTMS)

- magnetic seizure therapy (MST)

- deep brain stimulation (DBS)

This chapter includes text excerpted from "Brain Stimulation Therapies," National Institute of Mental Health (NIMH), June 2016.

A treatment plan may also include medication and psychotherapy. Choosing the right treatment plan should be based on a person's individual needs and medical situation, and under a doctor's care.

Electroconvulsive Therapy

Electroconvulsive therapy (ECT) uses an electric current to treat serious mental disorders. This type of therapy is usually considered only if a patient's illness has not improved after other treatments (such as antidepressant medication or psychotherapy) are tried, or in cases where rapid response is needed (as in the case of suicide risk and catatonia, for example).

ECT: Why It's Done

ECT is most often used to treat severe, treatment-resistant depression, but it may also be medically indicated in other mental disorders, such as bipolar disorder or schizophrenia. It also may be used in life-threatening circumstances, such as when a patient is unable to move or respond to the outside world (e.g., catatonia), is suicidal, or is malnourished as a result of severe depression.

ECT can be effective in reducing the chances of relapse when patients undergo follow-up treatments. Two major advantages of ECT over medication are that ECT begins to work quicker, often starting within the first week, and older individuals respond especially quickly.

ECT: How It Works

Before ECT is administered, a person is sedated with general anesthesia and given a medication called a muscle relaxant to prevent movement during the procedure. An anesthesiologist monitors breathing, heart rate and blood pressure during the entire procedure, which is conducted by a trained medical team, including physicians and nurses. During the procedure:

Electrodes are placed at precise locations on the head.

Through the electrodes, an electric current passes through the brain, causing a seizure that lasts generally less than one minute. Because the patient is under anesthesia and has taken a muscle relaxant, it is not painful and the patient cannot feel the electrical impulses.

Five to ten minutes after the procedure ends, the patient awakens. He or she may feel groggy at first as the anesthesia wears off.

But after about an hour, the patient usually is alert and can resume normal activities.

A typical course of ECT is administered about three times a week until the patient's depression improves (usually within 6 to 12 treatments). After that, maintenance ECT treatment is sometimes needed to reduce the chances that symptoms will return. ECT maintenance treatment varies depending on the needs of the individual, and may range from one session per week to one session every few months. Frequently, a person who undergoes ECT also takes antidepressant medication or a mood stabilizing medication.

ECT Side Effects

The most common side effects associated with ECT include:

- headache
- upset stomach
- muscle aches
- memory loss

Some people may experience memory problems, especially of memories around the time of the treatment. Sometimes the memory problems are more severe, but usually they improve over the days and weeks following the end of an ECT course.

Research has found that memory problems seem to be more associated with the traditional type of ECT called bilateral ECT, in which the electrodes are placed on both sides of the head.

In unilateral ECT, the electrodes are placed on just one side of the head—typically the right side because it is opposite the brain's learning and memory areas. Unilateral ECT has been found to be less likely to cause memory problems and therefore is preferred by many doctors, patients and families.

Vagus Nerve Stimulation

Vagus nerve stimulation (VNS) works through a device implanted under the skin that sends electrical pulses through the left vagus nerve, half of a prominent pair of nerves that run from the brainstem through the neck and down to each side of the chest and abdomen. The vagus nerves carry messages from the brain to the body's major organs (e.g., heart, lungs and intestines) and to areas of the brain that control mood, sleep, and other functions.

VNS: Why It's Done

VNS was originally developed as a treatment for epilepsy. However, scientists noticed that it also had favorable effects on mood, especially depressive symptoms. Using brain scans, scientists found that the device affected areas of the brain that are involved in mood regulation. The pulses appeared to alter the levels of certain neurotransmitters (brain chemicals) associated with mood, including serotonin, norepinephrine, GABA and glutamate.

In 2005, the U.S. Food and Drug Administration (FDA) approved VNS for use in treating treatment-resistant depression in certain circumstances:

- if the patient is 18 years of age or over; and

- if the illness has lasted two years or more; and

- if it is severe or recurrent; and

- if the depression has not eased after trying at least four other treatments

According to the FDA, it is not intended to be a first-line treatment, even for patients with severe depression. And, despite FDA approval, VNS remains an infrequently used because results of early studies testing its effectiveness for major depression were mixed. But a newer study, which pooled together findings from only controlled clinical trials, found that 32% of depressed people responded to VSN and 14% had a full remission of symptoms after being treated for nearly 2 years.

VNS: How It Works

A device called a pulse generator, about the size of a stopwatch, is surgically implanted in the upper left side of the chest. Connected to the pulse generator is an electrical lead wire, which is connected from the generator to the left vagus nerve.

Typically, 30-second electrical pulses are sent about every five minutes from the generator to the vagus nerve. The duration and frequency of the pulses may vary depending on how the generator is programmed. The vagus nerve, in turn, delivers those signals to the brain. The pulse generator, which operates continuously, is powered by a battery that lasts around 10 years, after which it must be replaced. Normally, people do not feel pain or any other sensations as the device operates.

The device also can be temporarily deactivated by placing a magnet over the chest where the pulse generator is implanted. A person may want to deactivate it if side effects become intolerable, or before engaging in strenuous activity or exercise because it may interfere with breathing. The device reactivates when the magnet is removed.

VNS treatment is intended to reduce symptoms of depression. It may be several months before the patient notices any benefits and not all patients will respond to VNS. It is important to remember that VNS is intended to be given along with other traditional therapies, such as medications, and patients should not expect to discontinue these other treatments, even with the device in place.

Note: VNS should only be prescribed and monitored by doctors who have specific training and expertise in the management of treatment-resistant depression and the use of this device.

VNS: Side Effects

VNS is not without risk. There may be complications such as infection from the implant surgery, or the device may come loose, move around or malfunction, which may require additional surgery to correct. Some patients have no improvement in symptoms and some actually get worse.

Other potential side effects include:

* Voice changes or hoarseness

* Cough or sore throat

* Neck pain

* Discomfort or tingling in the area where the device is implanted

* Breathing problems, especially during exercise

* Difficulty swallowing

Long-term side effects are unknown.

Repetitive Transcranial Magnetic Stimulation

Repetitive transcranial magnetic stimulation (rTMS) uses a magnet to activate the brain. First developed in 1985, rTMS has been studied as a treatment for depression, psychosis, anxiety, and other disorders.

Unlike ECT, in which electrical stimulation is more generalized, rTMS can be targeted to a specific site in the brain. Scientists believe that focusing on a specific site in the brain reduces the chance for the types of side effects associated with ECT. But opinions vary as to what site is best.

rTMS: Why It's Done

In 2008, rTMS was approved for use by the FDA as a treatment for major depression for patients who do not respond to at least one antidepressant medication in the current episode. It is also used in other countries as a treatment for depression in patients who have not responded to medications and who might otherwise be considered for ECT.

The evidence supporting rTMS for depression was mixed until the first large clinical trial, funded by NIMH, was published in 2010. The trial found that 14% achieved remission with rTMS compared to 5% with an inactive (sham) treatment. After the trial ended, patients could enter a second phase in which everyone, including those who previously received the sham treatment, was given rTMS. Remission rates during the second phase climbed to nearly 30%. A sham treatment is like a placebo, but instead of being an inactive pill, it's an inactive procedure that mimics real rTMS.

rTMS: How It Works

A typical rTMS session lasts 30 to 60 minutes and does not require anesthesia.

During the procedure:

- An electromagnetic coil is held against the forehead near an area of the brain that is thought to be involved in mood regulation.

- Then, short electromagnetic pulses are administered through the coil. The magnetic pulses easily pass through the skull, and causes small electrical currents that stimulate nerve cells in the targeted brain region.

Because this type of pulse generally does not reach further than two inches into the brain, scientists can select which parts of the brain will be affected and which will not be. The magnetic field is about the same strength as that of a magnetic resonance imaging (MRI) scan. Generally, the person feels a slight knocking or tapping on the head as the pulses are administered.

Not all scientists agree on the best way to position the magnet on the patient's head or give the electromagnetic pulses. They also do not yet know if rTMS works best when given as a single treatment or combined with medication and/or psychotherapy. More research is underway to determine the safest and most effective uses of rTMS.

rTMS: Side Effects

Sometimes a person may have discomfort at the site on the head where the magnet is placed. The muscles of the scalp, jaw or face may contract or tingle during the procedure. Mild headaches or brief lightheadedness may result. It is also possible that the procedure could cause a seizure, although documented incidences of this are uncommon. Two large-scale studies on the safety of rTMS found that most side effects, such as headaches or scalp discomfort, were mild or moderate, and no seizures occurred. Because the treatment is relatively new, however, long-term side effects are unknown.

Magnetic Seizure Therapy

MST: How It Works

Magnetic seizure therapy (MST) borrows certain aspects from both ECT and rTMS. Like rTMS, MST uses magnetic pulses instead of electricity to stimulate a precise target in the brain. However, unlike rTMS, MST aims to induce a seizure like ECT. So the pulses are given at a higher frequency than that used in rTMS. Therefore, like ECT, the patient must be anesthetized and given a muscle relaxant to prevent movement. The goal of MST is to retain the effectiveness of ECT while reducing its cognitive side effects.

MST is in the early stages of testing for mental disorders, but initial results are promising. A recent review article that examined the evidence from eight clinical studies found that MST triggered remission from major depression or bipolar disorder in 30–40% of individuals.

MST: Side Effects

Like ECT, MST carries the risk of side effects that can be caused by anesthesia exposure and the induction of a seizure. Studies in both animals and humans have found that MST produces:

- fewer memory side effects
- shorter seizures
- allows for a shorter recovery time than ECT

Deep Brain Stimulation

Deep brain stimulation (DBS) was first developed as a treatment for Parkinson disease to reduce tremor, stiffness, walking problems and uncontrollable movements. In DBS, a pair of electrodes is implanted in the brain and controlled by a generator that is implanted in the chest. Stimulation is continuous and its frequency and level are customized to the individual.

DBS has been studied as a treatment for depression or obsessive compulsive disorder (OCD). Currently, there is a Humanitarian Device Exemption for the use of DBS to treat OCD, but its use in depression remains only on an experimental basis. A review of all 22 published studies testing DBS for depression found that only three of them were of high quality because they not only had a treatment group but also a control group which did not receive DBS. The review found that across the studies, 40–50% of people showed receiving DBS greater than 50% improvement.

DBS: How It Works

DBS requires brain surgery. The head is shaved and then attached with screws to a sturdy frame that prevents the head from moving during the surgery. Scans of the head and brain using MRI are taken. The surgeon uses these images as guides during the surgery. Patients are awake during the procedure to provide the surgeon with feedback, but they feel no pain because the head is numbed with a local anesthetic and the brain itself does not register pain.

Once ready for surgery, two holes are drilled into the head. From there, the surgeon threads a slender tube down into the brain to place electrodes on each side of a specific area of the brain. In the case of depression, the first area of the brain targeted by DBS is called Area 25, or the sub-genual cingulate cortex. This area has been found to be overactive in depression and other mood disorders. But later research targeted several other areas of the brain affected by depression. So DBS is now targeting several areas of the brain for treating depression. In the case of OCD, the electrodes are placed in an area of the brain (the ventral capsule/ventral striatum) believed to be associated with the disorder.

After the electrodes are implanted and the patient provides feedback about their placement, the patient is put under general anesthesia. The electrodes are then attached to wires that are run inside the body from the head down to the chest, where a pair of battery-operated generators are implanted. From here, electrical pulses are continuously delivered over the wires to the electrodes in the brain. Although it is unclear exactly how the device works to reduce depression or OCD, scientists believe that the pulses help to "reset" the area of the brain that is malfunctioning so that it works normally again.

DBS Side Effects

DBS carries risks associated with any type of brain surgery. For example, the procedure may lead to:

- Bleeding in the brain or stroke
- Infection
- Disorientation or confusion
- Unwanted mood changes
- Movement disorders
- Lightheadedness
- Trouble sleeping

Because the procedure is still being studied, other side effects not yet identified may be possible. Long-term benefits and side effects are unknown.

Chapter 51

Light Therapy for Seasonal Affective Disorder

Winter Blues

National Institute of Health (NIH)-funded researchers have been studying the "winter blues" and a more severe type of depression called seasonal affective disorder, or SAD, for more than 3 decades. They've learned about possible causes and found treatments that seem to help most people. Still, much remains unknown about these winter-related shifts in mood.

"Winter blues is a general term, not a medical diagnosis. It's fairly common, and it's more mild than serious. It usually clears up on its own in a fairly short amount of time," says Dr. Matthew Rudorfer, a mental health expert at NIH. The so-called winter blues are often linked to something specific, such as stressful holidays or reminders of absent loved ones.

"Seasonal affective disorder (SAD), though, is different. It's a well-defined clinical diagnosis that's related to the shortening of daylight hours," says Rudorfer. "It interferes with daily functioning over a significant period of time." A key feature of SAD is that it follows a regular pattern. It appears each year as the seasons change, and it goes away several months later, usually during spring and summer.

This chapter includes text excerpted from "Beat the Winter Blues," *NIH News in Health*, National Institute on Aging (NIA), January 2013. Reviewed November 2016.

SAD is more common in northern than in southern parts of the United States, where winter days last longer. "In Florida only about 1% of the population is likely to suffer from SAD. But in the northern-most parts of the United States, about 10% of people in Alaska may be affected," says Rudorfer.

As with other forms of depression, SAD can lead to a gloomy outlook and make people feel hopeless, worthless and irritable. They may lose interest in activities they used to enjoy, such as hobbies and spending time with friends.

Shorter days seem to be a main trigger for SAD. Reduced sunlight in fall and winter can disrupt your body's internal clock, or circadian rhythm. This 24-hour "master clock" responds to cues in your sur-roundings, especially light and darkness. During the day, your brain sends signals to other parts of the body to help keep you awake and ready for action. At night, a tiny gland in the brain produces a chemi-cal called melatonin, which helps you sleep. Shortened daylight hours in winter can alter this natural rhythm and lead to SAD in certain people.

NIH researchers first recognized the link between light and sea-sonal depression back in the early 1980s. These scientists pioneered the use of light therapy, which has since become a standard treatment for SAD. "Light therapy is meant to replace the missing daylight hours with an artificial substitute," says Rudorfer.

In light therapy, patients generally sit in front of a light box every morning for 30 minutes or more, depending on the doctor's recom-mendation. The box shines light much brighter than ordinary indoor lighting.

Studies have shown that light therapy relieves SAD symptoms for as much as 70% of patients after a few weeks of treatment. Some improvement can be detected even sooner. "Our research has found that patients report an improvement in depression scores after even the first administration of light," says Dr. Teodor Postolache, who treats anxiety and mood disorders at the University of Maryland School of Medicine. "Still, a sizable proportion of patients improve but do not fully respond to light treatment alone."

Once started, light therapy should continue every day well into spring. "Sitting 30 minutes or more in front of a light box every day can put a strain on some schedules," says Postolache. So some people tend to stop using the light boxes after a while. Other options have been tested, such as light-emitting visors that allow patients to move around during therapy. "But results with visors for treating SAD hav-en't been as promising as hoped," Postolache says.

Light therapy is usually considered a first line treatment for SAD, but it doesn't work for everyone. Studies show that certain antidepressant drugs can be effective in many cases of SAD. The antidepressant bupropion (Wellbutrin) has been approved by the U.S. Food and Drug Administration (FDA) for treating SAD and for preventing winter depression. Doctors sometimes prescribe other antidepressants as well.

Growing evidence suggests that cognitive behavioral therapy (CBT)—a type of talk therapy—an also help patients who have SAD. "For the 'cognitive' part of CBT, we work with patients to identify negative self-defeating thoughts they have," says Dr. Kelly Rohan, a SAD specialist at the University of Vermont. "We try to look objectively at the thought and then reframe it into something that's more accurate, less negative, and maybe even a little more positive. The 'behavioral' part of CBT tries to teach people new behaviors to engage in when they're feeling depressed, to help them feel better."

Behavioral changes might include having lunch with friends, going out for a walk or volunteering in the community. "We try to identify activities that are engaging and pleasurable, and we work with patients to try to schedule them into their daily routine," says Rohan.

A preliminary study by Rohan and colleagues compared CBT to light therapy. Both were found effective at relieving SAD symptoms over 6 weeks in the winter. "We also found that people treated with CBT have less depression and less return of SAD the following winter compared to people who were treated with light therapy," Rohan says. A larger NIH-funded study is now under way to compare CBT to light therapy over 2 years of follow up.

If you're feeling blue this winter, and if the feelings last for several weeks, talk to a healthcare provider. "It's true that SAD goes away on its own, but that could take 5 months or more. Five months of every year is a long time to be impaired and suffering," says Rudorfer. "SAD is generally quite treatable, and the treatment options keep increasing and improving."

Chapter 52

Alternative and Complementary Therapies Used for Depression

Chapter Contents

Section 52.1

Complementary and Alternative Medicine (CAM) for Depression

This section includes text excerpted from "5 Tips: What You Should Know about the Science behind Depression and Complementary Health Approaches," National Center for Complementary and Integrative Health (NCCIH), October 20, 2015.

Depression is a medical condition that affects about 1 in 10 adults in the United States. Depression can be treated with conventional medicine, including antidepressants and certain types of psychotherapy. For more information on depression, visit the National Institute of Mental Health (NIMH)'s Web site. Still, many people turn to complementary health approaches in addition to conventional treatment. Although complementary approaches are commonly used and readily available in the marketplace, many of these treatments have not been rigorously studied for depression. For this reason, it's important that you understand the benefits and risks of these complementary approaches to make informed decisions about your health.

Here are five things you should know about some complementary health approaches for depression:

1. Some studies suggest that omega-3 fatty acid supplements may provide a small improvement along with conventional treatment, such as antidepressants, in patients with major depressive disorder (MDD) and in depressed patients without a diagnosis of MDD. However, a lot of questions remain about how, or if, omega-3 supplements work in the body to produce such an effect.

2. Although some studies of St. John's wort (Hypericum perforatum) have shown benefits similar to standard antidepressants for depression in a limited number of patients, others have not. Research has shown that St. John's wort interacts with many medications in ways that can interfere with their intended effects, making its safety risks outweigh the benefit of any use of St. John's wort.

3. Current scientific evidence does not support the use of other dietary supplements, including SAMe or inositol, for depression.

4. Some studies on mind and body practices, when used along with standard treatment for depression in adults, have had modestly promising results. For example, there is limited evidence that music therapy may provide an improvement in mood. In addition, studies indicate that relaxation training is better than no treatment in reducing symptoms of depression, but is not as beneficial as psychological therapies such as cognitive-behavioral therapy.

5. Take charge of your health—talk with your healthcare providers about any complementary health approaches you use. Together, you can make shared, well-informed decisions.

Section 52.2

Meditation Can Help in Conquering Depression

This section includes text excerpted from "Meditation: In Depth," National Center for Complementary and Integrative Health (NCCIH), April 2016.

What Is Meditation?

Meditation is a mind and body practice that has a long history of use for increasing calmness and physical relaxation, improving psychological balance, coping with illness, and enhancing overall health and well-being. Mind and body practices focus on the interactions among the brain, mind, body, and behavior.

There are many types of meditation, but most have four elements in common: a quiet location with as few distractions as possible; a specific, comfortable posture (sitting, lying down, walking, or in other positions); a focus of attention (a specially chosen word or set of words, an object, or the sensations of the breath); and an open attitude (letting distractions come and go naturally without judging them).

How Much Do We Know about Meditation?

Many studies have been conducted to look at how meditation may be helpful for a variety of conditions, such as high blood pressure, certain psychological disorders, and pain. A number of studies also have helped researchers learn how meditation might work and how it affects the brain.

What Do We Know about the Effectiveness of Meditation?

Some research suggests that practicing meditation may reduce blood pressure, symptoms of irritable bowel syndrome (IBS), anxiety and depression, and insomnia. Evidence about its effectiveness for pain and as a smoking-cessation treatment is uncertain.

What Do We Know about the Safety of Meditation?

Meditation is generally considered to be safe for healthy people. However, people with physical limitations may not be able to participate in certain meditative practices involving movement.

What the Science Says about the Effectiveness of Meditation

Many studies have investigated meditation for different conditions, and there's evidence that it may reduce blood pressure as well as symptoms of irritable bowel syndrome and flare-ups in people who have had ulcerative colitis. It may ease symptoms of anxiety and depression, and may help people with insomnia.

Pain

- Research about meditation's ability to reduce pain has produced mixed results. However, in some studies scientists suggest that meditation activates certain areas of the brain in response to pain.

- A small 2016 study funded in part by the National Center for Complementary and Integrative Health (NCCIH) found that mindfulness meditation does help to control pain and doesn't use the brain's naturally occurring opiates to do so. This suggests that combining mindfulness with pain medications and other approaches that rely on the brain's opioid activity may be particularly effective for reducing pain.

- In another 2016 NCCIH-funded study, adults aged 20 to 70 who had chronic low-back pain received either mindfulness-based stress reduction (MBSR) training, cognitive-behavioral therapy (CBT), or usual care. The MBSR and CBT participants had a similar level of improvement, and it was greater than those who got usual care, including long after the training ended. The researchers found that participants in the MBSR and CBT groups had greater improvement in functional limitation and back pain at 26 and 52 weeks compared with those who had usual care. There were no significant differences in outcomes between MBSR and CBT.

For High Blood Pressure

- Results of a NCCIH-funded trial involving 298 university students suggest that practicing Transcendental Meditation may lower the blood pressure of people at increased risk of developing high blood pressure.

- The findings also suggested that practicing meditation can help with psychological distress, anxiety, depression, anger/hostility, and coping ability.

- A literature review and scientific statement from the American Heart Association suggest that evidence supports the use of Transcendental Meditation (TM) to lower blood pressure. However, the review indicates that it's uncertain whether TM is truly superior to other meditation techniques in terms of blood-pressure lowering because there are few head-to-head studies.

For Irritable Bowel Syndrome (IBS)

- The few studies that have looked at mindfulness meditation training for irritable bowel syndrome (IBS) found no clear effects, the American College of Gastroenterology stated in a 2014 report. But the authors noted that given the limited number of studies, they can't be sure that IBS doesn't help.

- Results of a NCCIH-funded trial that enrolled 75 women suggest that practicing mindfulness meditation for 8 weeks reduces the severity of IBS symptoms.

- A 2013 review concluded that mindfulness training improved IBS patients' pain and quality of life but not their depression or anxiety. The amount of improvement was small.

For Ulcerative Colitis

In a 2014 pilot study, 55 adults with ulcerative colitis in remission were divided into two groups. For 8 weeks, one group learned and practiced mindfulness-based stress reduction (MBSR) while the other group practiced a placebo procedure. Six and twelve months later, there were no significant differences between the two groups in the course of the disease, markers of inflammation, or any psychological measure except perceived stress during flare-ups. The researchers concluded that MBSR might help people in remission from moderate to moderately severe disease—and maybe reduce rates of flare-up from stress.

For Anxiety, Depression, and Insomnia

- 2014 literature review of 47 trials in 3,515 participants suggests that mindfulness meditation programs show moderate evidence of improving anxiety and depression. But the researchers found no evidence that meditation changed health-related behaviors affected by stress, such as substance abuse and sleep.

- A review of 36 trials found that 25 of them reported better outcomes for symptoms of anxiety in the meditation groups compared to control groups.

- In a small, NCCIH-funded study, 54 adults with chronic insomnia learned mindfulness-based stress reduction (MBSR), a form of MBSR specially adapted to deal with insomnia (mindfulness-based therapy for insomnia, or MBTI), or a self-monitoring program. Both meditation-based programs aided sleep, with MBTI providing a significantly greater reduction in insomnia severity compared with MBSR.

For Smoking Cessation

- The results of 13 studies of mindfulness-based interventions for stopping smoking had promising results regarding craving, smoking cessation, and relapse prevention, a 2015 research review found. However, the studies had many limitations.

- Findings from a 2013 review suggest that meditation-based therapies may help people quit smoking; however, the small number of available studies is insufficient to determine rigorously if meditation is effective for this.

- A trial comparing mindfulness training with a standard behavioral smoking cessation treatment found that individuals who received mindfulness training showed a greater rate of reduction in cigarette use immediately after treatment and at 17-week follow-up.

- Results of a 2013 brain imaging study suggest that mindful attention reduced the craving to smoke, and also that it reduced activity in a craving-related region of the brain.

- However, in a second 2013 brain imaging study, researchers observed that a 2-week course of meditation (5 hours total) significantly reduced smoking, compared with relaxation training, and that it increased activity in brain areas associated with craving.

Other Conditions

- Results from a NCCIH-funded study of 279 adults who participated in an 8-week Mindfulness-Based Stress Reduction (MBSR) program found that changes in spirituality were associated with better mental health and quality of life.

- Guidelines from the American College of Chest Physicians published in 2013 suggest that MBSR and meditation may help to reduce stress, anxiety, pain, and depression while enhancing mood and self-esteem in people with lung cancer.

- Clinical practice guidelines issued in 2014 by the Society for Integrative Oncology (SIC) recommend meditation as supportive care to reduce stress, anxiety, depression, and fatigue in patients treated for breast cancer. The SIC also recommends its use to improve quality of life in these people.

- Meditation-based programs may be helpful in reducing common menopausal symptoms, including the frequency and intensity of hot flashes, sleep and mood disturbances, stress, and muscle and joint pain. However, differences in study designs mean that no firm conclusions can be drawn.

- Because only a few studies have been conducted on the effects of meditation for attention deficit hyperactivity disorder (ADHD), there isn't sufficient evidence to support its use for this condition.

- A 2014 research review suggested that mind and body practices, including meditation, reduce chemical identifiers of inflammation and show promise in helping to regulate the immune system.

- Results from a 2013 NCCIH-supported study involving 49 adults suggest that 8 weeks of mindfulness training may reduce stress-induced inflammation better than a health program that includes physical activity, education about diet, and music therapy.

Section 52.3

St. John's Wort and Depression

This section includes text excerpted from "St. John's Wort and Depression: In Depth," National Center for Complementary and Integrative Health (NCCIH), September 2013. Reviewed November 2016.

About Depression

Depression is a medical condition that affects about 1 in 10 U.S. adults. Mood, thoughts, physical health, and behavior all may be affected. The symptoms and severity of depression can vary from person to person. Depression can be treated with conventional medicine, including antidepressants and certain types of psychotherapy.

About St. John's Wort

Although St. John's wort (*Hypericum perforatum*) has been used for centuries for mental health conditions and is widely prescribed for depression in Europe, the herb can have serious side effects. In addition, current evidence that St. John's wort is effective for depression is not conclusive. It is also important to note that in the United States, the U.S. Food and Drug Administration (FDA) has not approved its use as an over-the-counter or prescription medicine for depression.

Side Effects and Cautions

St. John's wort is known to affect how the body uses and breaks down a number of drugs and can cause serious side effects.

- Serotonin is a brain chemical targeted by antidepressants. Combining St. John's wort and certain antidepressants can lead to a potentially life-threatening increase in serotonin levels—a condition called serotonin syndrome. Symptoms range from tremor and diarrhea to very dangerous confusion, muscle stiffness, drop in body temperature, and even death.

- Psychosis is a rare but possible side effect of taking St. John's wort, particularly in people who have or are at risk for mental health disorders, including bipolar disorder.

- Taking St. John's wort can weaken many prescription medicines, such as:

  - Antidepressants

  - Birth control pills

  - Cyclosporine, which prevents the body from rejecting transplanted organs

  - Digoxin, a heart medication

  - Some HIV drugs including indinavir

  - Some cancer medications including irinotecan

  - Warfarin and similar medications used to thin the blood.

- Other side effects of St. John's wort are usually minor and uncommon and may include upset stomach and sensitivity to sunlight. Also, St. John's wort is a stimulant and may worsen feelings of anxiety in some people.

What the Science Says about St. John's Wort for Depression

Study results on the effectiveness of St. John's wort for depression are mixed.

- A 2009 systematic review of 29 international studies suggested that St. John's wort may be better than a placebo (an inactive substance that appears identical to the study substance) and as effective as standard prescription antidepressants for major depression of mild to moderate severity. St. John's wort also appeared to have fewer side effects than standard antidepressants. The studies—conducted in German-speaking countries where St. John's wort has a long history of use by medical professionals—reported more positive results than those done in other countries, including the United States.

- Two studies, both sponsored by National Center for Complementary and Integrative Health (NCCIH) and the National Institute of Mental Health (NIMH), did not have positive results. Neither St. John's wort nor a standard antidepressant medication decreased symptoms of minor depression better than a placebo in a 2011 study. The herb was no more effective than placebo in treating major depression of moderate severity in a large 2002 study.

- Preliminary studies suggest that St. John's wort may prevent nerve cells in the brain from reabsorbing certain chemical messengers, including dopamine and serotonin. Scientists have found that these naturally occurring chemicals are involved in regulating mood, but they are unsure exactly how they work.

If You Are Considering St. John's Wort for Depression

- Do not use St. John's wort to replace conventional care or to postpone seeing a healthcare provider about a medical problem. If not adequately treated, depression can become severe. Consult a healthcare provider if you or someone you know may be depressed.

- Keep in mind that dietary supplements can cause medical problems if not used correctly or if used in large amounts, and some may interact with medications you take. Your healthcare provider can advise you.

- Many dietary supplements have not been tested in pregnant women, nursing mothers, or children. Little safety information on St. John's wort for pregnant women or children is available, so it is especially important to talk with health experts if you are pregnant or nursing or are considering giving a dietary supplement to a child.

- Tell all your healthcare providers about any complementary health approaches you use. Give them a full picture of what you do to manage your health. This will help ensure coordinated and safe care.

Section 52.4

Valerian

This section includes text excerpted from "Valerian,"
National Center for Complementary and Integrative
Health (NCCIH), November 1, 2016.

- Valerian is a plant native to Europe and Asia; it also grows in North America.

- Valerian has been used medicinally since the times of early Greece and Rome; Hippocrates wrote about its uses. Historically, valerian was used to treat nervousness, trembling, headaches, and heart palpitations.

- Today, valerian is used as a dietary supplement for insomnia, anxiety, and other conditions such as depression and menopause symptoms.

- The roots and rhizomes (underground stems) of valerian are used to make capsules, tablets, and liquid extracts, as well as teas.

How Much Do We Know?

- Knowledge about valerian is limited because there have been only a small number of high-quality studies in people.

What Have We Learned?

- The evidence on whether valerian is helpful for sleep problems is inconsistent.

- There's not enough evidence to allow any conclusions about whether valerian can relieve anxiety, depression, or menopausal symptoms.

What Do We Know about Safety?

- Studies suggest that valerian is generally safe for use by most healthy adults for short periods of time.

- No information is available about the long-term safety of valerian or its safety in children younger than age 3, pregnant women, or nursing mothers.

- Few side effects have been reported in studies of valerian. Those that have occurred include headache, dizziness, itching, and digestive disturbances.

- Because it is possible (though not proven) that valerian might have a sleep-inducing effect, it should not be taken along with alcohol or sedatives.

Keep in Mind

- Tell all your healthcare providers about any complementary or integrative health approaches you use. Give them a full picture of what you do to manage your health. This will help ensure coordinated and safe care.

Chapter 53

Treating Depression in Children and Adolescents

Chapter Contents

Section 53.1

Don't Leave Childhood Depression Untreated

This section includes text excerpted from "Don't Leave Childhood Depression Untreated," U.S. Food and Drug Administration (FDA), September 10, 2014.

Depression in Children

Every psychological disorder, including depression, has some behavioral components. Depressed children often lack energy and enthusiasm. They become withdrawn, irritable and sulky. They may feel sad, anxious and restless. They may have problems in school, and frequently lose interest in activities they once enjoyed.

Some parents might think that medication is the solution for depression-related problem behaviors. In fact, that's not the case. The U.S. Food and Drug Administration (FDA) hasn't approved any drugs solely for the treatment of "behavior problems." When FDA approves a drug for depression—whether for adults or children—it's to treat the illness, not the behavior associated with it.

"There are multiple parts to mental illness, and the symptoms are usually what drug companies study and what parents worry about. But it's rare for us at FDA to target just one part of the illness," says Mitchell Mathis, M.D., a psychiatrist who is the Director of FDA's Division of Psychiatry Products.

Depression Is Treatable

The first step to treating depression is to get a professional diagnosis; most children who are moody, grouchy or feel that they are misunderstood are not depressed and don't need any drugs.

Only about 11 percent of adolescents have a depressive disorder by age 18, according to the National Institute of Mental Health (NIMH). Before puberty, girls and boys have the same incidence of depression. After adolescence, girls are twice as likely to have depression as boys. The trend continues until after menopause. "That's a clue that depression might be hormonal, but so far, scientists haven't found out exactly how hormones affect the brain," says child and adolescent psychiatrist Tiffany R. Farchione, M.D., the Acting Deputy Director of FDA's Division of Psychiatry Products.

It's hard to tell if a child is depressed or going through a difficult time because the signs and symptoms of depression change as children grow and their brains develop. Also, it can take time to get a correct diagnosis because doctors might be getting just a snapshot of what's going on with the young patient.

"In psychiatry, it's easier to take care of adults because you have a lifetime of patient experience to draw from, and patterns are more obvious" says Mathis. "With kids, you don't have that information. Because we don't like to label kids with lifelong disorders, we first look for any other reason for those symptoms. And if we diagnose depression, we assess the severity before treating the patient with medications."

Getting the Proper Care

The second step is to decide on a treatment course, which depends on the severity of the illness and its impact on the child's life. Treatments for depression often include psychotherapy and medication. FDA has approved two drugs—fluoxetine (Prozac) and escitalopram (Lexapro)—to treat depression in children. Prozac is approved for ages 8 and older; Lexapro for kids 12 and older.

"We need more pediatric studies because many antidepressants approved for adults have not been proven to work in kids," Farchione says. "When we find a treatment that has been shown to work in kids, we're encouraged because that drug can have a big impact on a child who doesn't have many medication treatment options."

FDA requires that all antidepressants include a boxed warning about the increased risks of suicidal thinking and behavior in children, adolescents and young adults up to age 24. "All of these medicines work in the brain and the central nervous system, so there are risks. Patients and their doctors have to weigh those risks against the benefits," Mathis says.

Depression can lead to suicide. Children who take antidepressants might have more suicidal thoughts, which is why the labeling includes a boxed warning on all antidepressants. But the boxed warning does not say not to treat children, just to be aware of, and to monitor them for, signs of suicidality.

"A lot of kids respond very well to drugs. Oftentimes, young people can stop taking the medication after a period of stability, because some of these illnesses are not a chronic disorder like a major depression," Mathis adds. "There are many things that help young psychiatric patients get better, and drugs are just one of them."

It's important that patients and their doctors work together to taper off the medications. Abruptly stopping a treatment without gradually reducing the dose might lead to problems, such as mood disturbance, agitation and irritability.

Depression in children shouldn't be left untreated. Untreated acute depression may get better on its own, but it relapses and the patient is not cured. Real improvement can take six months or more, and may not be complete without treatment. And the earlier the treatment starts, the better the outcome.

"Kids just don't have time to leave their depression untreated," Farchione says. "The social and educational consequences of a lengthy recovery are huge. They could fail a grade. They could lose all of their friends."

Medications help patients recover sooner and more completely.

Section 53.2

Taking Your Child to a Therapist

Text in this section is excerpted from "Taking Your Child to a Therapist," © 1995–2016. The Nemours Foundation/KidsHealth®. Reprinted with permission.

Sometimes kids, like adults, can benefit from therapy. Therapy can help kids develop problem-solving skills and also teach them the value of seeking help. Therapists can help kids and families cope with stress and a variety of emotional and behavioral issues.

Many kids need help dealing with school stress, such as homework, test anxiety, bullying, or peer pressure. Others need help to discuss their feelings about family issues, particularly if there's a major transition, such as a divorce, move, or serious illness.

Should My Child See a Therapist?

Significant life events—such as the death of a family member, friend, or pet; divorce or a move; abuse; trauma; a parent leaving on military deployment; or a major illness in the family—can cause stress that might lead to problems with behavior, mood, sleep, appetite, and academic or social functioning.

In some cases, it's not as clear what's caused a child to suddenly seem withdrawn, worried, stressed, sulky, or tearful. But if you feel your child might have an emotional or behavioral problem or needs help coping with a difficult life event, trust your instincts.

Signs that a child may benefit from seeing a psychologist or licensed therapist include:

- developmental delay in speech, language, or toilet training
- learning or attention problems (such as Attention-deficit hyperactivity disorder (ADHD))
- behavioral problems (such as excessive anger, acting out, bedwetting or eating disorders)
- a significant drop in grades, particularly if your child normally maintains high grades
- episodes of sadness, tearfulness, or depression
- social withdrawal or isolation
- being the victim of bullying or bullying other children
- decreased interest in previously enjoyed activities
- overly aggressive behavior (such as biting, kicking, or hitting)
- sudden changes in appetite (particularly in adolescents)
- insomnia or increased sleepiness
- excessive school absenteeism or tardiness
- mood swings (e.g., happy one minute, upset the next)
- development of or an increase in physical complaints (such as headache, stomachache, or not feeling well) despite a normal physical exam by your doctor
- management of a serious, acute, or chronic illness
- signs of alcohol, drug, or other substance use (such as solvents or prescription drug abuse)
- problems in transitions (following separation, divorce, or relocation)
- bereavement issues

- custody evaluations
- therapy following sexual, physical, or emotional abuse or other traumatic events

Kids who aren't yet school-age could benefit from seeing a developmental or clinical psychologist if there's a significant delay in achieving developmental milestones such as walking, talking, and potty training, and if there are concerns regarding autism or other developmental disorders.

Talk to Caregivers, Teachers, and the Doctor

It's also helpful to speak to caregivers and teachers who interact regularly with your child. Is your child paying attention in class and turning in assignments on time? What's his or her behavior like at recess and with peers? Gather as much information as possible to determine the best course of action.

Discuss your concerns with your child's doctor, who can offer perspective and evaluate your child to rule out any medical conditions that could be having an effect. The doctor also may be able to refer you to a qualified therapist for the help your child needs.

Finding the Right Therapist

How do you find a qualified clinician who has experience working with kids and teens? While experience and education are important, it's also important to find a counselor your child feels comfortable talking to. Look for one who not only has the right experience, but also the best approach to help your child in the current circumstances.

Your doctor can be a good source of a referral. Most doctors have working relationships with mental health specialists such as child psychologists or clinical social workers. Friends, colleagues, or family members might also be able to recommend someone.

Consider a number of factors when searching for the right therapist for your child. A good first step is to ask if the therapist is willing to meet with you for a brief consultation or to talk with you during a phone interview before you commit to regular visits. Not all therapists are able to do this, given their busy schedules. Most therapists charge a fee for this type of service; others consider it a free visit.

Factors to Consider

Consider the following factors when evaluating a potential therapist:

- Is the therapist licensed to practice in your state? (You can check with the state board for that profession or check to see if the license is displayed in the office.)

- Is the therapist covered by your health insurance plan's mental health benefits? If so, how many sessions are covered by your plan? What will your co-pay be?

- What are his or her credentials?

- What type of experience does the therapist have?

- How long has the therapist worked with children and adolescents?

- Would your child find the therapist friendly?

- What is the cancellation policy if you're unable to keep an appointment?

- Is the therapist available by phone during an emergency?

- Who will be available to your child during the therapist's vacation or illness or during off-hours?

- What types of therapy does the therapist specialize in?

- Is the therapist willing to meet with you in addition to working with your child?

The right therapist–client match is critical, so you might need to meet with a few before you find one who clicks with both you and your child.

As with other medical professionals, therapists may have a variety of credentials and specific degrees. As a general rule, your child's therapist should hold a professional degree in the field of mental health (psychology, social work, or psychiatry) and be licensed by your state. Psychologists, social workers, and psychiatrists all diagnose and treat mental health disorders.

It's also a good idea to know what those letters that follow a therapist's name mean:

Psychiatrists: Psychiatrists (MDs or DOs) are medical doctors who have advanced training and experience in psychotherapy and pharmacology. They can also prescribe medications.

Clinical Psychologists: Clinical psychologists (PhDs, PsyDs, or EdDs) are therapists who have a doctorate degree that includes advanced training in the practice of psychology, and many specialize in treating children and teens and their families. Psychologists may help clients manage medications but do not prescribe medication.

Clinical Social Workers: A licensed clinical social worker (LCSW) has a master's degree, specializes in clinical social work, and is licensed in the state in which he or she practices. An LICSW is also a licensed clinical social worker. A CSW is a certified social worker. Many social workers are trained in psychotherapy, but the credentials vary from state to state. Likewise, the designations (i.e., LCSW, LICSW, CSW) can vary from state to state.

Different Types of Therapy

There are many types of therapy. Therapists choose the strategies that are most appropriate for a particular problem and for the individual child and family. Therapists will often spend a portion of each session with the parents alone, with the child alone, and with the family together.

Any one therapist may use a variety of strategies, including:

Cognitive Behavioral Therapy (CBT). This type of therapy is often helpful with kids and teens who are depressed, anxious, or having problems coping with stress. Cognitive behavioral therapy restructures negative thoughts into more positive, effective ways of thinking. It can include work on stress management strategies, relaxation training, practicing coping skills, and other forms of treatment.

Psychoanalytic therapy is less commonly used with children but can be used with older kids and teens who may benefit from more in-depth analysis of their problems. This is the quintessential "talk therapy" and does not focus on short-term problem-solving in the same way as CBT and behavioral therapies.

In some cases, kids benefit from **individual therapy,** one-on-one work with the therapist on issues they need guidance on, such as depression, social difficulties, or worry. In other cases, the right option is group therapy, where kids meet in groups of 6 to 12 to solve problems and learn new skills (such as social skills or anger management).

Family therapy can be helpful in many cases, such as when family members aren't getting along; disagree or argue often; or when a child or teen is having behavior problems. Family therapy involves counseling sessions with some, or all, family members, helping to improve communication skills among them. Treatment focuses on problem-solving techniques and can help parents re-establish their role as authority figures.

Preparing for the First Visit

You may be concerned that your child will become upset when told of an upcoming visit with a therapist. Although this is sometimes the case, it's essential to be honest about the session and why your child (or family) will be going. The issue will come up during the session, but it's important for you to prepare your child for it.

Explain to young kids that this type of visit to the doctor doesn't involve a physical exam or shots. You may also want to stress that this type of doctor talks and plays with kids and families to help them solve problems and feel better. Kids might feel reassured to learn that the therapist will be helping the parents and other family members too.

Older kids and teens may be reassured to hear that anything they say to the therapist is confidential and cannot be shared with anyone else, including parents or other doctors, without their permission—the exception is if they indicate that they're having thoughts of suicide or otherwise hurting themselves or others.

Giving kids this kind of information before the first appointment can help set the tone, prevent your child from feeling singled out or isolated, and provide reassurance that the family will be working together on the problem.

Providing Additional Support

While your child copes with emotional issues, be there to listen and care, and offer support without judgment. Patience is critical, too, as many young children are unable to verbalize their fears and emotions.

Try to set aside some time to discuss your child's worries or concerns. To minimize distractions, turn off the TV and let voice mail answer your phone calls. This will let your child know that he or she is your first priority.

Other ways to communicate openly and problem-solve include:

- Talk openly and as frequently with your child as you can.

- Show love and affection to your child, especially during troubled times.

- Set a good example by taking care of your own physical and emotional needs.

- Enlist the support of your partner, immediate family members, your child's doctor, and teachers.

- Improve communication at home by having family meetings that end with a fun activity (e.g., playing a game, making ice-cream sundaes).

- No matter how hard it is, set limits on inappropriate or problematic behaviors. Ask the therapist for some strategies to encourage your child's cooperation.

- Communicate frequently with the therapist.

- Be open to all types of feedback from your child and from the therapist.

- Respect the relationship between your child and the therapist. If you feel threatened by it, discuss this with the therapist (it's nothing to be embarrassed about).

- Enjoy favorite activities or hobbies with your child.

By recognizing problems and seeking help early on, you can help your child—and your entire family—move through the tough times toward happier, healthier times ahead.

Section 53.3

Therapy for Teens

This section includes text excerpted from "Going to Therapy,"
Office on Women's Health (OWH), U.S. Department of
Health and Human Services (HHS), January 7, 2015.

Lots of teens have some kind of emotional problem. In fact, almost half of U.S. teens will have a mental health problem before they turn 18. The good news is that therapy can really help.

Sometimes, people are embarrassed or afraid to see a therapist. But getting help from a therapist because you're feeling sad or anxious is really not different from seeing a doctor because you broke a bone. In fact, you can feel proud for being brave enough to do what you need to do to get your life back on track.

Here are the answers to some common questions about therapy.

What Is Therapy?

Therapy is when you talk about your problems with someone who is a professional counselor, such as a psychiatrist, psychologist, or social worker. Therapy sometimes is called psychotherapy. That is because it helps with your psychology—the mental and emotional parts of your life.

If you are going through a rough time, talking to a caring therapist can be a great relief. A therapist can help you cope with sadness, worry, and other strong or scary feelings. Here are some other ways therapy can help:

- It can teach you specific skills for handling difficult situations, such as problems with your family or school.

- It can help you find healthy ways to deal with stress or anger.

- It can teach you how to build healthy relationships.

- It can help you figure out how to think about things in more positive ways.

- It can help you figure out how to boost your self-confidence.

- It can help you decide where you want to go in life and how to deal with any obstacles that may come up along the way.

Therapy may feel great right away, or it might feel strange at first. It can take a little time getting used to talking with someone new about your problems. But therapists are trained to listen well, and they want to help.

As time goes on, you should feel comfortable with your therapist. If you don't feel comfortable, or if you think you're not getting better, tell your parent or guardian. Another therapist or type of therapy might work better.

Therapists protect people's privacy. They can share what you say only in very special cases, such as if they think you are in danger. If you're concerned, though, ask about the privacy policy. It's important to feel like you can tell the truth in therapy. It works best if you are honest about any problems you're facing, including problems with drugs or alcohol or any behaviors that can hurt your body or mind.

Just because you start to see a therapist doesn't mean that you will see one forever. You should be able to learn skills that let you handle your problems on your own. Sometimes, a few sessions are all you need to learn skills and feel better.

Why Do Teens Go for Therapy?

Many young people develop mental health conditions, like depression, eating disorders, or anxiety disorders. If you have a mental health problem, remember there are treatments that work, and you can feel better. Also, some teens go to therapy to get help through a tough time, like their parents' getting divorced or having too much stress at school.

If you feel out of control, or you feel like a mental health problem keeps you from enjoying life, get help. Reach out to a parent or guardian or another trusted adult.

What Should I Do to Get Started with Therapy?

If you need help finding a therapist, you can start by talking to your doctor, school nurse, or school counselor. If your family has insurance, the insurance company can tell you which therapists are covered under your plan. You and your parent or guardian also can look online for mental health treatment.

If you need help paying for therapy, you can ask a parent or guardian if they have health insurance that might help pay for therapy. If your family doesn't have insurance, they can find out about getting it through healthcare.gov. You also may be able to get free or low-cost therapy at a mental health clinic, hospital, university, or other places.

What Are Some Kinds of Therapy?

There are different kinds of therapy to help you feel better. The best treatment depends on the type of problem that you are facing.

You may have one-on-one talk therapy. This is when you talk to a therapist alone. Or you may join group therapy, where you work with a therapist and other people who are having similar issues. You may also do art therapy, where you paint or draw.

One kind of talk therapy that tends to work well for depression, anxiety, and several other problems is cognitive behavioral therapy. This type of therapy teaches you how to think and act in healthier ways.

Sometimes, your therapist will suggest that you take medicine in addition to therapy, which often can be a helpful combination.

What about Online Support Groups?

There are lots of support groups available on the Internet, including ones to help you handle your feelings. Chat rooms and other online options may help you feel less alone. But if you are having trouble coping, it's important to work with a therapist or other mental health professional.

Remember to be careful about getting info online. Some people use the Internet to promote unhealthy behaviors, like cutting and dangerous eating habits.

Section 53.4

Antidepressant Medications for Children and Adolescents

This section includes text excerpted from "Child and Adolescent Mental Health," National Institute of Mental Health (NIMH), May 3, 2016.

Antidepressants for Children and Adolescents

Depression is a serious disorder that can cause significant problems in mood, thinking, and behavior at home, in school, and with peers. It is estimated that major depressive disorder (MDD) affects about 5 percent of adolescents.

Research has shown that, as in adults, depression in children and adolescents is treatable. Certain antidepressant medications, called selective serotonin reuptake inhibitors (SSRIs), can be beneficial to children and adolescents with MDD. Certain types of psychological therapies also have been shown to be effective. However, our knowledge of antidepressant treatments in youth, though growing substantially, is limited compared to what we know about treating depression in adults.

Recently, there has been some concern that the use of antidepressant medications themselves may induce suicidal behavior in youths. Following a thorough and comprehensive review of all the available published and unpublished controlled clinical trials of antidepressants in children and adolescents, the U.S. Food and Drug Administration (FDA) issued a public warning in October 2004 about an increased risk of suicidal thoughts or behavior (suicidality) in children and adolescents treated with SSRI antidepressant medications. In 2006, an advisory committee to the FDA recommended that the agency extend the warning to include young adults up to age 25.

A comprehensive review of pediatric trials suggested that the benefits of antidepressant medications likely outweigh their risks to children and adolescents with major depression and anxiety disorders. The study, partially funded by National Institute of Mental Health (NIMH), was published in the April 18, 2007, issue of the Journal of the American Medical Association.

What Did the FDA Review Find?

In the FDA review, no completed suicides occurred among nearly 2,200 children treated with SSRI medications. However, about 4 percent of those taking SSRI medications experienced suicidal thinking or behavior, including actual suicide attempts—twice the rate of those taking placebo, or sugar pills.

In response, the FDA adopted a "black box" label warning indicating that antidepressants may increase the risk of suicidal thinking and behavior in some children and adolescents with MDD. A black-box warning is the most serious type of warning in prescription drug labeling.

The warning also notes that children and adolescents taking SSRI medications should be closely monitored for any worsening in depression, emergence of suicidal thinking or behavior, or unusual changes in behavior, such as sleeplessness, agitation, or withdrawal from normal social situations. Close monitoring is especially important during the first four weeks of treatment. SSRI medications usually have few side effects in children and adolescents, but for unknown reasons, they may trigger agitation and abnormal behavior in certain individuals.

What Do We Know about Antidepressant Medications?

The SSRIs include:

- fluoxetine (Prozac)

- sertraline (Zoloft)

- paroxetine (Paxil)

- citalopram (Celexa)

- escitalopram (Lexapro)

- fluvoxamine (Luvox)

Another antidepressant medication, venlafaxine (Effexor), is not an SSRI but is closely related.

SSRI medications are considered an improvement over older antidepressant medications because they have fewer side effects and are less likely to be harmful if taken in an overdose, which is an issue for patients with depression already at risk for suicide. They have been shown to be safe and effective for adults.

However, use of SSRI medications among children and adolescents ages 10 to 19 has risen dramatically in the past several years. Fluoxetine (Prozac) is the only medication approved by the FDA for use in treating depression in children ages 8 and older. The other SSRI medications and the SSRI-related antidepressant venlafaxine have not been approved for treatment of depression in children or adolescents, but doctors still sometimes prescribe them to children on an "off-label" basis. In June 2003, however, the FDA recommended that paroxetine not be used in children and adolescents for treating MDD.

Fluoxetine can be helpful in treating childhood depression, and can lead to significant improvement of depression overall. However, it may increase the risk for suicidal behaviors in a small subset of adolescents. As with all medical decisions, doctors and families should weigh the risks and benefits of treatment for each individual patient.

What Should You Do for a Child with Depression?

A child or adolescent with MDD should be carefully and thoroughly evaluated by a doctor to determine if medication is appropriate. Psychotherapy often is tried as an initial treatment for mild depression. Psychotherapy may help to determine the severity and persistence of the depression and whether antidepressant medications may be warranted. Types of psychotherapies include "cognitive behavioral therapy," which helps people learn new ways of thinking and behaving, and "interpersonal therapy," which helps people understand and work through troubled personal relationships.

Those who are prescribed an SSRI medication should receive ongoing medical monitoring. Children already taking an SSRI medication should remain on the medication if it has been helpful, but should be carefully monitored by a doctor for side effects. Parents should promptly seek medical advice and evaluation if their child or adolescent experiences suicidal thinking or behavior, nervousness, agitation, irritability, mood instability, or sleeplessness that either emerges or worsens during treatment with SSRI medications.

Once started, treatment with these medications should not be abruptly stopped. Although they are not habit-forming or addictive, abruptly ending an antidepressant can cause withdrawal symptoms or lead to a relapse. Families should not discontinue treatment without consulting their doctor.

All treatments can be associated with side effects. Families and doctors should carefully weigh the risks and benefits, and maintain appropriate follow-up and monitoring to help control for the risks.

What Does Research Tell Us?

An individual's response to a medication cannot be predicted with certainty. It is extremely difficult to determine whether SSRI medications increase the risk for completed suicide, especially because depression itself increases the risk for suicide and because completed suicides, especially among children and adolescents, are rare. Most controlled trials are too small to detect for rare events such as suicide (thousands of participants are needed). In addition, controlled trials typically exclude patients considered at high risk for suicide.

One major clinical trial, the NIMH-funded Treatment for Adolescents with Depression Study (TADS), has indicated that a combination of medication and psychotherapy is the most effective treatment for adolescents with depression. The clinical trial of 439 adolescents ages 12 to 17 with MDD compared four treatment groups—one that received a combination of fluoxetine and CBT, one that received fluoxetine only, one that received CBT only, and one that received a placebo only. After the first 12 weeks, 71 percent responded to the combination treatment of fluoxetine and CBT, 61 percent responded to the fluoxetine only treatment, 43 percent responded to the CBT only treatment, and 35 percent responded to the placebo treatment.

At the beginning of the study, 29 percent of the TADS participants were having clinically significant suicidal thoughts. Although the rate of suicidal thinking decreased among all the treatment groups, those in the fluoxetine/CBT combination treatment group showed the greatest reduction in suicidal thinking.

Researchers are working to better understand the relationship between antidepressant medications and suicide. So far, results are mixed. One study, using national Medicaid files, found that among adults, the use of antidepressants does not seem to be related to suicide attempts or deaths. However, the analysis found that the use of antidepressant medications may be related to suicide attempts and deaths among children and adolescents.

Another study analyzed health plan records for 65,103 patients treated for depression. It found no significant increase among adults and young people in the risk for suicide after starting treatment with newer antidepressant medications.

A third study analyzed suicide data from the National Vital Statistics and commercial prescription data. It found that among children ages five to 14, suicide rates from 1996 to 1998 were actually lower in areas of the country with higher rates of SSRI antidepressant prescriptions. The relationship between the suicide rates and the SSRI use rates, however, is unclear.

Chapter 54

Treatment-Resistant and Relapsed Depression

Chapter Contents

Section 54.1

Treatment-Resistant Depression: An Overview

This section includes text excerpted from "Nonpharmacologic Interventions for Treatment-Resistant Depression in Adults," Agency for Healthcare Research and Quality (AHRQ), U.S. Department of Health and Human Services (HHS), November 10, 2011. Reviewed November 2016.

Major depressive disorder (MDD) is common and costly. Over the course of a year, between 13.1 million and 14.2 million people will experience MDD. Approximately half of these people seek help for this condition, and only 20 percent of those receive adequate treatment. For those who do initiate treatment for their depression, approximately 50 percent will not adequately respond following acute-phase treatment; this refractory group has considerable clinical and research interest. Patients with only one prior treatment failure are sometimes included in this group, but patients with two or more prior treatment failures are a particularly important and poorly understood group and are considered to have treatment-resistant depression (TRD). These TRD patients represent a complex population with a disease that is difficult to manage.

Economic Burden of TRD

Patients with TRD incur the highest direct and indirect medical costs among those with MDD. These costs increase with the severity of TRD. Treatment-resistant patients are twice as likely to be hospitalized, and their cost of hospitalization is more than six times the mean total costs of depressed patients who are not treatment resistant. After considering both medical and disability claims from an employer's perspective, one study found that TRD employees cost $14,490 per employee per year, whereas the cost for non-TRD employees was $6,665 per employee per year. Given the burden of TRD generally, the uncertain prognosis of the disorder, and the high costs of therapy, clinicians and patients alike need clear evidence to guide their treatment decisions.

Criteria for TRD

Although TRD broadly is defined as inadequate response following adequate antidepressant therapy in MDD, treatment resistance is a complex phenomenon that is influenced by heterogeneity in depressive subtypes, psychiatric comorbidity, and comorbid medical illnesses. Major depression is usually considered treatment resistant when at least two antidepressant attempts have failed. However, criteria for treatment resistance have been variably defined in clinical research and practice. Important factors related to the definition of TRD include the number of failed treatments, the time between treatment attempts, and the adequacy of the dose and duration of antidepressant treatment. The term "pseudo-resistance" has been used to describe patients classified treatment-resistant even though they never actually received an adequate treatment course; pseudo-resistance may account for as many as 60 percent of patients initially classified as TRD.

Interventions for TRD

The choices are wide ranging, include both pharmacologic and non-pharmacologic interventions, and are fraught with incomplete, potentially conflicting evidence. Somatic treatments, which may involve use of a pharmacologic intervention or a device, are commonly considered for patients with TRD. Antidepressant medications, which are the most commonly used intervention, have decreasing efficacy for producing remission after patients have experienced two treatment failures. Such drugs also often have side effects, sometimes minor but sometimes quite serious. For these reasons, clinicians often look for alternative strategies for their TRD patients.

Nonpharmacologic Interventions for TRD

Nonpharmacologic somatic treatments and nonsomatic psychotherapy treatments offer alternatives to antidepressant medications, although the evidence base for many of these treatments is limited. Interventions that offer promising options for patients with TRD include ECT, rTMS, VNS, and evidence-based psychotherapy (e.g., cognitive therapy, such as cognitive behavioral therapy [CBT or IPT]). In some cases, these therapies or procedures can be used in combination (e.g., ECT and rTMS). They are described in more detail below. Generally, although these interventions may be safe and effective options for TRD, little evidence exists to guide decisions about their comparative efficacy. Further, how the nonpharmacologic options compare with pharmacologic treatments remains unclear.

Electroconvulsive Therapy (ECT)

ECT has been available for use in the United States since the 1930s. Current evidence indicates that ECT has a role in the treatment of people with depression and in certain subgroups of people with schizophrenia, catatonia, and mania. Its primary current role in depression is for treatment resistance or intolerance. ECT involves passing an electric current through the brain to produce a convulsion. Electrodes are usually placed at the bifrontal, bilateral, or right unilateral position. It is not commonly used as a first-line therapy or in primary care practice. The exceptions are uses in an emergency in which the person's life is at risk because of refusing to eat or drink or being in a catatonic state or in cases of attempted suicide. The effectiveness of ECT may be related to the stimulus parameters used, including position of electrodes, dosage, and waveform of electricity.

ECT shows greater improvement in patients with suicidal intent than other antidepressant treatments; thus, it may be used as an early therapeutic option in suicidal patients.Research also indicates that despite physical illness, coexisting diseases, or cognitive impairment, older patients tolerate ECT as well as younger patients and may demonstrate better response. Because ECT is a procedure that involves anesthesia, it also poses slight risks to patients from the procedure itself. Other potential risks include seizure and adverse cognitive effects.

Repetitive Transcranial Magnetic Stimulation (rTMS)

rTMS involves magnetic focal stimulation through the scalp. The current elicited by the electromagnetic coil stimulates nerve cells in the region of the brain involved in mood regulation and depression. It can be administered in an office setting without the use of anesthesia. Patients may perceive it as less threatening than ECT. Patients having conductive, ferromagnetic, or other magnetic-sensitive metals in the head or within 30cm of the treatment coil should not undergo this procedure. Sessions are usually 40 minutes in length, administered daily (usually only weekdays) for 2 to 6 weeks.

rTMS is usually considered a reasonable option for acute treatment of TRD as opposed to VNS and pharmacotherapy, which are predominantly used as long-term treatments for TRD. The FDA states that rTMS is "indicated for the treatment of Major Depressive Disorder in adult patients who have failed to achieve satisfactory improvement from one prior antidepressant medication at or above the minimal effective dose and duration in the current episode.Possible side effects with rTMS include mild headaches, syncope, and transient hearing changes. Although rTMS does pose a risk of seizure, it reportedly does not have the cognitive risks of ECT.

Vagus Nerve Stimulation (VNS)

VNS involves surgically placed electrodes around the left vagus nerve. The VNS device consists of a round battery-powered generator that is implanted into the chest wall and attached to wires threaded along the vagus nerve. The therapy includes minor surgery, lasting approximately 30 to 60 minutes. Once implanted, the generator pulses the nerve for 30 seconds once every 5 minutes. The total duration of this intervention is generally 10 weeks, although the stimulation can be extended for longer intervals. VNS was first used in patients with epilepsy; it was also found simultaneously to improve mood. The FDA approved VNS for TRD in July 2005, with labeled indication for "adjunctive long-term treatment of chronic or recurrent depression for patients 18 years of age or older who are experiencing a major depressive episode and have not had an adequate response to four or more adequate antidepressant treatments.

The place in therapy for VNS may be for patients who have four or more adequate antidepressant treatment failures. Considerations also include a longer onset of antidepressant action than other treatments, as VNS benefits for TRD may not be fully realized for 6 to 12 months. Further, VNS poses surgical risks and is associated with several side effects such as voice alteration, cough, neck pain, paresthesia, and dyspnea.

Cognitive Behavioral Therapy (CBT) or Interpersonal Psychotherapy (IPT)

Use of CBT began in the 1960s. It is a type of psychotherapy that aims to modify distorted, maladaptive, and depressogenic cognitions and related behavioral dysfunction. The therapist first introduces the patient to the cognitive model. Agendas, feedback, and psychoeducational procedures are used to structure sessions. To treat depressed patients with CBT, therapists emphasize negatively distorted thinking and deficits in learning and memory functioning.

413

Developed in the 1970s, IPT helps patients explore social and interpersonal issues that relate to depressive symptoms. Depressive symptoms identified are related to one of the four key problem areas: grief, disputes, transitions, and deficits. After selecting a focus area, later sessions help the patient develop strategies to deal with the problem. Both CBT and IPT have been studied extensively for depression, eating disorders, anxiety, and personality disorders, but understanding of their role in the treatment of TRD is more limited. Both therapies involve weekly sessions with the therapist, which last for 30 to 60 minutes. CBT may be carried out in a group setting if deemed beneficial for the patient. The therapy generally lasts from 3 to 4 months for acute phase treatment, although treatment duration may be for longer periods.

CBT and IPT do not have any risks or side effects associated with them. Patients need to have normal cognitive functioning to comprehend the therapist's questions. CBT and IPT are comparable psychotherapies for major depression and appear to be as effective as antidepressant medication treatment, although CBT may be more effective in patients with severe depression.

Section 54.2

Teens Who Recover from Hard-to-Treat Depression Still at Risk for Relapse

This section includes text excerpted from "Teens Who Recover from Hard-to-treat Depression Still at Risk for Relapse," National Institute of Mental Health (NIMH), December 3, 2010. Reviewed November 2016.

Teens with hard-to-treat depression who reach remission after 24 weeks of treatment are still at a significant risk for relapse, according to long-term, follow-up data from an National Institute of Mental Health (NIMH)-funded study published online ahead of print November 16, 2010, in the *Journal of Clinical Psychiatry*. The long-term data reiterate the need for aggressive treatment decisions for teens with stubborn depression.

A Study on Resistant Depression in Adolescents

In the Treatment of Resistant Depression in Adolescents (TOR-DIA) study, teens whose depression had not improved after an initial course of selective serotonin reuptake inhibitor (SSRI) antidepressant treatment were randomly assigned to one of four interventions for 12 weeks:

- Switch to another SSRI-paroxetine (Paxil), citalopram (Celexa) or fluoxetine (Prozac)

- Switch to a different SSRI plus cognitive behavioral therapy (CBT), a type of psychotherapy that emphasizes problem-solving and behavior change

- Switch to venlafaxine (Effexor), a different type of antidepressant called a serotonin and norepinephrine reuptake inhibitor (SNRI)

- Switch to venlafaxine plus CBT

As reported in May 2010, nearly 40 percent of those who completed 24 weeks of treatment achieved remission, regardless of the treatment to which they had initially been assigned. However, those who achieved remission were more likely to have responded to treatment early—during the first 12 weeks.

After 24 weeks of treatment, the participants were discharged from the study and urged to continue care within their community. They were then asked to return for an assessment at 72 weeks.

Results of the Study

Of the 334 original TORDIA participants, about 61 percent had reached remission by week 72. Symptoms of depression steadily decreased after the initial 24 weeks of treatment. But at 72 weeks, many participants still reported having residual symptoms of depression, such as irritability, fatigue and low self-esteem.

Those with more severe depression at baseline were less likely to reach remission. Those who responded early to treatment—within the first six weeks of treatment—were more likely to reach remission. Initial treatment assignment during the study did not appear to influence the remission rate or time to remission.

However, of the 130 participants who had remitted by week 24, 25 percent had relapsed by week 72. Ethnic minorities tended to have a higher risk for relapse than whites.

Significance

Because more than one-third of the teens did not recover and the relapse rate was high, the authors conclude that more effective interventions early in the treatment process are needed. In addition, the higher risk of relapse for ethnic minorities suggests that cultural factors may influence the long-term course of depression and recovery, but it is unclear what those factors may be.

What's Next

The findings indicate that new methods are needed to accurately identify those who may not respond early in treatment so that patients unlikely to reach remission using a particular treatment may be offered alternative treatments earlier in the process. More data is needed, however, to be able to predict who might be more likely to remit and who may not.

Section 54.3

Rapidly-Acting Treatments for Treatment-Resistant Depression (RAPID)

This section includes text excerpted from "Rapidly-Acting Treatments for Treatment-Resistant Depression (RAPID)," National Institute of Mental Health (NIMH), November 19, 2012. Reviewed November 2016.

Rapidly-Acting Treatments for Treatment-Resistant Depression (RAPID) is an National Institute of Mental Health (NIMH)-funded research project that promotes development of speedier therapies for severe, treatment-resistant depression. The initiative is supporting a team of researchers, led by Maurizio Fava, M.D., of Massachusetts General Hospital, who are identifying and testing promising pharmacological and/or non-pharmacological treatments that lift depression within a few days.

By contrast, current antidepressant medications usually take a few weeks to work—and half of patients fail to fully respond. While a proven brain stimulation technique, electroconvulsive therapy (ECT), works faster, it runs a risk of cognitive side-effects and requires anesthesia and a surgical setting. The urgent need for improved, faster acting antidepressant treatments is underscored by the fact that severe depression can be life-threatening, due to heightened risk of suicide.

Recent studies have shown that ketamine, a drug known previously as an anesthetic, can lift depression in many patients within hours. Researchers are making significant progress in pinpointing its mechanism of action and in identifying biomarkers that predict response.

It's unlikely that ketamine itself will become a practical treatment for most cases of depression. It must be administered through infusion, requiring a hospital setting, and can potentially trigger adverse side effects. Patients also typically relapse after treatment ends. But such research provides clues to potentially discoverable fast-acting antidepressant brain mechanisms, and the RAPID team is collaborating with investigators in NIMH's Intramural Research Program, who have pioneered studies of fast-acting antidepressant mechanisms in trials of ketamine and scopolamine. The project aims to translate such evidence into practical treatments by evaluating interventions that show efficacy in proof of concept trials in humans, and following up, if warranted, with randomized clinical trials.

The RAPID team, which incorporates several research sites, is planning to test new compounds that work through the same brain mechanisms as ketamine, as well as non-pharmacological treatments such as magnetic brain stimulation therapies. Through this research, we will enhance our understanding of the underlying mechanisms of depression and guide the development of new ways to quickly help patients who have not responded to current antidepressant medications.

Part Seven

Strategies for Managing Depression

Chapter 55

Understanding Mental Illness Stigma and Depression Triggers

Chapter Contents

Section 55.1

Stigmas about Mental Illness Contribute to Depression

This section includes text excerpted from "Stigma and Mental Illness," Centers for Disease Control and Prevention (CDC), June 18, 2015.

Stigma and Mental Illness

Stigma has been defined as an attribute that is deeply discrediting. This stigmatized trait sets the bearer apart from the rest of society, bringing with it feelings of shame and isolation. Often, when a person with a stigmatized trait is unable to perform an action because of the condition, other people view the person as the problem rather than viewing the condition as the problem. More recent definitions of stigma focus on the results of stigma—the prejudice, avoidance, rejection and discrimination directed at people believed to have an illness, disorder or other trait perceived to be undesirable. Stigma causes needless suffering, potentially causing a person to deny symptoms, delay treatment and refrain from daily activities. Stigma can exclude people from access to housing, employment, insurance, and appropriate medical care. Thus, stigma can interfere with prevention efforts, and examining and combating stigma is a public health priority.

The Substance Abuse and Mental Health Services Administration (SAMHSA) and the Centers for Disease Control and Prevention (CDC) have examined public attitudes toward mental illness in two surveys. In the 2006 HealthStyles survey, only one-quarter of young adults between the ages of 18–24 believed that a person with mental illness can eventually recover. In 2007, adults in 37 states and territories were surveyed about their attitudes toward mental illness, using the 2007 Behavioral Risk Factor Surveillance System (BRFSS) Mental Illness and Stigma module. This study found that:

- 78% of adults with mental health symptoms and 89% of adults without such symptoms agreed that treatment can help persons with mental illness lead normal lives.

- 57% of adults without mental health symptoms believed that people are caring and sympathetic to persons with mental illness.

- Only 25% of adults with mental health symptoms believed that people are caring and sympathetic to persons with mental illness.

These findings highlight both the need to educate the public about how to support persons with mental illness and the need to reduce barriers for those seeking or receiving treatment for mental illness.

Section 55.2

Depression Triggers: How to Prevent Them

"Depression Triggers: How to Prevent Them,"
© 2017 Omnigraphics. Reviewed November 2016.

Depression affects between 15 and 20 million Americans each year. It is a medical condition that should be taken seriously. Some forms of depression are related to malfunctions in brain circuits that transmit signal-carrying chemicals called neurotransmitters, which help regulate mood. Although these cases may not be preventable, they often respond well to treatment. However, studies suggest that it may be possible to prevent some depressive episodes by learning to recognize and avoid common situations that serve as depression triggers. Potential environmental triggers include stressful life events, such as divorce or job loss, as well as unexpected factors that can impact emotional well-being, such as being a caregiver or spending too much time on social media.

The following list describes situations that have been shown to correlate with depression and offers tips for how to avoid or cope with them:

Stress

Nearly 25 percent of American adults reported feeling "extreme stress" in 2015, according to the American Psychological Association

423

(APA), ranking their overall stress levels above 5 on a 10-point scale. Some of the main sources of stress included economic worries, job security, family responsibilities, health concerns, and discrimination or harassment. Many other people simply feel overwhelmed by daily chores, obligations, and deadlines that seem to get in the way of their enjoyment of life. To prevent stress from turning into depression, experts recommend keeping a positive attitude, recognizing your own limits, and setting and enforcing personal boundaries. When tasks seem overwhelming, breaking them down into steps may make them seem more manageable. Finally, building an emotional support network, discussing problems and concerns, and leaning on others for help as needed are important means of coping with stress.

Job Loss

Losing a job can cause a serious blow to a person's sense of identity and self-esteem, especially for older and highly paid workers who are likely to have more trouble finding equivalent positions. People who are fired or laid off may feel rejected, frightened, and uncertain about the future. In addition, unemployment often causes financial difficulties, which in turn can create strain in family relationships. The combination of these factors means that job loss is a leading trigger for depression. Experts recommend that people affected by job loss build a support network consisting of friends and colleagues, and take advantage of career-related courses and job-search resources. It is also important to stay busy and connected, structuring free time by scheduling lunches, walks, classes, or volunteer activities. Finally, after taking time to process the emotional impact of the job loss, it may be helpful to identify its positive aspects. For instance, losing a job might offer an unexpected opportunity to make a career change, pursue a new business idea, or move to a different geographic area.

Financial Problems

Money concerns and accumulated debts are a source of stress and worry for many people, especially those who feel as if they are struggling with financial problems alone. Common emotions associated with financial stress—such as shame, fear, anxiety, uncertainty—can negatively impact self-esteem and trigger depression. Research has shown that one of the key methods of combating financial stress involves formulating a plan and taking positive action. Reviewing sources of income and expenses and establishing a budget are important first steps toward increasing financial stability. People who are not good with money can take advantage of free financial services offered by many communities or borrow books on financial management from a local library. To avoid becoming overwhelmed, experts recommend focusing on areas you can control and creating a long-term plan to pay down debt and build savings. Finally, it is important to remain active and stay connected to friends and family by enjoying free activities, such as a concert in a park.

Divorce

Divorce creates a complicated mix of emotions for those affected by it, including anger, resentment, sadness, regret, guilt, and failure. It also causes a sudden change in social status from couple to single, which can generate feelings of loneliness, fear, and uncertainty. Finally, many divorces involve stressful conflict over financial settlements and custody of children. Taken together, the emotional upheaval of divorce becomes a potent depression trigger. Therapy—whether individual, couples, family, or support groups—can help people navigate the complicated emotions of divorce and move forward with greater confidence. It can also help resolve conflicts, reduce bitterness, and promote effective co-parenting.

Sexual Dysfunction

An active sex life is a proven outlet that helps relieve stress and improve mood. In addition, sexual performance is intricately tied to self-esteem and identity, especially for men. As a result, sexual dysfunction, loss of libido, and sexual health issues can trigger depression. These issues can arise due to age, underlying health problems, or even as side effects of common antidepressant medications, such as selective serotonin reuptake inhibitors (SSRIs). To address sexual problems that may trigger depression, see a healthcare professional for a complete medical examination. Although discussing sex is uncomfortable for many people, it is important not to allow shame or embarrassment to prevent you from getting help. Studies have shown that a satisfying sex life can improve relationships as well as release chemicals in the brain that improve mood.

Infertility

Inability to have a much-desired baby is a powerful depression trigger, especially for women who suffer multiple miscarriages or have age- or health-related fertility issues. Experts suggest that people who feel despair over infertility try to take charge of the situation by investigating alternative routes to parenthood, such as adoption. Single women whose fertility window is closing due to age or health might explore such options as preserving eggs or using a sperm donor. Even if you ultimately decide not to pursue the matter, simply researching the steps involved can make you feel less vulnerable and more empowered.

Caregiving

Serving as a caregiver for a person who is elderly or afflicted with a debilitating illness is another potential depression trigger. Caregiving demands tremendous time and energy, creates stress, and depletes emotional resources. Oftentimes caregivers struggle with conflicting emotions, such as love, concern, and compassion coupled with resentment, guilt, and inadequacy. People who must manage multiple responsibilities, such as job and family pressures, along with caregiving are most at risk for stress and depression. Experts recommend that caregivers establish firm boundaries around how much they can handle and ask for help as needed. In addition, it is vital for caregivers to build a support system, delegate or outsource some tasks, arrange for occasional breaks to replenish their reserves of energy and compassion, and take care of their own health and well-being.

"Empty Nest" Syndrome

Although a child leaving home to begin college or adult life can be a joyous event, it is also a major life change for parents who suddenly must face an empty nest. Many parents struggle with feelings of loss and uncertainty as they adjust to a new daily routine and a different self-identity. Divorced or single parents are particularly vulnerable to loneliness and depression, although it also affects married couples who built their lives around their children and suddenly find that they do not share many common interests. Experts suggest that parents plan in advance to help reduce the emotional impact of empty nest syndrome. Beginning a year or more before the child leaves home, it may be helpful to sign up for a class, join a book group, plan a vacation, or schedule regular activities with friends. Although taking time to adjust is normal, the key to avoiding depression is to remain active, discover new interests, and have things to look forward to outside of the parental role.

Serious Illness

Being diagnosed with a serious illness is a frightening and disorienting experience that can profoundly affect a person's sense of self and outlook for the future. While the physical symptoms can be difficult enough to deal with, the emotional impact can shake the foundations of relationships and trigger depression. One of the most important steps in coping with a serious illness diagnosis is taking a proactive role in establishing a treatment plan. Patients should seek second opinions, ask for referrals to specialists, and build an effective team that includes a patient advocate or social worker as well as doctors. Experts also recommend joining a support group to gain access to the insights and understanding of people who have dealt with the same illness or condition.

Alcohol Abuse

Research has shown that alcoholism and depression are intricately linked. Although many people use alcohol as a way of relaxing and forgetting their troubles, it actually serves as a depressant in the central nervous system. As a result, using alcohol to cope with depression symptoms only makes them worse. Depression can promote alcohol abuse in people who are susceptible to it, while alcohol abuse can trigger depression in people who are prone to it. In fact, studies have shown that up to 50% of alcoholics suffer from major depression. The only way to break the connection is to cut back on drinking and see whether depression symptoms improve over time. People who hide or deny their drinking, repeatedly try and fail to quit drinking, or find that their drinking has negative effects on their lives may need to seek help for alcohol addiction. Treatment options range from Alcoholics Anonymous to residential treatment programs and inpatient medical detoxification.

Hormone Imbalance

As people age, they experience fluctuation and decline in the levels of key hormones in the bloodstream. This natural process can cause a number of unpleasant symptoms, including fatigue, weight gain, hot flashes, low libido, anxiety, and depression. While the experiences of women undergoing menopause receive the most attention, men also go through midlife hormonal changes that can affect mood, energy, and sexual performance. Experts suggest that people age 45 and older keep a record of their symptoms and discuss them with a doctor. Hormonal imbalances can often be stabilized with hormone supplementation or replacement therapy. Some people also find that vitamins, herbal remedies, and stress-management techniques such as meditation and yoga can help combat mood swings associated with hormone fluctuations. Treating underlying conditions such as thyroid disorders can also help regulate hormone levels and reduce the risk of depression.

Unhealthy Habits

Obesity, an unhealthy diet full of refined carbohydrates, and poor sleep habits can also trigger depression. Fortunately, these triggers are among the easiest to avoid. Experts recommend evaluating your lifestyle and making gradual, long-term changes to improve your overall health and well-being. They warn against fad diets and instead suggest a diet that emphasizes fresh fruits and vegetables, whole grains, lean proteins, healthy fats, and drinking plenty of water. Consuming foods high in saturated fat or sugar—such as chips, cookies, white bread, and soda—has been shown to increase the risk of depressive episodes, so these should be avoided. In addition, experts recommend increasing physical fitness by walking or doing other activities to help maintain a healthy weight, improve mood, and stave off depression. Exercise also helps improve sleep, which is another aspect of general health that correlates to depression. Studies have shown that people who get the recommended six to eight hours of sleep per night are less likely to experience depression than those who receive more or less than the recommended amount. Some tips for improving sleep include maintaining a consistent schedule, avoiding use of electronics in the bedroom, creating a calm, relaxing sleep environment, and employing techniques such as reading or meditation to wind down after a busy day.

News and Social Media

Smartphones and other mobile devices make it easier to keep connected and up to date than ever before. Yet studies have shown that excessive consumption of bad news—which outweighs coverage of good news by a 17-1 margin in the modern media—can trigger anxiety and depression. Similarly, obsessive checking of social media like Facebook, where others tend to highlight only the best aspects of their lives, can create feelings of envy, loneliness, frustration, and guilt that can trigger or worsen depression symptoms. To reduce the impact of news and social media on mood, experts suggest spending less time online and more time socializing in real life with friends and family. Spending time talking with people who care has been shown to improve mood and increase life satisfaction.

References

1. Brabaw, Kasandra. "Five Strange, Surprising Depression Triggers," Prevention.com, October 26, 2015.

2. Haiken, Melanie. "Ten Biggest Depression Triggers, and How to Turn Them Off," Caring.com, September 5, 2016.

3. Theobald, Mikel. "Avoiding Ten Common Depression Triggers," EverydayHealth, 2016.

Chapter 56

Well-Being Concepts

Well-Being Concepts for Better Life

Well-being is a positive outcome that is meaningful for people and for many sectors of society, because it tells us that people perceive that their lives are going well. Good living conditions (e.g., housing, employment) are fundamental to well-being. Tracking these conditions is important for public policy. However, many indicators that measure living conditions fail to measure what people think and feel about their lives, such as the quality of their relationships, their positive emotions and resilience, the realization of their potential, or their overall satisfaction with life—i.e., their "well-being." Well-being generally includes global judgments of life satisfaction and feelings ranging from depression to joy.

Why Is Well-Being Useful for Public Health?

- Well-being integrates mental health (mind) and physical health (body) resulting in more holistic approaches to disease prevention and health promotion.

- Well-being is a valid population outcome measure beyond morbidity, mortality, and economic status that tells us how people perceive their life is going from their own perspective.

This chapter includes text excerpted from "Health-Related Quality of Life (HRQOL)," Centers for Disease Control and Prevention (CDC), May 22, 2016.

- Well-being is an outcome that is meaningful to the public.

- Advances in psychology, neuroscience, and measurement theory suggest that well-being can be measured with some degree of accuracy.

- Results from cross-sectional, longitudinal and experimental studies find that well-being is associated with:

- Self-perceived health

- Longevity

- Healthy behaviors

- Mental and physical illness

- Social connectedness

- Productivity

- Factors in the physical and social environment

- Well-being can provide a common metric that can help policy makers shape and compare the effects of different policies (e.g., loss of green space might impact well-being more so than commercial development of an area).

- Measuring, tracking and promoting well-being can be useful for multiple stakeholders involved in disease prevention and health promotion.

Well-being is associated with numerous health-, job-, family-, and economically-related benefits. For example, higher levels of well-being are associated with decreased risk of disease, illness, and injury; better immune functioning; speedier recovery; and increased longevity. Individuals with high levels of well-being are more productive at work and are more likely to contribute to their communities.

Previous research lends support to the view that the negative affect component of well-being is strongly associated with neuroticism and that positive affect component has a similar association with extraversion. This research also supports the view that positive emotions—central components of well-being—are not merely the opposite of negative emotions, but are independent dimensions of mental health that can, and should be fostered. Although a substantial proportion of the variance in well-being can be attributed to heritable factors, environmental factors play an equally if not more important role.

How Does Well-Being Relate to Health Promotion?

Health is more than the absence of disease; it is a resource that allows people to realize their aspirations, satisfy their needs and to cope with the environment in order to live a long, productive, and fruitful life. In this sense, health enables social, economic and personal development fundamental to well-being. Health promotion is the process of enabling people to increase control over, and to improve their health. Environmental and social resources for health can include: peace, economic security, a stable ecosystem, and safe housing. Individual resources for health can include: physical activity, healthful diet, social ties, resiliency, positive emotions, and autonomy. Health promotion activities aimed at strengthening such individual, environmental and social resources may ultimately improve well-being.

How Is Well-Being Defined?

There is no consensus around a single definition of well-being, but there is general agreement that at minimum, well-being includes the presence of positive emotions and moods (e.g., contentment, happiness), the absence of negative emotions (e.g., depression, anxiety), satisfaction with life, fulfillment and positive functioning. In simple terms, well-being can be described as judging life positively and feeling good. For public health purposes, physical well-being (e.g., feeling very healthy and full of energy) is also viewed as critical to overall well-being. Researchers from different disciplines have examined different aspects of well-being that include the following:

- Physical well-being
- Economic well-being
- Social well-being
- Development and activity
- Emotional well-being
- Psychological well-being
- Life satisfaction
- Domain specific satisfaction
- Engaging activities and work

How Is Well-Being Measured?

Because well-being is subjective, it is typically measured with self-reports. The use of self-reported measures is fundamentally different from using objective measures (e.g., household income, unemployment levels, and neighbourhood crime) often used to assess well-being. The use of both objective and subjective measures, when available, are desirable for public policy purposes.

There are many well-being instruments available that measure self-reported well-being in different ways, depending on whether one measures well-being as a clinical outcome, a population health outcome, for cost-effectiveness studies, or for other purposes. For example, well-being measures can be psychometrically-based or utility-based. Psychometrically-based measures are based on the relationship between, and strength among, multiple items that are intended to measure one or more domains of well-being. Utility-based measures are based on an individual or group's preference for a particular state, and are typically anchored between 0 (death) to 1 (optimum health). Some studies support use of single items (e.g., global life satisfaction) to measure well-being parsimoniously. Peer reports, observational methods, physiological methods, experience sampling methods, ecological momentary assessment, and other methods are used by psychologists to measure different aspects of well-being.

Chapter 57

Building Resilience

Chapter Contents

Section 57.1

Understanding Resilience

This section includes text excerpted from "Resilience and Stress
Management: Resilience," Substance Abuse and Mental Health
Services Administration (SAMHSA), December 10, 2015.

What Is Resilience?

Resilience is the ability to:

- Bounce back
- Take on difficult challenges and still find meaning in life
- Respond positively to difficult situations
- Rise above adversity
- Cope when things look bleak
- Tap into hope
- Transform unfavorable situations into wisdom, insight, and compassion
- Endure

Resilience refers to the ability of an individual, family, organization, or community to cope with adversity and adapt to challenges or change. It is an ongoing process that requires time and effort and engages people in taking a number of steps to enhance their response to adverse circumstances. Resilience implies that after an event, a person or community may not only be able to cope and recover, but also change to reflect different priorities arising from the experience and prepare for the next stressful situation.

- Resilience is the most important defense people have against stress.
- It is important to build and foster resilience to be ready for future challenges.
- Resilience will enable the development of a reservoir of internal resources to draw upon during stressful situations.

Research has shown that resilience is ordinary, not extraordinary, and that people regularly demonstrate this ability.

- Resilience is not a trait that people either have or do not have.
- Resilience involves behaviors, thoughts, and actions that can be learned and developed in anyone.
- Resilience is tremendously influenced by a person's environment.

Resilience changes over time. It fluctuates depending on how much a person nurtures internal resources or coping strategies. Some people are more resilient in work life, while others exhibit more resilience in their personal relationships. People can build resilience and promote the foundations of resilience in any aspect of life they choose.

What Is Individual or Personal Resilience?

Individual resilience is a person's ability to positively cope after failures, setbacks, and losses. Developing resilience is a personal journey. Individuals do not react the same way to traumatic or stressful life events. An approach to building resilience that works for one person might not work for another. People use varying strategies to build their resilience. Because resilience can be learned, it can be strengthened. Personal resilience is related to many factors including individual health and well-being, factors with and into which a person is born, life history and experience, and social support.

Factors That Influence Individual Health and Well Being

Factors with and into which a person is born

- Personality
- Ethnicity
- Cultural background
- Economic background

Life history and experience

These are past events and relationships that influence how people approach current stressors:

- Family history
- Previous physical health
- Previous mental health
- Trauma history
- Past social experiences
- Past cultural experiences

437

Social support

These are support systems provided by family, friends, and members of the community, work, or school environments:

- Feeling connected to others

- A sense of security

- Feeling connected to resources

Along with the factors listed above, there are several attributes that have been correlated with building and promoting resilience.

The American Psychological Association (APA) reports that resilience includes the following attributes:

- The capacity to make and carry out realistic plans

- Communication and problem-solving skills

- A positive or optimistic view of life

- Confidence in personal strengths and abilities

- The capacity to manage strong feelings, emotions, and impulses

What Is Family Resilience?

Family resilience is the coping process in the family as a functional unit. Crisis events and persistent stressors affect the whole family, posing risks not only for individual dysfunction, but also for relational conflict and family breakdown. Family processes mediate the impact of stress for all of its members and relationships, and the protective processes in place foster resilience by buffering stress and facilitating adaptation to current and future events. Following are the three key factors in family resilience:

- Family belief systems foster resilience by making meaning in adversity, creating a sense of coherence, and providing a positive outlook.

- Family organization promotes resilience by facilitating flexibility, capacity to adapt, connectedness and cohesion, emotional and structural bonding, and access to resources.

- Family communication enhances resilience by involving clear communication, open and emotional expressions, trust and collaborative problem solving, and conflict management.

What Is Organizational Resilience?

Organizational resilience is the ability and capacity of a workplace to withstand potential significant economic times, systemic risk, or systemic disruptions by adapting, recovering, or resisting being affected and resuming core operations or continuing to provide an acceptable level of functioning and structure.

- A resilient workforce and organization is important during major decisions or business changes.
- Companies and organizations, like individuals, need to be able to rebound from potentially disastrous changes.
- The challenge for the incorporation of resilience into a workplace is to identify what enhances the ability of an organization to rebound effectively.

Measuring workplace resilience involves identifying and evaluating the following:

- Past and present mitigative mechanisms and practices that increase safety
- Past and present mitigative mechanisms and practices that decrease error
- Necessary redundancy in systems
- Planning and programming that demonstrate collective mindfulness
- Anticipation of potential trouble and solutions to potential problems

What Is Community Resilience?

Community resilience is the individual and collective capacity to respond to adversity and change. A resilient community is one that takes intentional action to enhance the personal and collective capacity of its citizens and institutions to respond to and influence the course of social and economic change. For a community to be resilient, its members must put into practice early and effective actions so that they can respond to change. When responding to stressful events, a resilient community will be able to strengthen community bonds, resources, and the capacity to cope. Systems involved with building and maintaining community resilience must work together.

439

How Does Culture Influence Resilience?

Cultural resilience refers to a culture's capacity to maintain and develop cultural identity and critical cultural knowledge and practices. Along with an entire culture fostering resilience, the interaction of culture and resilience for an individual also is important. An individual's culture will have an impact on how the person communicates feelings and copes with adversity. Cultural parameters are often embedded deep in an individual. A person's cultural background may deeply influence in how he or she responds to different stressors. Assimilation could be a factor in cultural resilience, as it could be a positive way for a person to manage his/her environment. However, assimilation could create conflict between generations, so it could be seen as positive or negative depending on the individual and culture. Because of this, coping strategies are going to be different. With growing cultural diversity, the public has greater access to a number of different approaches to building resilience. It is something that can be built using approaches that make sense within each culture and are tailored to each individual.

Section 57.2

Factors That Promote Resilience

This section includes text excerpted from "Resilience and Stress Management: Resilience," Substance Abuse and Mental Health Services Administration (SAMHSA), December 10, 2015.

Resilience involves the modification of a person's response to a potentially risky situation. People who are resilient are able to maintain high self-esteem and self-efficacy in spite of the challenges they face. By fostering resilience, people are building psychological defenses against stress. The more resources and defenses available during a time of struggle, the better able to cope and bounce back from adverse circumstances people will be. A person's ability to regain a sense of normalcy or define a new normalcy after adverse circumstances will be partially based on the resources available to him/her. Resilience building can begin at any time. Following is information regarding types of resilience, the qualities of which each type consists, factors that can inhibit or enhance resilience, and people who help facilitate the growth of resilience.

Table 57.1. Resilience Factors

Signs of This Type of Resilience	Vulnerability Factors Inhibiting Resilience	Protective Factors Enhancing Resilience	Facilitators of Resilience
Individual Resilience—The ability for an individual to cope with adversity and change			
Optimism	Poor social skills	Social competence	Individuals
Flexibility	Poor problem solving	Problem-solving skills	Parents
Self-confidence	Lack of empathy	Good coping skills	Grandparents
Competence	Family violence	Empathy	Caregivers
Insightfulness	Abuse or neglect	Secure or stable family	Children
Perseverance	Divorce or partner breakup	Supportive relationships	Adolescents
Perspective	Death or loss	Intellectual abilities	Friends
Self-control	Lack of social support	Self-efficacy	Partners
Sociability		Communication skills	Spouses
			Teachers
			Faith Community
Organizational Resilience—The ability for a business or industry, including its employees, to cope with adversity and change			
Proactive employees	Unclear expectations	Open communication	Employers
Clear mission, goals, and values	Conflicted expectations	Supportive colleagues	Managers
Encourages opportunities to influence change	Threat to job security	Clear responsibilities	Directors
Clear communication	Lack of personal control	Ethical environment	Employees

Table 57.1. Continued

Signs of This Type of Resilience	Vulnerability Factors Inhibiting Resilience	Protective Factors Enhancing Resilience	Facilitators of Resilience
Nonjudgmental	Hostile atmosphere	Sense of control	Employee assistance programs
Emphasizes learning	Defensive atmosphere	Job security	Other businesses
Rewards high performance	Unethical environment	Supportive management	
	Lack of communication	Connectedness among departments	
		Recognition	
Community Resilience—The ability for an individual and the collective community to respond to adversity and change			
Connectedness	Lack of support services	Access to support services	Community leaders
Commitment to community	Social discrimination	Community networking	Faith-based organizations
Shared values	Cultural discrimination	Strong cultural identity	Volunteers
Structure, roles, and responsibilities exist throughout community	Norms tolerating violence	Strong social support systems	Nonprofit organizations
Supportive	Deviant peer group	Norms against violence	Churches/houses of worship
Good communication	Low socioeconomic status	Identification as a community	Support services staff
Resource sharing	Crime rate	Cohesive community leadership	Teachers
Volunteerism	Community disorganization		Youth groups
Responsive organizations	Civil rivalry		Boy/Girl Scouts
Strong schools			Planned social networking events

Section 57.3

Building Resilience in Children and Youth Dealing with Trauma

This section includes text excerpted from "Helping Children and Adolescents Cope with Violence and Disasters: What Parents Can Do," National Institute of Mental Health (NIMH), November 27, 2013. Reviewed November 2016.

Each year, children experience violence and disaster and face other traumas. Young people are injured, they see others harmed by violence, they suffer sexual abuse, and they lose loved ones or witness other tragic and shocking events. Parents and caregivers can help children overcome these experiences and start the process of recovery.

What Is Trauma?

"Trauma" is often thought of as physical injuries. Psychological trauma is an emotionally painful, shocking, stressful, and sometimes life-threatening experience. It may or may not involve physical injuries, and can result from witnessing distressing events. Examples include a natural disaster, physical or sexual abuse, and terrorism.

Disasters such as hurricanes, earthquakes, and floods can claim lives, destroy homes or whole communities, and cause serious physical and psychological injuries. Trauma can also be caused by acts of violence. The September 11, 2001 terrorist attack is one example. Mass shootings in schools or communities and physical or sexual assault are other examples. Traumatic events threaten our sense of safety.

Reactions (responses) to trauma can be immediate or delayed. Reactions to trauma differ in severity and cover a wide range of behaviors and responses. Children with existing mental health problems, past traumatic experiences, and/or limited family and social supports may be more reactive to trauma. Frequently experienced responses among children after trauma are loss of trust and a fear of the event happening again.

Commonly Experienced Responses to Trauma among Children

Children age 5 and under may react in a number of ways including:

- Showing signs of fear
- Clinging to parent or caregiver
- Crying or screaming
- Whimpering or trembling
- Moving aimlessly
- Becoming immobile
- Returning to behaviors common to being younger
- Thumbsucking
- Bedwetting
- Being afraid of the dark

Children age 6 to 11 may react by:

- Isolating themselves
- Becoming quiet around friends, family, and teachers
- Having nightmares or other sleep problems
- Refusing to go to bed
- Becoming irritable or disruptive
- Having outbursts of anger
- Starting fights
- Being unable to concentrate
- Refusing to go to school
- Complaining of physical problems
- Developing unfounded fears
- Becoming depressed
- Expressing guilt over what happened
- Feeling numb emotionally
- Doing poorly with school and homework

- Losing interest in fun activities

Adolescents age 12 to 17 may react by:

- Having flashbacks to the event (flashbacks are the mind reliving the event)
- Having nightmares or other sleep problems
- Avoiding reminders of the event
- Using or abusing drugs, alcohol, or tobacco
- Being disruptive, disrespectful, or behaving destructively
- Having physical complaints
- Feeling isolated or confused
- Being depressed
- Being angry
- Losing interest in fun activities
- Having suicidal thoughts

Adolescents may feel guilty. They may feel guilt for not preventing injury or deaths. They also may have thoughts of revenge.

What Can Parents Do to Help?

After violence or disaster, parents and family members should identify and address their own feelings—this will allow them to help others. Explain to children what happened and let them know:

- You love them
- The event was not their fault
- You will do your best to take care of them
- It's okay for them to feel upset

Do:

- Allow children to cry
- Allow sadness
- Let children talk about feelings
- Let them write about feelings

- Let them draw pictures about the event or their feelings

Don't:

- Expect children to be brave or tough

- Make children discuss the event before they are ready

- Get angry if children show strong emotions

- Get upset if they begin bedwetting, acting out, or thumbsucking

Other tips:

- If children have trouble sleeping give them extra attention, let them sleep with a light on, or let them sleep in your room (for a short time).

- Try to keep normal routines, for example, reading bedtime stories, eating dinner together, watching TV together, reading books, exercising, or playing games. If you can't keep normal routines, make new ones together.

- Help children feel in control when possible by letting them choose meals, pick out clothes, or make some decisions for themselves.

How Can I Help Young Children Who Experienced Trauma?

Helping children can start immediately, even at the scene of the event. Most children recover within a few weeks of a traumatic experience, while some may need help longer. Grief, a deep emotional response to loss, may take months to resolve. Children may experience grief over the loss of a loved one, teacher, friend, or pet. Grief may be re-experienced or worsened by news reports or the event's anniversary.

Some children may need help from a mental health professional. Some people may seek other kinds of help from community leaders. Identify children who need support and help them obtain it.

Examples of problematic behaviors could be:

- Refusing to go to places that remind them of the event

- Emotional numbness

- Behaving dangerously
- Unexplained anger/rage
- Sleep problems including nightmares

Adult helpers should:

Pay attention to children

- Listen to them
- Accept/do not argue about their feelings
- Help them cope with the reality of their experiences

Reduce effects of other stressors, such as:

- Frequent moving or changes in place of residence
- Long periods away from family and friends
- Pressures to perform well in school
- Transportation problems
- Fighting within the family
- Being hungry

Monitor healing:

- It takes time
- Do not ignore severe reactions
- Pay attention to sudden changes in behaviors, speech, language use, or strong emotions

Remind children that adults:

- Love them
- Support them
- Will be with them when possible

Parents and caregivers should also limit viewing of repetitive news reports about traumatic events. Young children may not understand that news coverage is about one event and not multiple similar events.

Help for All People in the First Days and Weeks

There are steps adults can take following a disaster that can help them cope, making it easier for them to provide better care for children. These include creating safe conditions, remaining calm and friendly, and connecting with others. Being sensitive to people under stress and respecting their decisions is important.

When possible, help people:

- Get food

- Get a safe place to live

- Get help from a doctor or nurse if hurt

- Contact loved ones or friends

- Keep children with parents or relatives

- Understand what happened

- Understand what is being done

- Know where to get help

Don't:

- Force people to tell their stories

- Probe for personal details

- Say things like "everything will be OK," or "at least you survived"

- Say what you think people should feel or how people should have acted

- Say people suffered because they deserved it

- Be negative about available help

- Make promises that you can't keep such as "you will go home soon."

Chapter 58

Building Self-Esteem and Body Image

Does any of this sound familiar? "I'm too tall." "I'm too short." "I'm too skinny." "If only I were shorter/taller/had curly hair/straight hair/a smaller nose/longer legs, I'd be happy."

Are you putting yourself down? If so, you're not alone. As a teen, you're going through lots of changes in your body. And, as your body changes, so does your image of yourself. It's not always easy to like every part of your looks, but when you get stuck on the negatives it can really bring down your self-esteem.

Why Are Self-Esteem and Body Image Important?

Self-esteem is all about how much you feel you are worth—and how much you feel other people value you. Self-esteem is important because feeling good about yourself can affect your mental health and how you behave. People with high self-esteem know themselves well. They're realistic and find friends that like and appreciate them for who they are. People with high self-esteem usually feel more in control of their lives and know their own strengths and weaknesses.

Body image is how you view your physical self—including whether you feel you are attractive and whether others like your looks. For many people, especially people in their early teens, body image can be closely linked to self-esteem.

Text in this chapter is excerpted from "Body Image and Self-Esteem," © 1995–2016. The Nemours Foundation/KidsHealth®. Reprinted with permission.

What Influences a Person's Self-Esteem?

Puberty and Development

Some people struggle with their self-esteem and body image when they begin puberty because it's a time when the body goes through many changes. These changes, combined with wanting to feel accepted by our friends, means it can be tempting to compare ourselves with others. The trouble with that is, not everyone grows or develops at the same time or in the same way.

Media Images and Other outside Influences

Our tweens and early teens are a time when we become more aware of celebrities and media images—as well as how other kids look and how we fit in. We might start to compare ourselves with other people or media images ("ideals" that are frequently airbrushed). All of this can affect how we feel about ourselves and our bodies even as we grow into our teens.

Families and School

Family life can sometimes influence our body image. Some parents or coaches might be too focused on looking a certain way or "making weight" for a sports team. Family members might struggle with their own body image or criticize their kids' looks ("why do you wear your hair so long?" or "how come you can't wear pants that fit you?"). This can all influence a person's self-esteem, especially if they're sensitive to others peoples' comments.

People also may experience negative comments and hurtful teasing about the way they look from classmates and peers. Although these often come from ignorance, sometimes they can affect body image and self-esteem.

Healthy Self-Esteem

If you have a positive body image, you probably like and accept yourself the way you are, even if you don't fit some media "ideal." This healthy attitude allows you to explore other aspects of growing up, such as developing good friendships, becoming more independent from your parents, and challenging yourself physically and mentally. Developing these parts of yourself can help boost your self-esteem.

A positive, optimistic attitude can help people develop strong self-esteem. For example, if you make a mistake, you might want to say, "Hey, I'm human" instead of "Wow, I'm such a loser" or not blame others when things don't go as expected.

Knowing what makes you happy and how to meet your goals can help you feel capable, strong, and in control of your life. A positive attitude and a healthy lifestyle (such as exercising and eating right) are a great combination for building good self-esteem.

Tips for Improving Body Image

Some people think they need to change how they look to feel good about themselves. But all you need to do is change the way you see your body and how you think about yourself. Here are some tips on doing that:

Recognize that your body is your own, no matter what shape or size it comes in. Try to focus on how strong and healthy your body is and the things it can do, not what's wrong with it or what you feel you want to change about it. If you're worried about your weight or size, check with your doctor to verify that things are ok. But it's no one's business but your own what your body is like—ultimately, you have to be happy with yourself.

Identify which aspects of your appearance you can realistically change and which you can't. Humans, by definition, are imperfect. It's what makes each of us unique and original! Everyone (even the most perfect-seeming celeb) has things that they can't change and need to accept—like their height, for example, or their shoe size. Remind yourself that "real people aren't perfect and perfect people aren't real (they're usually airbrushed!)".

If there are things about yourself that you want to change and can, do this by making goals for yourself. For example, if you want to get fit, make a plan to exercise every day and eat healthy. Then keep track of your progress until you reach your goal. Meeting a challenge you set for yourself is a great way to boost self-esteem!

When you hear negative comments coming from within, tell yourself to stop. Appreciate that each person is more than just how he or she looks on any given day. We're complex and constantly changing. Try to focus on what's unique and interesting about yourself.

Try building your self-esteem by giving yourself three compliments every day. While you're at it, every evening list three things in your day that really gave you pleasure. It can be anything from the way the sun felt on your face, the sound of your favorite band, or the way someone laughed at your jokes. By focusing on the good things you do and the positive aspects of your life, you can change how you feel about yourself.

Some people with physical disabilities or differences may feel they are not seen for their true selves because of their bodies and what they can and can't do. Other people may have such serious body image issues that they need a bit more help. Working with a counselor or therapist can help some people gain perspective and learn to focus on their individual strengths as well as develop healthier thinking.

Where Can I Go If I Need Help?

Sometimes low self-esteem and body image problems are too much to handle alone. A few teens may become depressed, and lose interest in activities or friends. Some go on to develop eating disorders or body image disorders, or use alcohol or drugs to escape feelings of low worth.

If you're feeling this way, it can help to talk to a parent, coach, religious leader, guidance counselor, therapist, or friend. A trusted adult—someone who supports you and doesn't bring you down—can help you put your body image in perspective and give you positive feedback about your body, your skills, and your abilities.

If you can't turn to anyone you know, call a teen crisis hotline (an online search can give you the information for national and local hotlines). The most important thing is to get help if you feel like your body image and self-esteem are affecting your life.

Chapter 59

Dealing with the Effects of Trauma

Coping with Trauma

When trauma survivors take direct action to cope with their stress reactions, they put themselves in a position of power. Active coping with the trauma makes you begin to feel less helpless.

- Active coping means accepting the impact of trauma on your life and taking direct action to improve things.

- Active coping occurs even when there is no crisis. Active coping is a way of responding to everyday life. It is a habit that must be made stronger.

Know That Recovery Is a Process

Following exposure to a trauma most people experience stress reactions. Understand that recovering from the trauma is a process and takes time. Knowing this will help you feel more in control.

- Having an ongoing response to the trauma is normal.

- Recovery is an ongoing, daily process. It happens little by little. It is not a matter of being cured all of a sudden.

This chapter includes text excerpted from "Coping with Traumatic Stress Reactions," U.S. Department of Veterans Affairs (VA), August 14, 2015.

- Healing doesn't mean forgetting traumatic events. It doesn't mean you will have no pain or bad feelings when thinking about them.

- Healing may mean fewer symptoms and symptoms that bother you less.

- Healing means more confidence that you will be able to cope with your memories and symptoms. You will be better able to manage your feelings.

Positive Coping Actions

Certain actions can help to reduce your distressing symptoms and make things better. Plus, these actions can result in changes that last into the future. Here are some positive coping methods:

Learn about Trauma and Posttraumatic Stress Disorder (PTSD)

It is useful for trauma survivors to learn more about common reactions to trauma and about PTSD. Find out what is normal. Find out what the signs are that you may need assistance from others. When you learn that the symptoms of PTSD are common, you realize that you are not alone, weak, or crazy. It helps to know your problems are shared by hundreds of thousands of others. When you seek treatment and begin to understand your response to trauma, you will be better able to cope with the symptoms of PTSD.

Talk to Others for Support

When survivors talk about their problems with others, something helpful often results. It is important not to isolate yourself. Instead make efforts to be with others. Of course, you must choose your support people with care. You must also ask them clearly for what you need. With support from others, you may feel less alone and more understood. You may also get concrete help with a problem you have.

Practice Relaxation Methods

Try some different ways to relax, including:

- Muscle relaxation exercises
- Breathing exercises

- Meditation
- Swimming, stretching, yoga
- Prayer
- Listening to quiet music
- Spending time in nature

While relaxation techniques can be helpful, in a few people they can sometimes increase distress at first. This can happen when you focus attention on disturbing physical sensations and you reduce contact with the outside world. Most often, continuing with relaxation in small amounts that you can handle will help reduce negative reactions. You may want to try mixing relaxation in with music, walking, or other activities.

Distract Yourself with Positive Activities

Pleasant recreational or work activities help distract a person from his or her memories and reactions. For example, art has been a way for many trauma survivors to express their feelings in a positive, creative way. Pleasant activities can improve your mood, limit the harm caused by PTSD, and help you rebuild your life.

Talking to Your Doctor or a Counselor about Trauma and PTSD

Part of taking care of yourself means using the helping resources around you. If efforts at coping don't seem to work, you may become fearful or depressed. If your PTSD symptoms don't begin to go away or get worse over time, it is important to reach out and call a counselor who can help turn things around. Your family doctor can also refer you to a specialist who can treat PTSD. Talk to your doctor about your trauma and your PTSD symptoms. That way, he or she can take care of your health better.

Many with PTSD have found treatment with medicines to be helpful for some symptoms. By taking medicines, some survivors of trauma are able to improve their sleep, anxiety, irritability, and anger. It can also reduce urges to drink or use drugs.

Coping with the Symptoms of PTSD

Here are some direct ways to cope with these specific PTSD symptoms:

Unwanted distressing memories, images, or thoughts

- Remind yourself that they are just that, memories.

- Remind yourself that it's natural to have some memories of the trauma(s).

- Talk about them to someone you trust.

- Remember that, although reminders of trauma can feel overwhelming, they often lessen with time.

Sudden feelings of anxiety or panic

Traumatic stress reactions often include feeling your heart pounding and feeling lightheaded or spacey. This is usually caused by rapid breathing. If this happens, remember that:

- These reactions are not dangerous. If you had them while exercising, they most likely would not worry you.

- These feelings often come with scary thoughts that are not true. For example, you may think, "I'm going to die," "I'm having a heart attack," or "I will lose control." It is the scary thoughts that make these reactions so upsetting.

- Slowing down your breathing may help.

- The sensations will pass soon and then you can go on with what you were doing.

Each time you respond in these positive ways to your anxiety or panic, you will be working toward making it happen less often. Practice will make it easier to cope.

Feeling like the trauma is happening again (flashbacks)

- Keep your eyes open. Look around you and notice where you are.

- Talk to yourself. Remind yourself where you are, what year you're in, and that you are safe. The trauma happened in the past, and you are in the present.

- Get up and move around. Have a drink of water and wash your hands.

- Call someone you trust and tell them what is happening.

- Remind yourself that this is a common response after trauma.

- Tell your counselor or doctor about the flashback(s).

Dreams and nightmares related to the trauma

- If you wake up from a nightmare in a panic, remind yourself that you are reacting to a dream. Having the dream is why you are in a panic, not because there is real danger now.

- You may want to get up out of bed, regroup, and orient yourself to the here and now.

- Engage in a pleasant, calming activity. For example, listen to some soothing music.

- Talk to someone if possible.

- Talk to your doctor about your nightmares. Certain medicines can be helpful.

Difficulty falling or staying asleep

- Keep to a regular bedtime schedule.

- Avoid heavy exercise for the few hours just before going to bed.

- Avoid using your sleeping area for anything other than sleeping or sex.

- Avoid alcohol, tobacco, and caffeine. These harm your ability to sleep.

- Do not lie in bed thinking or worrying. Get up and enjoy something soothing or pleasant. Read a calming book, drink a glass of warm milk or herbal tea, or do a quiet hobby.

Irritability, anger, and rage

- Take a time out to cool off or think things over. Walk away from the situation.

- Get in the habit of exercise daily. Exercise reduces body tension and relieves stress.

- Remember that staying angry doesn't work. It actually increases your stress and can cause health problems.

- Talk to your counselor or doctor about your anger. Take classes in how to manage anger.

- If you blow up at family members or friends, find time as soon as you can to talk to them about it. Let them know how you feel and what you are doing to cope with your reactions.

Difficulty concentrating or staying focused

- Slow down. Give yourself time to focus on what it is you need to learn or do.

- Write things down. Making "to do" lists may be helpful.

- Break tasks down into small do-able chunks.

- Plan a realistic number of events or tasks for each day.

- You may be depressed. Many people who are depressed have trouble concentrating. Again, this is something you can discuss with your counselor, doctor, or someone close to you.

Trouble feeling or expressing positive emotions

- Remember that this is a common reaction to trauma. You are not doing this on purpose. You should not feel guilty for something you do not want to happen and cannot control.

- Make sure to keep taking part in activities that you enjoy or used to enjoy. Even if you don't think you will enjoy something, once you get into it, you may well start having feelings of pleasure.

- Take steps to let your loved ones know that you care. You can express your caring in little ways: write a card, leave a small gift, or phone someone and say hello.

A Final Word

Try using all these ways of coping to find which ones are helpful to you. Then practice them. Like other skills, they work better with practice. Be aware that there are also behaviors that don't help.

Chapter 60

Grief, Bereavement, and Coping with Loss

Coping with Loss

People cope with the loss of a loved one in different ways. Most people who experience grief will cope well. Others will have severe grief and may need treatment. There are many things that can affect the grief process of someone who has lost a loved one to cancer. They include:

- The personality of the person who is grieving.

- The relationship with the person who died.

- The loved one's cancer experience and the way the disease progressed.

- The grieving person's coping skills and mental health history.

- The amount of support the grieving person has.

- The grieving person's cultural and religious background.

- The grieving person's social and financial position.

This chapter includes text excerpted from "Grief, Bereavement, and Coping with Loss (PDQ®)—Patient Version," National Cancer Institute (NCI), March 6, 2013. Reviewed November 2016.

This chapter defines grief and bereavement and describes the different types of grief reactions, treatments for grief, important issues for grieving children, and cultural responses to grief and loss. It is intended as a resource to help caregivers of cancer patients.

Bereavement and Grief

Bereavement is the period of sadness after losing a loved one through death. Grief and mourning occur during the period of bereavement. Grief and mourning are closely related. Mourning is the way we show grief in public. The way people mourn is affected by beliefs, religious practices, and cultural customs. People who are grieving are sometimes described as bereaved.

Grief is the normal process of reacting to the loss. Grief is the emotional response to the loss of a loved one. Common grief reactions include the following:

- Feeling emotionally numb.

- Feeling unable to believe the loss occurred.

- Feeling anxiety from the distress of being separated from the loved one.

- Mourning along with depression.

- A feeling of acceptance.

Types of Grief Reactions

Anticipatory Grief

Anticipatory grief may occur when a death is expected. Anticipatory grief occurs when a death is expected, but before it happens. It may be felt by the families of people who are dying and by the person dying. Anticipatory grief helps family members get ready emotionally for the loss. It can be a time to take care of unfinished business with the dying person, such as saying "I love you" or "I forgive you."

Like grief that occurs after the death of a loved one, anticipatory grief involves mental, emotional, cultural, and social responses. However, anticipatory grief is different from grief that occurs after the death. Symptoms of anticipatory grief include the following:

- Depression.

- Feeling a greater than usual concern for the dying person.

- Imagining what the loved one's death will be like.

- Getting ready emotionally for what will happen after the death.

Anticipatory grief may help the family but not the dying person. Anticipatory grief helps family members cope with what is to come. For the patient who is dying, anticipatory grief may be too much to handle and may cause him or her to withdraw from others.

Anticipatory grief does not always occur. Some researchers report that anticipatory grief is rare. Studies showed that periods of acceptance and recovery usually seen during grief are not common before the patient's actual death. The bereaved may feel that trying to accept the loss of a loved one before death occurs may make it seem that the dying patient has been abandoned.

Also, grief felt before the death will not decrease the grief felt afterwards or make it last a shorter time.

Normal Grief

Normal or common grief begins soon after a loss and symptoms go away over time. During normal grief, the bereaved person moves toward accepting the loss and is able to continue normal day-to-day life even though it is hard to do. Common grief reactions include:

- Emotional numbness, shock, disbelief, or denial. These often occur right after the death, especially if the death was not expected.

- Anxiety over being separated from the loved one. The bereaved may wish to bring the person back and become lost in thoughts of the deceased. Images of death may occur often in the person's everyday thoughts.

- Distress that leads to crying; sighing; having dreams, illusions, and hallucinations of the deceased; and looking for places or things that were shared with the deceased.

- Anger.

- Periods of sadness, loss of sleep, loss of appetite, extreme tiredness, guilt, and loss of interest in life. Day-to-day living may be affected.

In normal grief, symptoms will occur less often and will feel less severe as time passes. Recovery does not happen in a set period of time. For most bereaved people having normal grief, symptoms lessen between 6 months and 2 years after the loss.

Many bereaved people will have grief bursts or pangs. Grief bursts or pangs are short periods (20–30 minutes) of very intense distress. Sometimes these bursts are caused by reminders of the deceased person. At other times they seem to happen for no reason.

Grief is sometimes described as a process that has stages. There are several theories about how the normal grief process works. Experts have described different types and numbers of stages that people go through as they cope with loss. At this time, there is not enough information to prove that one of these theories is more correct than the others.

Although many bereaved people have similar responses as they cope with their losses, there is no typical grief response. The grief process is personal.

Complicated Grief

There is no right or wrong way to grieve, but studies have shown that there are patterns of grief that are different from the most common. This has been called complicated grief.

Complicated grief reactions that have been seen in studies include:

- **Minimal grief reaction:** A grief pattern in which the person has no, or only a few, signs of distress or problems that occur with other types of grief.

- **Chronic grief:** A grief pattern in which the symptoms of common grief last for a much longer time than usual. These symptoms are a lot like ones that occur with major depression, anxiety, or posttraumatic stress.

Factors That Affect Complicated Grief

Researchers study grief reactions to try to find out what might increase the chance that complicated grief will occur.

Studies have looked at how the following factors affect the grief response:

Whether the death is expected or unexpected.

It may seem that any sudden, unexpected loss might lead to more difficult grief. However, studies have found that bereaved people with high self-esteem and/or a feeling that they have control over life are likely to have a normal grief reaction even after an unexpected loss. Bereaved people with low self-esteem and/or a sense that life cannot be controlled are more likely to have complicated grief after an unexpected loss. This includes more depression and physical problems.

The personality of the bereaved.

Studies have found that people with certain personality traits are more likely to have long-lasting depression after a loss. These include people who are very dependent on the loved one (such as a spouse), and people who deal with distress by thinking about it all the time.

The religious beliefs of the bereaved.

Some studies have shown that religion helps people cope better with grief. Other studies have shown it does not help or causes more distress. Religion seems to help people who go to church often. The positive effect on grief may be because church-goers have more social support.

Whether the bereaved is male or female.

In general, men have more problems than women do after a spouse's death. Men tend to have worse depression and more health problems than women do after the loss. Some researchers think this may be because men have less social support after a loss.

The age of the bereaved.

In general, younger bereaved people have more problems after a loss than older bereaved people do. They have more severe health problems, grief symptoms, and other mental and physical symptoms. Younger bereaved people, however, may recover more quickly than older bereaved people do, because they have more resources and social support.

The amount of social support the bereaved has.

Lack of social support increases the chance of having problems coping with a loss. Social support includes the person's family, friends, neighbors, and community members who can give psychological, physical, and financial help. After the death of a close family member, many people have a number of related losses. The death of a spouse, for example, may cause a loss of income and changes in lifestyle and day-to-day living. These are all related to social support.

Treatment of Grief

Normal grief may not need to be treated.

Most bereaved people work through grief and recover within the first 6 months to 2 years. Researchers are studying whether bereaved people experiencing normal grief would be helped by formal treatment. They are also studying whether treatment might prevent complicated grief in people who are likely to have it.

For people who have serious grief reactions or symptoms of distress, treatment may be helpful.

Complicated grief may be treated with different types of psychotherapy (talk therapy).

Researchers are studying the treatment of mental, emotional, social, and behavioral symptoms of grief. Treatment methods include discussion, listening, and counseling.

Complicated grief treatment (CGT) is a type of grief therapy that was helpful in a clinical trial.

Complicated grief treatment (CGT) has three phases:

- The first phase includes talking about the loss and setting goals toward recovery. The bereaved are taught to work on these two things.

- The second phase includes coping with the loss by retelling the story of the death. This helps bereaved people who try not to think about their loss.

- The last phase looks at progress that has been made toward recovery and helps the bereaved make future plans. The bereaved's feelings about ending the sessions are also discussed.

In a clinical trial of patients with complicated grief, CGT was compared to interpersonal psychotherapy (IPT). IPT is a type of psychotherapy that focuses on the person's relationships with others and is helpful in treating depression. In patients with complicated grief, the CGT was more helpful than IPT.

Cognitive behavioral therapy (CBT) for complicated grief was helpful in a clinical trial. Cognitive behavioral therapy (CBT) works with the way a person's thoughts and behaviors are connected. CBT helps the patient learn skills that change attitudes and behaviors by replacing negative thoughts and changing the rewards of certain behaviors. A clinical trial compared CBT to counseling for complicated grief. Results showed that patients treated with CBT had more improvement in symptoms and general mental distress than those in the counseling group.

Depression related to grief is sometimes treated with drugs. There is no standard drug therapy for depression that occurs with grief. Some healthcare professionals think depression is a normal part of grief and doesn't need to be treated. Whether to treat grief-related depression with drugs is up to the patient and the healthcare professional to decide.

Clinical trials of antidepressants for depression related to grief have found that the drugs can help relieve depression. However, they give less relief and take longer to work than they do when used for depression that is not related to grief.

Chapter 61

Coping with the Holiday Blues

Why do people get the holiday blues? Some people feel stressed from being overbooked or left out. Some people worry about affording all the travel and gifts. Others might be facing their first major holiday without a loved one whom they recently lost. There are a million different reasons that holiday stressors can turn into the holiday blues. If you're feeling down this season, here are some simple steps you can take to lift your spirits.

Why Do People Get Holiday Blues and How to Manage Them?

Some people feel stressed from being overbooked or left out. Some people worry about affording all the travel and gifts. Others might be facing their first major holiday without a loved one whom they recently lost. There are a million different reasons that holiday stressors can turn into the holiday blues. If you're feeling down this season, here are some simple steps you can take to lift your spirits.

- **Spend time with people you care about.** I get it—sometimes staying at home is the more appealing option. But spending time with those you care about can help you feel connected to others.

This chapter includes text excerpted from "Beat the Holiday Blues," Office on Women's Health (OWH), U.S. Department of Health and Human Services (HHS), December 11, 2015.

Reach out to the people with whom you can be yourself for one-on-one or small group gatherings. If the people you love don't live nearby, schedule a time for a video call. Just seeing a loved one's smiling face can make a big difference in your mood.

- **Give back.** If you're feeling isolated or lonely, try volunteering in your community. Stock shelves at the local food bank, help out at a nursing home, or spend time at a nearby animal shelter. It feels good to help others, and you might find you have a skill that your community really needs. Plus, volunteering is a great way to surround yourself with other people and take your mind off of your worries for a while.

- **Don't compare yourself to others.** A recent article encouraged people to avoid looking at social media during the holidays. Pictures can be misleading and make it look like people are having a lot more fun than they actually are. Social media allows people to share their best moments, which aren't always an accurate representation of everyday life. Try to remember that your friend with the "perfect" life has bad times, too—they just don't share those pictures.

- **Sweat it out.** You probably see exercise as a must—do on every health—related list you ever read. It's there for a reason. Exercise has a long list of benefits, including helping you deal with stress and anxiety. If it's too cold in your area to enjoy a walk or run, now is a good time to see what workout DVDs are available at your local library. There are smartphone apps that can also guide you through a workout.

- **Get some sun.** For some people, the winter season means seasonal affective disorder (SAD) brought on by lack of sunlight. People with SAD experience many of the same symptoms as people with depression. If you find that you have these kinds of symptoms every year or for months at a time over the winter season, talk to your doctor. People with light to moderate SAD may find relief by spending extra hours outdoors, while people with moderate to severe SAD often benefit from light therapy and/or antidepressants.

- **Have fun without overdoing it.** Enjoying good food and drink is part of what the holidays are all about, but set limits for yourself, especially with alcohol. In the moment, it may seem like a stress reliever, but alcohol is only putting any feelings of stress or anxiety on hold. It doesn't solve any problems, and it can make things worse.

- **Be honest about how you're feeling.** Sometimes the hardest part of this season is thinking you should feel a certain way, even when you don't. Don't force it. When friends or family ask how you're doing, be honest. You never know who else might be feeling the same way.

- **Ask for help.** If there's something your friends and family can do to make the holidays more enjoyable for you, tell them. No one but you knows what you need. But if you feel like you've tried everything and you still feel down, consider getting help from a professional. Talking to a therapist, even for a few weeks, might be just the boost you need to get over your holiday blues and feel yourself again.

The holidays can be stressful under the best of circumstances. My goal every year is to enjoy them for what they are rather than imagining what they should be. And when all else fails, remember that in just a few weeks, the holidays will be over and you'll get a fresh start with a new year!

Chapter 62

Peer Support and Social Inclusion

By sharing their experiences, peers bring hope to people in recovery and promote a sense of belonging within the community.

Peer support services are delivered by individuals who have common life experiences with the people they are serving. People with mental and/or substance use disorders have a unique capacity to help each other based on a shared affiliation and a deep understanding of this experience. In self-help and mutual support, people offer this support, strength, and hope to their peers, which allows for personal growth, wellness promotion, and recovery.

Research has shown that peer support facilitates recovery and reduces healthcare costs. Peers also provide assistance that promotes a sense of belonging within the community. The ability to contribute to and enjoy one's community is key to recovery and well-being. Another critical component that peers provide is the development of self-efficacy through role modeling and assisting peers with ongoing recovery through mastery of experiences and finding meaning, purpose, and social connections in their lives.

Through the Recovery Community Services Program (RCSP), Substance Abuse and Mental Health Services Administration (SAMHSA) recognizes that social support includes informational, emotional,

---

This chapter includes text excerpted from "Peer Support and Social Inclusion," Substance Abuse and Mental Health Services Administration (SAMHSA), July 2, 2015.

and intentional support. Examples of peer recovery support services include:

- **Peer mentoring or coaching**—developing a one-on-one relationship in which a peer leader with recovery experience encourages, motivates, and supports a peer in recovery

- **Peer recovery resource connecting**—connecting the peer with professional and nonprofessional services and resources available in the community

- **Recovery group facilitation**—facilitating or leading recovery-oriented group activities, including support groups and educational activities

- **Building community**—helping peers make new friends and build healthy social networks through emotional, instrumental, informational, and affiliation types of peer support

Community Living and Participation

Recovery for individuals with behavioral health conditions is greatly enhanced by social connection. Yet, many people with mental and/or substance use disorders are not fully engaged in their communities either through personal relationships, social events, or civic activities. Unfortunately, many individuals often remain socially isolated and excluded. Negative perceptions, prejudice, and discrimination contribute to the social exclusion of people living with behavioral health disorders.

People living with mental and/or substance use conditions can increase social connections greatly when they have access to recovery-oriented services and establish positive relationships with family and friends. Greater social connections lead to improved economic, educational, recreational, and cultural opportunities that are generally available.

In a socially inclusive society, people in recovery have the opportunity and necessary supports to contribute to their community as citizens, parents, employees, students, volunteers, and leaders. Prevention activities help create communities in which people have an improved quality of life that includes healthier environments at work and in school, and supportive neighborhoods and work environments. Social connections and understanding also help people in recovery from addictions benefit from alcohol- and tobacco-free activities in the community.

Part Eight

Suicide

Chapter 63

Understanding Suicide

Suicide is when people direct violence at themselves with the intent to end their lives, and they die as a result of their actions. Suicide is a leading cause of death in the United States. A suicide attempt is when people harm themselves with the intent to end their lives, but they do not die as a result of their actions. Many more people survive suicide attempts than die, but they often have serious injuries. However, a suicide attempt does not always result in a physical injury.

Why Is Suicide a Public Health Problem?

Suicide is a significant problem in the United States:

- 41,149 people killed themselves in 2013.

- Over 494,169 people with self-inflicted injuries were treated in U.S. emergency departments in 2013.

- Suicides result in an estimated $44.6 billion in combined medical and work loss costs.

These numbers underestimate this problem. Many people who have suicidal thoughts or make suicide attempts never seek services.

How Does Suicide Affect Health?

Suicide, by definition, is fatal and is a problem throughout the lifespan. In 2013, suicide was the second leading cause of death among

This chapter includes text excerpted from "Understanding Suicide," Centers for Disease Control and Prevention (CDC), June 15, 2015.

persons aged 15–24 years, the second among persons aged 25–34 years, the fourth among person aged 35–54 years, the eighth among persons aged 55–64 years, the seventeenth among persons 65 years and older, and the tenth leading cause of death across all ages.

People who attempt suicide and survive may experience serious injuries, such as broken bones, brain damage, or organ failure. These injuries may have long-term effects on their health. People who survive suicide attempts may also have depression and other mental health problems.

Suicide also affects the health of others and the community. When people die by suicide, their family and friends often experience shock, anger, guilt, and depression. The medical costs and lost wages associated with suicide also take their toll on the community.

Who Is at Risk for Suicide?

There is no single cause of suicide. Several factors can increase a person's risk for attempting or dying by suicide. However, having these risk factors does not always mean that suicide will occur. Risk factors for suicide include:

- Previous suicide attempt(s)
- History of depression or other mental illness
- Alcohol or drug abuse
- Family history of suicide or violence
- Physical illness
- Feeling alone

Suicide affects everyone, but some groups are at higher risk than others. Men are about four times more likely than women to die from suicide. However, women are more likely to express suicidal thoughts and to make nonfatal attempts than men. The prevalence of suicidal thoughts, suicide planning, and suicide attempts is significantly higher among young adults aged 18–29 years than it is among adults aged ≥30 years. Other groups with higher rates of suicidal behavior include American Indian and Alaska Natives, rural populations, and active or retired military personnel.

How Can We Prevent Suicide?

Suicide is a significant public health problem, and there is a lot to learn about how to prevent it. One strategy is to learn about the warning signs of suicide, which can include individuals talking about wanting to hurt themselves, increasing substance use, and having changes in their mood, diet, or sleeping patterns. When these warning signs appear, quickly connecting the person to supportive services is critical. Promoting opportunities and settings that strengthen connections among people, families, and communities is another suicide prevention goal.

Chapter 64

Suicide in the United States

Suicide Statistics

- Suicide was the tenth leading cause of death for all ages in 2013.

- There were 41,149 suicides in 2013 in the United States—a rate of 12.6 per 100,000 is equal to 113 suicides each day or one every 13 minutes.

- Based on data about suicides in 16 National Violent Death Reporting System (NVDRS) states in 2010, 33.4% of suicide decedents tested positive for alcohol, 23.8% for antidepressants, and 20.0% for opiates, including heroin and prescription painkillers.

- Suicide results in an estimated $51 billion in combined medical and work loss costs.

Nonfatal Suicidal Thoughts and Behavior

- Among adults aged ≥18 years in the United States during 2013:

    - An estimated 9.3 million adults (3.9% of the adult U.S. population) reported having suicidal thoughts in the past year.

    - The percentage of adults having serious thoughts about suicide was highest among adults aged 18 to 25 (7.4%), followed

This chapter includes text excerpted from "Suicide," Centers for Disease Control and Prevention (CDC), September 11, 2015.

by adults aged 26 to 49 (4.0%), then by adults aged 50 or older (2.7%).

- An estimated 2.7 million people (1.1%) made a plan about how they would attempt suicide in the past year.

- The percentage of adults who made a suicide plan in the past year was higher among adults aged 18 to 25 (2.5%) than among adults aged 26 to 49 (1.35%) and those aged 50 or older (0.6%).

- An estimated 1.3 million adults aged 18 or older (0.6%) attempted suicide in the past year. Among these adults who attempted suicide, 1.1 million also reported making suicide plans (0.2 million did not make suicide plans).

Among students in grades 9–12 in the United States during 2013:

- 17.0% of students seriously considered attempting suicide in the previous 12 months (22.4% of females and 11.6% of males).

- 13.6% of students made a plan about how they would attempt suicide in the previous 12 months (16.9% of females and 10.3% of males).

- 8.0% of students attempted suicide one or more times in the previous 12 months (10.6% of females and 5.4% of males).

- 2.7% of students made a suicide attempt that resulted in an injury, poisoning, or an overdose that required medical attention (3.6% of females and 1.8% of males).

Gender Disparities

- Males take their own lives at nearly four times the rate of females and represent 77.9% of all suicides.

- Females are more likely than males to have suicidal thoughts.

- Suicide is the seventh leading cause of death for males and the fourteenth leading cause for females.

- Firearms are the most commonly used method of suicide among males (56.9%).

- Poisoning is the most common method of suicide for females (34.8%).

Racial and Ethnic Disparities

- Suicide is the eighth leading cause of death among American Indians/Alaska Natives across all ages.

- Among American Indians/Alaska Natives aged 10 to 34 years, suicide is the second leading cause of death.

- The suicide rate among American Indian/Alaska Native adolescents and young adults ages 15 to 34 (19.5 per 100,000) is 1.5 times higher than the national average for that age group (12.9 per 100,000).

- The percentages of adults aged 18 or older having suicidal thoughts in the previous 12 months were 2.9% among blacks, 3.3% among Asians, 3.6% among Hispanics, 4.1% among whites, 4.6% among Native Hawaiians /Other Pacific Islanders, 4.8% among American Indians/Alaska Natives, and 7.9% among adults reporting two or more races.

- Among Hispanic students in grades 9–12, the prevalence of having seriously considered attempting suicide (18.9%), having made a plan about how they would attempt suicide (15.7%), having attempted suicide (11.3%), and having made a suicide attempt that resulted in an injury, poisoning, or overdose that required medical attention (4.1%) was consistently higher than white and black students.

Age Group Differences

- Suicide is the third leading cause of death among persons aged 10–14, the second among persons aged 15–34 years, the fourth among persons aged 35–44 years, the fifth among persons aged 45–54 years, the eighth among person 55–64 years, and the seventeenth among persons 65 years and older.

- In 2011, middle-aged adults accounted for the largest proportion of suicides (56%), and from 1999–2010, the suicide rate among this group increased by nearly 30%.

- Among adults aged 18–22 years, similar percentages of full-time college students and other adults in this age group had suicidal thoughts (8.0 and 8.7%, respectively) or made suicide plans (2.4 and 3.1%).

- Full-time college students aged 18–22 years were less likely to attempt suicide (0.9 vs. 1.9 percent) or receive medical attention as a result of a suicide attempt in the previous 12 months (0.3 vs. 0.7%).

Nonfatal, Self-Inflicted Injuries

- In 2013, 494,169 people were treated in emergency departments for self-inflicted injuries.

- Nonfatal, self-inflicted injuries (including hospitalized and emergency department treated and released) resulted in an estimated $10.4 billion in combined medical and work loss costs.

Chapter 65

Suicidal Behavior, Risk, and Protective Factors

Suicidal Behavior[1]

Suicide causes immeasurable pain, suffering, and loss to individuals, families, and communities nationwide. On average, 112 Americans die by suicide each day. Suicide is the second leading cause of death among 15–24 year olds and more than 9.4 million adults in the United States had serious thoughts of suicide within the past 12 months. But suicide is preventable, so it's important to know what to do.

Risk Factors for Suicide[2]

A combination of individual, relationship, community, and societal factors contribute to the risk of suicide. Risk factors are those characteristics associated with suicide—they might not be direct causes.

- Family history of suicide
- Family history of child maltreatment

This chapter includes text excerpted from documents published by two public domain sources. Text under headings marked 1 are excerpted from "Suicidal Behavior," MentalHealth.gov, U.S. Department of Health and Human Services (HHS), October 11, 2015; Text under headings marked 2 are excerpted from "Suicide: Risk and Protective Factors," Centers for Disease Control and Prevention (CDC), August 15, 2016.

- Previous suicide attempt(s)
- History of mental disorders, particularly clinical depression
- History of alcohol and substance abuse
- Feelings of hopelessness
- Impulsive or aggressive tendencies
- Cultural and religious beliefs (e.g., belief that suicide is noble resolution of a personal dilemma)
- Local epidemics of suicide
- Isolation, a feeling of being cut off from other people
- Barriers to accessing mental health treatment
- Loss (relational, social, work, or financial)
- Physical illness
- Easy access to lethal methods
- Unwillingness to seek help because of the stigma attached to mental health and substance abuse disorders or to suicidal thoughts

Warning Signs of Suicide[1]

If someone you know is showing one or more of the following behaviors, he or she may be thinking about suicide. Don't ignore these warning signs. Get help immediately.

- Talking about wanting to die or to kill oneself
- Looking for a way to kill oneself
- Talking about feeling hopeless or having no reason to live
- Talking about feeling trapped or in unbearable pain
- Talking about being a burden to others
- Increasing the use of alcohol or drugs
- Acting anxious or agitated; behaving recklessly
- Sleeping too little or too much
- Withdrawing or feeling isolated
- Showing rage or talking about seeking revenge

- Displaying extreme mood swings

Protective Factors for Suicide[2]

Protective factors buffer individuals from suicidal thoughts and behavior. To date, protective factors have not been studied as extensively or rigorously as risk factors. Identifying and understanding protective factors are, however, equally as important as researching risk factors.

- Effective clinical care for mental, physical, and substance abuse disorders
- Easy access to a variety of clinical interventions and support for help seeking
- Family and community support (connectedness)
- Support from ongoing medical and mental healthcare relationships
- Skills in problem solving, conflict resolution, and nonviolent ways of handling disputes
- Cultural and religious beliefs that discourage suicide and support instincts for self-preservation

Chapter 66

Relationship between Posttraumatic Stress Disorder (PTSD) and Suicide

This chapter explores the relation between posttraumatic stress disorder (PTSD) and suicide and provides information that helps with understanding suicide.

How Common Is Suicide?

It is challenging to determine an exact number of suicides. Many times, suicides are not reported and it can be very difficult to determine whether or not a particular individual's death was intentional. For a suicide to be recognized, examiners must be able to say that the deceased meant to die. Other factors that contribute to the difficulty are differences among states as to who is mandated to report a death, as well as changes over time in the coding of mortality data.

Data from the National Vital Statistics System (NVSS), a collaboration between the National Center for Health Statistics (NCHS) of the U.S. Department of Health and Human Services (HHS) and each U.S. state, provides the best estimate of suicides. Overall, men have significantly higher rates of suicide than women. This is true whether or not they are Veterans. For comparison: From 1999–2010, the suicide

This chapter includes text excerpted from "The Relationship between PTSD and Suicide," U.S. Department of Veterans Affairs (VA), July 7, 2016.

rate in the U.S. population among males was 19.4 per 100,000, compared to 4.9 per 100,000 in females. Based on the most recent data available, in fiscal year 2009, the suicide rate among male Veteran VA users was 38.3 per 100,000, compared to 12.8 per 100,000 in females.

Does Trauma Increase an Individual's Suicide Risk?

A body of research indicates that there is a correlation between many types of trauma and suicidal behaviors. For example, there is evidence that traumatic events such as childhood abuse may increase a person's suicide risk. A history of military sexual trauma (MST) also increases the risk for suicide and intentional self-harm, suggesting a need to screen for suicide risk in this population.

Does PTSD Increase an Individual's Suicide Risk?

Considerable debate exists about the reason for the heightened risk of suicide in trauma survivors. Whereas some studies suggest that suicide risk is higher among those who experienced trauma due to the symptoms of PTSD, others claim that suicide risk is higher in these individuals because of related psychiatric conditions. However, a study analyzing data from the National Comorbidity Survey, a nationally representative sample, showed that PTSD alone out of six anxiety diagnoses was significantly associated with suicidal ideation or attempts. While the study also found an association between suicidal behaviors and both mood disorders and antisocial personality disorder, the findings pointed to a robust relationship between PTSD and suicide after controlling for comorbid disorders.

A later study using the Canadian Community Health Survey data also found that respondents with PTSD were at higher risk for suicide attempts after controlling for physical illness and other mental disorders. Some studies that point to PTSD as a precipitating factor of suicide suggest that high levels of intrusive memories can predict the relative risk of suicide. Anger and impulsivity have also been shown to predict suicide risk in those with PTSD. Further, some cognitive styles of coping such as using suppression to deal with stress may be additionally predictive of suicide risk in individuals with PTSD.

Can PTSD Treatment Help?

Current practice guidelines for treatment of PTSD indicate that trauma-focused therapies are not recommended for individuals with "significant suicidality". Because "suicidality" is a vague term and there is no guidance for what significant suicidality means, we interpret this recommendation to pertain to actively suicidal patients, or those in an acute clinical emergency for whom suicidality should be addressed without delay. Providers must therefore use clinical judgment prior to initiating and throughout trauma-focused therapy.

Individuals with PTSD who present with intermittent but manageable suicidal thoughts may benefit from trauma-focused therapy. Two effective treatments for PTSD, cognitive processing therapy (CPT) and prolonged exposure (PE) have been shown to reduce suicidal ideation. A recent study that randomized women who experienced rape into CPT or PE treatment found that reductions in PTSD symptoms were associated with decreases in suicidal ideation throughout treatment. The reductions were maintained over a 5–10 year follow-up period. The effect of PTSD treatment on suicidal ideation was greater for women who completed CPT. Further research is needed to provide additional evidence in other populations.

Suicide as a Traumatic Event

Researchers have also examined exposure to suicide as a traumatic event. Studies show that trauma from exposure to suicide can contribute to PTSD. In particular, adults and adolescents are more likely to develop PTSD as a result of exposure to suicide if one or more of the following conditions are true: if they witness the suicide, if they are very connected with the person who dies, or if they have a history of psychiatric illness. Studies also show that traumatic grief is more likely to arise after exposure to traumatic death such as suicide. Traumatic grief refers to a syndrome in which individuals experience functional impairment, a decline in physical health, and suicidal ideation. These symptoms occur independently of other conditions such as depression and anxiety.

To help prevent suicide. Know about the suicide warning signs and the National Suicide Prevention Lifeline: 1-800-273-TALK (1-800-273-8255). To be routed to the Veterans Crisis Line, dial 1 after being connected.

You can also. While helping a suicidal person can be a difficult process, remember that the assistance you provide could save someone's life. If you think someone may be suicidal, you should directly ask him or her. Contrary to popular belief, asking someone if they are suicidal will not put the idea in their head.

Often the most difficult part of obtaining treatment is the initial call to a mental health professional. It is usually easier for a suicidal individual to accept professional help if they have assistance with this part of the process.

Chapter 67

Suicide among Youth and Older Adults

Chapter Contents

Section 67.1

Teen Suicide

Ethan felt like there was no point going on with life. Things had been tough since his mom died. His dad was working two jobs and seemed frazzled and angry most of the time. Whenever he and Ethan talked, it usually ended in yelling.

Ethan had just found out he'd failed a math test, and he was afraid of how mad and disappointed his dad would be. In the past, he always talked things over with his girlfriend—the only person who seemed to understand. But they'd broken up the week before, and now Ethan felt he had nowhere to turn.

Ethan knew where his dad kept his guns. But as he was unlocking the cabinet, he heard his kid sister arriving home from school. He didn't want Grace to be the person to find him, so he put the gun back and went to watch TV with her instead.

Later, when he realized how close he'd come to ending his life, Ethan was terrified. He summoned the courage to talk to his dad. After a long conversation, he realized how much his dad cared. All he could think of was how he'd almost thrown it all away.

Why Do Teens Try to Kill Themselves?

Most teens interviewed after making a suicide attempt say that they did it because they were trying to escape from a situation that seemed impossible to deal with or to get relief from really bad thoughts or feelings. Like Ethan, they didn't want to die as much as they wanted to escape from what was going on. And at that particular moment dying seemed like the only way out.Some people who end their lives or attempt suicide might be trying to escape feelings of rejection, hurt, or loss. Others might feel angry, ashamed, or guilty about something. Some people may be worried about disappointing friends or family members. And some may feel unwanted, unloved, victimized, or like they're a burden to others.

We all feel overwhelmed by difficult emotions or situations sometimes. But most people get through it or can put their problems in perspective and find a way to carry on with determination and hope. So why does one person try suicide when another person in the same tough situation does not? What makes some people more resilient (better able to deal with life's setbacks and difficulties) than others? What makes a person unable to see another way out of a bad situation besides ending his or her life? The answer to those questions lies in the fact that most people who commit suicide have depression.

Depression

Depression leads people to focus mostly on failures and disappointments, to emphasize the negative side of their situations, and to downplay their own capabilities or worth. Someone with severe depression is unable to see the possibility of a good outcome and may believe they will never be happy or things will never go right for them again. Depression affects a person's thoughts in such a way that the person doesn't see when a problem can be overcome. It's as if the depression puts a filter on the person's thinking that distorts things. That's why depressed people don't realize that suicide is a permanent solution to a temporary problem in the same way that other people do. A teen with depression may feel like there's no other way out of problems, no other escape from emotional pain, or no other way to communicate a desperate unhappiness.

Sometimes people who feel suicidal may not even realize they are depressed. They're unaware that it is the depression—not the situation—that's influencing them to see things in a "there's no way out," "it will never get better," "there's nothing I can do" kind of way. When depression lifts because someone gets the proper therapy or treatment, the distorted thinking is cleared. The person can find pleasure, energy, and hope again. But while someone is seriously depressed, suicidal thinking is a real concern. People with a condition called bipolar disorder are also more at risk for suicide because their condition can cause them to go through times when they are extremely depressed as well as times when they have abnormally high or frantic energy (called mania or manic). Both of these extreme phases of bipolar disorder affect and distort a person's mood, outlook, and judgment. For people with this condition, it can be a challenge to keep problems in perspective and act with good judgment.

493

Substance Abuse

Teens with alcohol and drug problems are also more at risk for suicidal thinking and behavior. Alcohol and some drugs have depressive effects on the brain. Misuse of these substances can bring on serious depression. That's especially true for some teens who already have a tendency to depression because of their biology, family history, or other life stressors. The problem can be made worse because many people who are depressed turn to alcohol or drugs as an escape. But they may not realize that the depressive effects alcohol and drugs have on the brain can actually intensify depression in the long run.

In addition to their depressive effects, alcohol and drugs alter a person's judgment. They interfere with the ability to assess risk, make good choices, and think of solutions to problems. Many suicide attempts occur when someone is under the influence of alcohol or drugs.

This doesn't mean that everyone who is depressed or who has an alcohol or drug problem will try to kill themselves, of course. But these conditions—especially both together—increase a person's risk for suicide.

Suicide Is Not Always Planned

Sometimes a depressed person plans a suicide in advance. Many times, though, suicide attempts happen impulsively, in a moment of feeling desperately upset. A situation like a breakup, a big fight with a parent, an unintended pregnancy, being outed by someone else, or being victimized in any way can cause someone to feel desperately upset. Often, a situation like this, on top of an existing depression, acts like the final straw. Some people who attempt suicide mean to die and some aren't completely sure they want to die. For some, a suicide attempt is a way to express deep emotional pain. They can't say how they feel, so, for them, attempting suicide feels like the only way to get their message across. Sadly, many people who really didn't mean to kill themselves end up dead or critically ill.

Warning Signs

There are often signs that someone may be thinking about or planning a suicide attempt. Here are some of them:

- talking about suicide or death in general
- talking about "going away"

- referring to things they "won't be needing," and giving away possessions
- talking about feeling hopeless or feeling guilty
- pulling away from friends or family and losing the desire to go out
- having no desire to take part in favorite things or activities
- having trouble concentrating or thinking clearly
- experiencing changes in eating or sleeping habits
- engaging in self-destructive behavior (drinking alcohol, taking drugs, or cutting, for example)

What If This Is You?

If you have been thinking about suicide, get help now. Depression is powerful. You can't wait and hope that your mood might improve. When a person has been feeling down for a long time, it's hard to step back and be objective.

Talk to someone you trust as soon as you can. If you can't talk to a parent, talk to a coach, a relative, a school counselor, a religious leader, or a teacher. Call a suicide crisis line (such as 1-800-SUICIDE) or your local emergency number (911).

These toll-free lines are staffed 24 hours a day, 7 days a week by trained professionals who can help you without ever knowing your name or seeing your face. All calls are confidential—no one you know will find out that you've called. They are there to help you figure out how to work through tough situations.

What If It's Someone You Know?

It is always a good thing to start a conversation with someone you think may be considering suicide. It allows you to get help for the person, and just talking about it may help the person to feel less alone and more cared about and understood.Talking things through also may give the person an opportunity to consider other solutions to problems. Most of the time, people who are considering suicide are willing to talk if someone asks them out of concern and care. Because people who are depressed are not as able to see answers as well as others, it can help to have someone work with them in coming up with at least one other way out of a bad situation.

Even if a friend or classmate swears you to secrecy, you must get help as soon as possible—your friend's life could depend on it. Someone who is seriously thinking about suicide may have sunk so deeply into an emotional hole that the person could be unable to recognize that he or she needs help. Tell an adult you trust as soon as possible. If necessary, you can also call a suicide crisis line (such as 1-800-SUICIDE) or your local emergency number (911). These are confidential resources and the people at any of these places are happy to talk to you to help you figure out what to do.

Sometimes, teens who make a suicide attempt—or who die as a result of suicide—seem to give no clue beforehand. This can leave loved ones feeling not only grief stricken but guilty and wondering if they missed something. It is important for family members and friends of those who die by suicide to know that sometimes there is no warning and they should not blame themselves. When someone dies by suicide, the people left behind can wrestle with a terrible emotional pain. Teens who have had a recent loss or crisis or who had a family member or classmate who committed suicide may be especially vulnerable to suicidal thinking and behavior themselves.

If you've been close to someone who has attempted or committed suicide, it can help to talk with a therapist or counselor—someone who is trained in dealing with this complex issue. Or, you could join a group for survivors where you can share your feelings and get the support of people who have been in the same situation as you.

Coping with Problems

Being a teen is not easy. There are many new social, academic, and personal pressures. And for teens who have additional problems to deal with, such as living in violent or abusive environments, life can feel even more difficult. Some teens worry about sexuality and relationships, wondering if their feelings and attractions are normal, or if they will be loved and accepted. Others struggle with body image and eating problems; trying to reach an impossible ideal leaves them feeling bad about themselves.

Some teens have learning problems or attention problems that make it hard for them to succeed in school. They may feel disappointed in themselves or feel they are a disappointment to others. These problems can be difficult and draining—and can lead to depression if they go on too long without relief or support. We all struggle with painful problems and events at times. How do people get through it without becoming depressed? Part of it is staying connected to family, friends, school, faith, and other support networks.

People are better able to deal with tough circumstances when they have at least one person who believes in them, wants the best for them, and in whom they can confide. People also cope better when they keep in mind that most problems are temporary and can be overcome.

When struggling with problems, it helps to:

- Tell someone you trust what's going on with you.

- Be around people who are caring and positive.

- Ask someone to help you figure out what to do about a problem you're facing.

- Work with a therapist or counselor if problems are getting you down and depressed—or if you don't have a strong support network or feel you can't cope.

Counselors and therapists can provide emotional support and can help teens build their own coping skills for dealing with problems. It can also help to join a support network for people who are going through the same problems—for example, anorexia and body image issues, living with an alcoholic family member, or sexuality and sexual health concerns. These groups can help provide a caring environment where you can talk through problems with people who share your concerns. Check your phone book or look online to find local support groups, or ask a school counselor or a youth group leader to help you find what you need.

Section 67.2

Suicide among Young Adults

This section contains text excerpted from the following sources: Text beginning with the heading "Youth Suicide" is excerpted from "Violence Prevention," Centers for Disease Control and Prevention (CDC), March 10, 2015; Text under the heading "Maintain Mental Health" is excerpted from "College Health and Safety," Centers for Disease Control and Prevention (CDC), August 9, 2016.

Youth Suicide

Suicide (i.e., taking one's own life) is a serious public health problem that affects even young people. For youth between the ages of 10 and 24, suicide is the third leading cause of death. It results in approximately 4600 lives lost each year. The top three methods used in suicides of young people include firearm (45%), suffocation (40%), and poisoning (8%).

Deaths from youth suicide are only part of the problem. More young people survive suicide attempts than actually die. A nationwide survey of youth in grades 9–12 in public and private schools in the U.S. found that 16% of students reported seriously considering suicide, 13% reported creating a plan, and 8% reporting trying to take their own life in the 12 months preceding the survey. Each year, approximately 157,000 youth between the ages of 10 and 24 receive medical care for self-inflicted injuries at Emergency Departments across the United States.

Suicide affects all youth, but some groups are at higher risk than others. Boys are more likely than girls to die from suicide. Of the reported suicides in the 10 to 24 age group, 81% of the deaths were males and 19% were females. Girls, however, are more likely to report attempting suicide than boys. Cultural variations in suicide rates also exist, with Native American/Alaskan Native youth having the highest rates of suicide-related fatalities. A nationwide survey of youth in grades 9–12 in public and private schools in the United States found Hispanic youth were more likely to report attempting suicide than their black and white, non-Hispanic peers.

Several factors can put a young person at risk for suicide. However, having these risk factors does not always mean that suicide will occur.

Risk factors:

- History of previous suicide attempts
- Family history of suicide
- History of depression or other mental illness
- Alcohol or drug abuse
- Stressful life event or loss
- Easy access to lethal methods
- Exposure to the suicidal behavior of others
- Incarceration

Most people are uncomfortable with the topic of suicide. Too often, victims are blamed, and their families and friends are left stigmatized. As a result, people do not communicate openly about suicide. Thus an important public health problem is left shrouded in secrecy, which limits the amount of information available to those working to prevent suicide.

The good news is that research over the last several decades has uncovered a wealth of information on the causes of suicide and on prevention strategies.

Maintain Your Mental Health

Anxiety is a normal reaction to stress, and can help you deal with a tense situation, study harder for an exam, or keep your focus during an important speech. But if you cannot shake your worries and concerns, or if the feelings make you want to avoid everyday activities, you may have an anxiety disorder. Everybody has the blues, feels anxious, or gets stressed at times. But depression is more than a bad day. Depression often goes unrecognized and untreated and may lead to tragic results, such as suicide. For youth between ages 10 and 24, suicide is the third leading cause of death. Suicide is a serious—but preventable—problem that can have lasting harmful effects on individuals, families, and communities.

Quick tips

- Develop a support network of friends. Campus and extracurricular activities such as athletics and student clubs are great ways to meet new friends.

- If you have concerns about your study habits or coursework load, talk with teachers, counselors, family members, and friends for advice and support.

- Stay active. Regular physical activity can help keep your thinking, learning, and judgment skills sharp. It can also reduce your risk for depression, and it may help you sleep better.

- Visit your school or local health clinic, and discuss your concerns with a health professional. If the health professional advises treatment, follow instructions. Attend follow-up appointments to track your progress, and watch for side effects from any medications that may be prescribed.

- If you or someone you know is thinking about suicide, get help from a counselor or healthcare provider. Call the national suicide hotline at 1-800-273-TALK (8255).

Section 67.3

Older Adults: Depression and Suicide Facts

This section includes text excerpted from "Older Adults and Depression," National Institute of Mental Health (NIMH), September 10, 2016.

- Do you feel very tired, helpless, and hopeless?

- Have you lost interest in many of the activities and interests you previously enjoyed?

- Are you having trouble working, sleeping, eating, and functioning?

- Have you felt this way day after day?

- If you answered yes, you may be experiencing depression.

As you get older, you may go through a lot of changes—death of loved ones, retirement, stressful life events, or medical problems. It's normal to feel uneasy, stressed, or sad about these changes. But after adjusting, many older adults feel well again.

Depression is different. It is a medical condition that interferes with daily life and normal functioning. It is not a normal part of aging, a sign of weakness, or a character flaw. Many older adults with depression need treatment to feel better.

Types of Depression

There are several types of depression. The most common include:

- **Major Depression**—severe symptoms that interfere with your ability to work, sleep, concentrate, eat, and enjoy life. Some people may experience only a single episode within their lifetime, but more often, a person may experience multiple episodes.

- **Persistent Depressive Disorder (Dysthymia)**—depression symptoms that are less severe than those of major depression, but last a long time (at least two years).

- **Minor Depression**—depression symptoms that are less severe than those of major depression and dysthymia, and symptoms do not last long.

Do You Know the Signs?

Depression may sometimes be undiagnosed or misdiagnosed in some older adults because sadness is not their main symptom. They may have other, less obvious symptoms of depression or they may not be willing to talk about their feelings. It is important to know the signs and seek help if you are concerned.

Depression has many symptoms, including physical ones. If you have been experiencing several of the following symptoms for at least two weeks, you may be suffering from depression:

- Persistent sad, anxious, or "empty" mood

- Loss of interest or pleasure in hobbies and activities

- Feelings of hopelessness, pessimism

- Feelings of guilt, worthlessness, helplessness

- Decreased energy, fatigue, being "slowed down"

- Difficulty concentrating, remembering, making decisions
- Difficulty sleeping, early-morning awakening, or oversleeping
- Appetite and/or unintended weight changes
- Thoughts of death or suicide, suicide attempts
- Restlessness, irritability
- Aches or pains, headaches, cramps, or digestive problems without a clear physical cause and/or that do not ease even with treatment

Risk Factors

Although most cases of depression are diagnosed in young adults, depression can occur at any age. Certain people are at a higher risk for developing depression. If you are an older adult, you may be at a higher risk if you:

- are female
- have a chronic medical illness, such as cancer, diabetes or heart disease
- have a disability
- sleep poorly
- are lonely or socially isolated

You may also be at a higher risk if you:
- have a personal or family history of depression
- use certain medications
- suffer from a brain disease
- misuse alcohol or drugs
- have experienced stressful life events such as loss of a spouse, divorce, or taking care of someone with a chronic illness

How Do I Get Help?

If you think that you or a loved one may have depression, it is important to seek treatment. A person with depression cannot simply "snap out of it"—it is a medical condition that affects your quality of life. Depression can also lead to suicide, particularly if left untreated, and you are more likely to develop a physical illness if you have depression.

The good news is that, in most cases, depression is treatable in older adults. The right treatment may help improve your overall health and quality of life. With the right treatment, you may begin to see improvements as early as two weeks from the start of your therapy. Some symptoms may start to improve within a week or two, but it may be several weeks before you feel the full effect.

Talking to Your Doctor

If you think you have depression, the first step is to talk to your doctor or healthcare provider. Your doctor will review your medical history and do a physical exam to rule out other conditions that may be causing or contributing to your depression symptoms. He or she may also ask you a series of questions about how you're feeling. It is important to be open and honest about your symptoms, even if you feel embarrassed or shy.

If other factors can be ruled out, the doctor may refer you to a mental health professional, such as a psychologist, counselor, social worker, or psychiatrist. Some providers are specially trained to treat depression and other emotional problems in older adults.

Chapter 68

Warning Signs of Suicide and How to Deal with It

Chapter Contents

Section 68.1

Warning Signs of Suicide

Text in this section is excerpted from "My Friend Is
Talking about Suicide," © 1995–2016. The Nemours
Foundation/KidsHealth®. Reprinted with permission.

Everyone feels sad, depressed, or angry sometimes—especially when dealing with the pressures of school, friends, and family. But some people may feel sadness or hopelessness that just won't go away, and even small problems may seem like too much to handle.

Depression can affect many areas of a person's life and outlook. Someone who has very intense feelings of depression, emotional pain, or irritability may begin to think about suicide.

You may have heard that people who talk about suicide won't actually go through with it. **That's not true. People who talk about suicide may be likely to try it.**

Other warning signs that someone may be thinking of suicide include:

- talking about suicide or death in general

- talking about "going away"

- talking about feeling hopeless or feeling guilty

- pulling away from friends or family and losing the desire to go out

- having no desire to take part in favorite activities

- having trouble concentrating or thinking clearly

- experiencing changes in eating or sleeping habits

- engaging in self-destructive behavior (drinking alcohol, taking drugs, or driving too fast, for example)

As a friend, you may also know if the person is going through some tough times. Sometimes, a specific event, stress, or crisis—like a relationship breaking up or a death in the family—can trigger suicidal behavior in someone who is already feeling depressed and showing the warning signs listed above.

What You Can Do

Ask

If you have a friend who is talking about suicide or showing other warning signs, don't wait to see if he or she starts to feel better. Talk about it. Most of the time, people who are considering suicide are willing to discuss it if someone asks them out of concern and care.

Some people (both teens and adults) are reluctant to ask teens if they have been thinking about suicide or hurting themselves. That's because they're afraid that, by asking, they may plant the idea of suicide. This is not true. It is always a good thing to ask.

Starting the conversation with someone you think may be considering suicide helps in many ways. First, it allows you to get help for the person. Second, just talking about it may help the person to feel less alone, less isolated, and more cared about and understood—the opposite of the feelings that may have led to suicidal thinking to begin with. Third, talking may provide a chance to consider that there may be another solution.

Asking someone if he or she is having thoughts about suicide can be difficult. Sometimes it helps to let your friend know why you are asking. For instance, you might say, "I've noticed that you've been talking a lot about wanting to be dead. Have you been having thoughts about trying to kill yourself?"

Listen

Listen to your friend without judging and offer reassurance that you're there and you care. If you think your friend is in immediate danger, stay close—make sure he or she isn't left alone.

Tell

Even if you're sworn to secrecy and you feel like you'll be betraying your friend if you tell, you should still get help. Share your concerns with an adult you trust as soon as possible. You can also call the toll-free number for a suicide crisis line (like 1-800-SUICIDE) or a local emergency number (911).

The important thing is to notify a responsible adult. Although it may be tempting to try to help your friend on your own, it's always safest to get help.

After Suicide

Sometimes even if you get help and adults intervene, a friend or classmate may attempt or die by suicide. When this happens, it's common to have many different emotions. Some teens say they feel guilty—especially if they felt they could have interpreted their friend's actions and words better. Others say they feel angry with the person for doing something so selfish. Still others say they feel nothing at all—they are too filled with grief to process their emotions.

When someone attempts suicide, those who know that person may feel afraid or uncomfortable about talking to him or her. Try to overcome these feelings of discomfort—this is a time when someone absolutely needs to feel connected to others.

If you are having difficulty dealing with a friend or classmate's suicide, it's best to talk to an adult you trust. Feeling grief after a friend dies by suicide is normal. But if that sadness begins to interfere with your everyday life, it's a sign that you may need to speak with someone about your feelings.

Section 68.2

Preventing Suicide

This section contains text excerpted from the following sources:
Text in this section begins with excerpts from "Preventing Suicide,"
Centers for Disease Control and Prevention (CDC), September 9,
2016; Text under the heading "How You Can Help" is excerpted
from "Suicide Prevention," Substance and Mental Health Services
Administration (SAMHSA), October 29, 2015; Text under the
heading "Five Action Steps for Helping Someone in Emotional Pain"
is excerpted from "Suicide Prevention," National Institute of Mental
Health (NIMH), August 2016.

Suicide can be prevented. In 2014, more than 42,000 Americans took their own lives and almost half a million Americans received medical care for self-inflicted injuries. September 10th is World Suicide Prevention Day, and the entire month is dedicated to suicide prevention awareness in the United States. Help prevent suicide in your community by knowing the facts, warning signs, and where to get help. Suicide is a serious public health problem that affects people of all ages. It is the tenth leading cause of death for Americans. The top three methods used in suicides include firearms (49.9%), suffocation (26.7%), and poisoning (15.9%).

Deaths from suicide are only part of the problem. Many more people survive suicide attempts than actually die. In 2014, nearly half a million people (469,096) received medical care for self-inflicted injuries at emergency departments across the United States. More than one million adults self-reported a suicide attempt, and 9.4 million adults self-reported serious thoughts of suicide. People rarely communicate openly about suicide, which hinders effective prevention. Suicide is often the result of multiple risk factors. Having these risk factors, however, does not mean that suicide will occur. Some of the risk factors researchers identified include the following:

- History of previous suicide attempts

- Family history of suicide

- History of depression or other mental illness

- History of alcohol or drug abuse

- Stressful life event or loss (e.g., job, financial, relationship)

- Easy access to lethal methods

- History of interpersonal violence

- Stigma associated with mental illness and help-seeking

Protective factors buffer individuals from suicidal thoughts and behavior. Some of the protective factors researchers identified are listed below:

- Skills in problem solving, conflict resolution, and nonviolent ways of handling disputes

- Effective clinical care for mental, physical, and substance abuse disorders

- Easy access to various clinical interventions and support

- Family and community support (connectedness)

- Cultural or religious beliefs that discourage suicide and support seeking help

Many people are uncomfortable with the topic of suicide. Too often, victims are blamed and their families and friends are left stigmatized. As a result, people rarely communicate openly about suicide. Thus, an important public health problem is left hidden in secrecy, which hinders effective prevention. Effective care for mental, physical, and substance abuse disorders has been identified as a protective factor.

How You Can Help

If you believe someone may be thinking about suicide:

- Ask them if they are thinking about killing themselves. (This will not put the idea into their head or make it more likely that they will attempt suicide.)

- Listen without judging and show you care.

- Stay with the person (or make sure the person is in a private, secure place with another caring person) until you can get further help.

- Remove any objects that could be used in a suicide attempt.

- Call Substance and Mental Health Services Administration (SAMHSA) National Suicide Prevention Lifeline at 1-800-273-TALK (8255) and follow their guidance.

- If danger for self-harm seems imminent, call 911.

Everyone has a role to play in preventing suicide. For instance, faith communities can work to prevent suicide simply by fostering cultures and norms that are life-preserving, providing perspective and social support to community members, and helping people navigate the struggles of life to find a sustainable sense of hope, meaning, and purpose.

Five Action Steps for Helping Someone in Emotional Pain

- **Ask:** "Are you thinking about killing yourself?" It's not an easy question but studies show that asking at-risk individuals if they are suicidal does not increase suicides or suicidal thoughts.

- **Keep them safe:** Reducing a suicidal person's access to highly lethal items or places is an important part of suicide prevention. While this is not always easy, asking if the at-risk person has a plan and removing or disabling the lethal means can make a difference.

- **Be there:** Listen carefully and learn what the individual is thinking and feeling. Findings suggest acknowledging and talking about suicide may in fact reduce rather than increase suicidal thoughts.

- **Help them connect:** Save the National Suicide Prevention Lifeline's number in your phone so it's there when you need it: 1-800-8255 (TALK). You can also help make a connection with a trusted individual like a family member, friend, spiritual advisor, or mental health professional.

- **Stay connected:** Staying in touch after a crisis or after being discharged from care can make a difference. Studies have shown the number of suicide deaths goes down when someone follows up with the at-risk person.

Section 68.3

Treating People with Suicidal Thoughts

This section includes text excerpted from "Suicide Prevention," National Institute of Mental Health (NIMH), August 2016.

Research has shown that there are multiple risk factors for suicide and that these factors may vary with age, gender, physical, and mental well-being, and with individual experiences. Treatments and therapies for people with suicidal thoughts or actions will vary as well.

Psychotherapies

Multiple types of psychosocial interventions have been found to be beneficial for individuals who have attempted suicide. These types of interventions may prevent someone from making another attempt. Psychotherapy, or "talk therapy," is one type of psychosocial intervention and can effectively reduce suicide risk.

One type of psychotherapy is called cognitive behavioral therapy (CBT). CBT can help people learn new ways of dealing with stressful experiences through training. CBT helps individuals recognize their own thought patterns and consider alternative actions when thoughts of suicide arise.

Another type of psychotherapy, called dialectical behavior therapy (DBT), has been shown to reduce the rate of suicide among people with borderline personality disorder, a serious mental illness characterized by unstable moods, relationships, self-image, and behavior. A therapist trained in DBT helps a person recognize when his or her feelings or actions are disruptive or unhealthy, and teaches the skills needed to deal better with upsetting situations.

Medication

Some individuals at risk for suicide might benefit from medication. Doctors and patients can work together to find the best medication or medication combination, as well as the right dose.

Clozapine, is an antipsychotic medication used primarily to treat individuals with schizophrenia. However, it is the only medication with a specific U.S. Food and Drug Administration (FDA) indication for reducing the risk of recurrent suicidal behavior in patients with schizophrenia or schizoaffective disorder who are at risk for ongoing suicidal behavior. Because many individuals at risk for suicide often have psychiatric and substance use problems, individuals might benefit from medication along with psychosocial intervention.

If you are prescribed a medication, be sure you:

- Talk with your doctor or a pharmacist to make sure you understand the risks and benefits of the medications you're taking.

- Do not stop taking a medication without talking to your doctor first. Suddenly stopping a medication may lead to "rebound" or worsening of symptoms. Other uncomfortable or potentially dangerous withdrawal effects also are possible.

- Report any concerns about side effects to your doctor right away. You may need a change in the dose or a different medication.

- Report serious side effects to the U.S. Food and Drug Administration (FDA) MedWatch Adverse Event Reporting program online or by phone at 1-800-332-1088. You or your doctor may send a report.

Other medications have been used to treat suicidal thoughts and behaviors but more research is needed to show the benefit for these options.

Chapter 69

Recovering from a Suicide Attempt

How Did It Get to This Point?

The time right after your suicide attempt can be the most confusing and emotional part of your entire life. In some ways, it may be even more difficult than the time preceding your attempt. Not only are you still facing the thoughts and feelings that led you to consider suicide, but now you may be struggling to figure out what to do since you survived. It's likely that your decision to try to kill yourself didn't come out of the blue. It probably developed over time, perhaps from overwhelming feelings that seemed too much to bear. Experiencing these emotions might have been especially difficult if you had to deal with them alone. A variety of stressful situations can lead to suicidal feelings, including the loss of a loved one, relationship issues, financial difficulties, health problems, trauma, depression, or other mental health concerns. It's possible that you were experiencing some of these problems when you started to think about suicide.

While the events that lead to a suicide attempt can vary from person to person, a common theme that many suicide attempt survivors report is the need to feel relief. At desperate moments, when it feels like nothing else is working, suicide may seem like the only way to get relief from unbearable emotional pain.

This chapter includes text excerpted from "A Journey toward Health and Hope," Substance and Mental Health Services Administration (SAMHSA), 2015.

Just as it took time for the pain that led to your suicide attempt to become unbearable, it may also take some time for it to subside. That's okay. The important thing is that you're still here; you're alive, which means you have time to find healthier and more effective ways to cope with your pain.

What Am I Feeling Right Now?

Right now, you're probably experiencing many conflicting emotions. You may be thinking:

- "Why am I still here? I wish I were dead. I couldn't even do this right."

- "I don't know if I can get through this. I don't even have the energy to try."

- "I can't do this alone."

- "How do I tell anyone about this? What do I say to them? What will they think of me?"

- "Maybe someone will pay attention to me now; maybe someone will help me."

- "Maybe there is a reason I survived. How do I figure out what that reason is?"

Right after a suicide attempt, many survivors have said that the pain that led them to harm themselves was still present. Some felt angry that they survived their attempt. Others felt embarrassed, ashamed, or guilty that they put their family and friends through a difficult situation. Most felt alone and said they had no idea how to go on living. They didn't know what to expect and even questioned whether they had the strength to stay alive. Still others felt that if they survived their attempt, there must be some reason they were still alive, and they wanted to discover why. You're probably experiencing some of the same feelings and may be wondering how others have faced these challenges.

Am I the Only One Who Feels This Way?

Knowing how others made it through can help you learn new ways to recover from your own suicide attempt. It's estimated that more than one million people attempt suicide each year in the United States, from all parts of society. In other words, you're not alone. However, it can be hard to know how other survivors recovered because suicide is a personal topic that often is not discussed openly and honestly. This can leave those affected feeling like they don't know where to turn.

Shame, dreading the reaction of others, or fear of being hospitalized are some of the reasons that prevent people from talking about suicide. This is unfortunate, because direct and open communication about suicide can help prevent people from acting on suicidal thoughts. Hopefully, reading about the experiences of other survivors in this chapter will make it easier for you to talk about your own attempt, learn ways to keep yourself safe, know when to ask for help, and most importantly, find hope as you think about what happens next on your journey.

It's okay if you feel conflicting emotions right now. Other suicide attempt survivors know that what you're experiencing is normal. They understand that your concerns are real. Going on won't be easy, and finding a way to ease your emotional pain may be challenging, but this can be a time to start down a new path toward a better life—to start your journey toward help and hope. Those who have recovered from a suicide attempt want you to know that:

You are not alone. You matter. Life can get better. It may be difficult, but the effort you invest in your recovery will be worth it. Right now, moving forward may seem impossible. And while it probably won't be easy, many other survivors will tell you that they're glad they held on and worked for a better life. By taking a few steps now, and then a few more when you're ready, you can regain your strength. Sometimes it can be helpful just to take a few steps forward, even when you don't feel like it. In fact, you might start to remember that others care about you. You might discover that suicide is not the only way to relieve your pain. You may find that your feelings will change, either on your own or by working with a counselor. You could wake up one day surprised to feel less pain than you do today.

Taking the First Steps

Making big changes right now might be out of the question for you. You may not even know where to begin. That's okay. Recovery is a process, and it's important that you move at your own pace. There are a few things you might want to do to ease your transition back to everyday life. Some important steps that others have found helpful are listed below.

First, it might be less stressful to decide in advance how to deal with others' questions about your suicide attempt. The people around you may be surprised by your suicide attempt and have questions or comments about what happened. Thinking about what you might say in advance can help you prepare for their reactions.

Second, re-establishing connections may help you feel better. Often, the stress or depression that leads to a suicide attempt can cause people to disconnect from others who care about them or the things they used to enjoy doing. Reconnecting with the people and things you love or loved can help instill hope.

Third, because suicidal thoughts might return, you'll want to be prepared with a plan to stay safe. A safety plan is a tool that can help you identify triggers (like events or experiences) that lead to suicidal thoughts and can help you cope if the pain that led to your suicide attempt returns.

Fourth, finding and working with a counselor can help you start to recover. Unlike friends or family, a counselor is an unbiased listener who won't be personally affected by your suicide attempt. The counselor's role is to help you sort through your feelings and find ways to feel better. You may find it helpful to use this chapter with your counselor to begin discussing your experiences and feelings about your suicide attempt. A counselor can be a peer supporter, psychiatrist, social worker, psychologist, or other skilled person. If counseling isn't possible, there are also ways you can help yourself, but please remember that you don't have to go through this alone.

Re-Establishing Connections

It's likely that the overwhelming life events, stress, and depression that led to your suicide attempt affected your ability to enjoy life. Struggling with suicidal thoughts can be exhausting and leave you with little energy to do the things you once loved. It also can put stress on your relationships with friends and family. The irony of depression and suicidal thinking is that they may cause you to give up the things in life that help you feel better, just when you need them the most.

Establishing Your Connections. It may be hard to answer some of these questions right now. It's okay if you can't answer them immediately.

- Who are the important people in my life? (Friends, family, colleagues, counselors, clergy, pets, etc.)

- What are my plans for the future? What things have i always wanted to do in life?

- What have i come to believe about suicide?

- What are the things i cherish in life?

- What things do i enjoy doing? What did i used to enjoy?

- What gives me a sense of purpose in life?

- What are my other reasons for living?

Even up until the moment of their attempts, many suicide attempt survivors report that there was an internal struggle going on inside them. One side argued that suicide was the best way to end the pain they were experiencing. The other side struggled to find another way to feel better. To put it another way, most people with suicidal thoughts had reasons for dying and reasons for living. Before your suicide attempt, you might have lost connections to your reasons for living, but it's important to re-establish those connections because they can help instill hope. They can remind you about the things you love in life. The exercise on the previous page will help you consider reasons for living. Personalizing this can help remind you of where you were before you started to feel suicidal and where you would like to be again.

Planning to Stay Safe

You might still have thoughts of suicide after your attempt, even if you've decided that you want to stay alive. Perhaps the pain that led to your suicide attempt is still there. It's okay to have suicidal thoughts. Everyone needs to feel relief from unbearable pain, and suicidal thoughts may be one of the ways you've learned to cope.

What's important is that you don't act on those thoughts and that you try to find other, safer ways to ease your pain. A safety plan can help you do this.

What Is a Safety Plan?

In times of trouble, you may not see that you have options other than harming yourself. A safety plan is a written list of coping strategies and resources to help you survive a suicidal crisis. A safety plan can help you discover other ways to ease your pain so you don't feel tempted to act on suicidal thoughts you may experience.

Your plan will be a personalized list of strategies to help you cope. You can use these strategies before or during a suicidal crisis. By writing them down, you'll always know what they are, even if you're upset or not thinking clearly. You can complete your plan by yourself or with the help of a counselor, peer, family member, or friend. The following pages will help you brainstorm elements of your safety plan.

What Do I Write in My Safety Plan?

- Things that lead to suicidal thoughts

- Things I can do to take my mind off my problems

- People and places that distract me from my problems

- People I can ask for help

- Doctors, counselors, peer specialists, or other professionals to contact in a crisis

- The number for the local crisis line or National Suicide Prevention Lifeline (1-800-273-TALK)

- Items to remove so that I won't use them to hurt myself

- Reminders of hope and reasons for living

Have People Ready to Help

You will feel more secure with someone you can trust as your supporter in times of crisis. It may be a family member, friend, peer support or health professional. Try to select a person you can trust to respect you and stay level-headed in an emergency. To cover all your bases, you may want to ask a second person to serve as a backup contact. It's important that those you ask to be your primary support person and backup support person feel comfortable in these roles and know what to do. Share your safety plan with them and keep them aware of how you are feeling. Don't forget to thank them for their help.

Moving toward a Hopeful Future

After you've taken your first steps back into daily life, it might be time to consider taking on a few more challenges. You've already made it through the toughest part. Now it's time to think about doing some things that can give you a greater sense of wellbeing and happiness.

Many survivors talk about a "second chance," or slowly coming to value what would have been lost if their attempt had resulted in their death. Over time, they begin to reclaim a sense of purpose in their lives, a new sense of identity, and real reasons for hope.

Maintaining Hope

When you made your suicide attempt, you felt as if suicide was a way to end your pain. At that moment, in your mind, your reasons for dying outweighed your reasons for living. As you've learned, reconnecting with your reasons for living can help you build hope. Some survivors recommend putting together a "hope box" that can serve as a physical reminder of the things in your life that bring you joy. When you begin to feel bad about yourself or your life and feel depressed, the contents of your hope box can help lift your spirits. It also is a good place to keep your safety plan.

Staying in Control by Being Organized

Dealing with stress or emotional pain can feel overwhelming and lead you to neglect day-to-day tasks and responsibilities. Feeling like life is out of control can make anyone feel anxious. It might help to make a list of the things you have to do each day. That way, you won't forget important events or get distracted and not complete things you need to get done.

Checking items off a to-do list can also help you feel a sense of accomplishment. Keep it simple and short to begin with; you can always add more when you have more energy. Keeping a calendar and using a daily planner are great ways to help yourself stay organized and maintain a sense of control over your life.

Getting in Touch with Your Spirituality

Some suicide attempt survivors find comfort in spirituality. Spirituality can mean different things to different people, and for some it can provide a feeling of being connected to something larger than themselves. Some may experience this by attending churches, temples, synagogues, mosques, and other places of worship. Others discover deeper meanings in nature, philosophy, or music. Would getting in touch with your spirituality bring you comfort and peace? Only you can answer that, but it does help some people.

Maintaining a Healthy Lifestyle

Maintaining a healthy lifestyle can affect the way you feel, not only physically, but emotionally. If you feel depressed or overwhelmed emotionally, it's easy to forget the basics of taking care of yourself physically. It will make a difference if you maintain a healthy life-style during your recovery. Of course this means limiting your use of alcohol and eliminating other drugs, as these can negatively affect your emotions, but it's more than just that. Getting enough sleep, eating well, and exercising are also crucial to your recovery.

Sleep

A link between sleep and depression is well-documented. When depressed, many people find themselves sleeping a lot more than usual, while others are unable to sleep adequately. Poor sleep can lead to fatigue, inactivity, anxiety, and irritability, making depression or other mental health issues even worse. Insomnia can also be associated with suicidal thoughts and actions. If you have depression that includes sleep disturbances, certain kinds of talk therapy (like CBT) can help, as well as medication. So it is important to discuss sleep problems with your counselor or psychiatrist.

Getting enough sleep is crucial because your body restores itself during sleep.

Diet

Appetite changes—either poor appetite with weight loss or increased appetite with weight gain—also can be symptoms of major depression. If your appetite has changed and you have low, depressed mood, please talk with your psychiatrist or counselor about whether you should consider medication.

While no particular diet has been proven to decrease depression and anxiety or improve emotional health, there does seem to be a correlation between what we eat and how we feel. A healthy diet is recommended as a key part of the overall treatment for depression. Additionally, ensuring that your body has the nutrients it needs can increase your energy level. Enrolling in a healthy cooking class can help you find ways to eat well and meet new people. You also can find out how to prepare healthy food online.

Exercise

When you exercise, your body releases endorphins, a chemical that affects how people perceive pain. It's believed that the release of endorphins can help people feel more energized and even improve their emotional states, allowing them to be more hopeful about life. In fact, some studies suggest that exercise can be an effective treatment for depression. Given that exercise can improve your mood, you might want to join a local gym, take a walk every day with a friend, or do exercises at home. Incorporating an exercise plan into your daily life (exercising three or more times each week) is highly recommended.

Taking Medication

If you choose to go to counseling, your counselor may recommend taking medication to improve your mood, especially if maintaining a healthy lifestyle and counseling aren't giving you the results you're looking for. You may struggle with the decision to take medication and feel as though it's a sign of weakness. It's important to remember that people take medications for all sorts of illnesses, and there is no reason to be embarrassed if you choose to try medications to alleviate depression, anxiety, or another mental health concern that causes you pain.

Certainly, only you can decide if you want to take medication; however, many people have felt that their depression and anxiety improved after taking medication. Most people (including researchers) indicate that counseling combined with medication provides the best results.

If you do choose to try medication, here are a few important things to remember:

- It can take some time for medication to have an effect. While some medications (for instance, sleep medication) may work immediately, medications for depression may take up to 8 weeks to reach their full effect. Your psychiatrist or doctor can tell you what to expect.

- You must take your medication as directed, without skipping dosages, for it to be effective.

- It's important to continue taking your medication for the entire period it is prescribed. You may be tempted to stop taking medication when you start to feel better. Stopping too soon can cause a relapse. Always work with your psychiatrist or doctor if you want to stop or change your medication.

- If your thoughts of suicide increase after you start taking medication, be sure to contact your psychiatrist or doctor immediately.

- Different medications work for different people. Be patient; sometimes it can take time to find the medications that work best for you. If one medication doesn't work, that doesn't mean none of them will. Finding the right medication can take persistence.

Advocating for Others to Support Your Recovery

When you're feeling stronger, you may find that helping others who are facing suicide can help you, too. Sharing your experiences and wisdom might save other lives. And saving lives can be a source of pride and accomplishment for you. Speaking about your experience also helps to break the guilt and shame that can be associated with suicide and lets others know they're not alone. You should give serious consideration to whether you're ready to talk openly about your suicide attempt before deciding to advocate for others. It's important to ensure that you've given yourself enough time to heal and learn from your experience before using it to help others. Some questions you might ask yourself include:

- Am I ready to speak? Have I healed enough to speak?

- Am I prepared for my family's reactions to going public?

- Am I prepared for the possible social effects of going public with my story?

- Am I familiar with the resources available to help others?

- How will I take care of myself?

Hopes for a Safe Journey

The time after your suicide attempt is an important one. It can be a turning point in your life. Often, your suicide attempt can break the silence that surrounded the problems you were experiencing and your suicidal thoughts. Making a choice to be open about how you're feeling and seeking help, when you're ready, can be the first step on the path to a more fulfilling life.

As discussed, recovering from your suicide attempt is a process. It will likely have its ups and downs. You may feel overwhelmed or sad at times, and you may experience suicidal thoughts again. However, it's important to remember that feelings change. Finding ways to cope with those negative feelings while staying alive will give you a chance to enjoy the positive things life has in store for you. The content of this chapter can help you feel better. They've worked for other people, and they may work for you, too. We ask you always to remember our message:

- You are not alone
- You matter
- Life can get better
- It may be difficult, but the effort you invest in your recovery will be worth it

Part Nine

Additional Help and Information

Chapter 70

Glossary of Terms Related to Depression

agitation: A condition in which a person is unable to relax and be still. The person may be very tense and irritable, and become easily annoyed by small things.

anticonvulsant: A drug or other substance used to prevent or stop seizures or convulsions. Also called antiepileptic.

antidepressant: Medication used to treat depression and other mood and anxiety disorders.

antipsychotic: Medication used to treat psychosis.

anxiety disorder: Any of a group of illnesses that fill people's lives with overwhelming anxieties and fears that are chronic and unremitting. Anxiety disorders include panic disorder, obsessive-compulsive disorder, posttraumatic stress disorder, phobias, and generalized anxiety disorder.

anxiety: An abnormal sense of fear, nervousness, and apprehension about something that might happen in the future.

auditory hallucinations: Hearing something that is not real. Hearing voices is an example of auditory hallucinations.

This glossary contains terms excerpted from documents produced by several sources deemed reliable.

avoidance: One of the symptoms of posttraumatic stress disorder (PTSD). Those with PTSD avoid situations and reminders of their trauma.

behavioral therapy: Behavioral therapy focuses on a person's actions and aims to change unhealthy behavior patterns.

benzodiazepine: A type of CNS depressant prescribed to relieve anxiety and sleep problems. Valium and Xanax are among the most widely prescribed medications.

bipolar disorder: A depressive disorder in which a person alternates between episodes of major depression and mania (periods of abnormally and persistently elevated mood). Also referred to as manic depression.

cognition: Conscious mental activities (such as thinking, communicating, understanding, solving problems, processing information and remembering) that are associated with gaining knowledge and understanding.

cognitive behavioral therapy (CBT): CBT helps people focus on how to solve their current problems. The therapist helps the patient learn how to identify distorted or unhelpful thinking patterns, recognize and change inaccurate beliefs, relate to others in more positive ways, and change behaviors accordingly.

cognitive impairment: Experiencing difficulty with cognition. Examples include having trouble paying attention, thinking clearly or remembering new information.

delirium: A mental state in which a person is confused, disoriented, and not able to think or remember clearly. The person may also be agitated and have hallucinations, and extreme excitement.

delusions: Beliefs that have no basis in reality.

dementia: Loss of brain function that occurs with certain diseases. It affects memory, thinking, language, judgment and behavior.

depression: Used to describe an emotional state involving sadness, lack of energy, and low self-esteem.

dysthymia: A depressive disorder that is less severe than major depressive disorder but is more persistent.

eating disorder: Eating disorders, such as anorexia nervosa, bulimia nervosa, and binge-eating disorder, involve serious problems with eating. This could include an extreme decrease of food or severe over-eating, as well as feelings of distress and concern about body shape or weight.

hallucinations: Hearing, seeing, touching, smelling or tasting things that are not real.

hypertension: Also called high blood pressure, it is having blood pressure greater than 0 over 90 mmHg (millimeters of mercury). Long-term high blood pressure can damage blood vessels and organs, including the heart, kidneys, eyes, and brain.

hypnosis: An altered state of consciousness characterized by increased responsiveness to suggestion. The procedure is used to effect positive changes and to treat numerous health conditions including ulcers, chronic pain, respiratory ailments, stress, and headaches.

insomnia: Not being able to sleep

interpersonal therapy: This therapy is based on the idea that improving communication patterns and the ways people relate to others will effectively treat depression. IPT helps identify how a person interacts with other people. When a behavior is causing problems, IPT guides the person to change the behavior.

ischemia: Lack of blood supply to a part of the body. Ischemia may cause tissue damage due to the lack of oxygen and nutrients.

light therapy: Light therapy is used to treat seasonal affective disorder (SAD), a form of depression that usually occurs during the autumn and winter months, when the amount of natural sunlight decreases. During light therapy, a person sits in front of a "light box" for periods of time, usually in the morning. The box emits a full spectrum light, and sitting in front of it appears to help reset the body's daily rhythms.

major depressive disorder: Also called major depression, this is a combination of symptoms that interfere with a person's ability to work, sleep, study, eat, and enjoy once-pleasurable activities.

mania: Feelings of intense mental and physical hyperactivity, elevated mood, and agitation.

meditation: Meditation is a mind and body practice. There are many types of meditation, most of which originated in ancient religious and spiritual traditions. Some forms of meditation instruct the practitioner to become mindful of thoughts, feelings, and sensations and to observe them in a nonjudgmental way.

mental illness: A health condition that changes a person's thinking, feelings, or behavior (or all three) and that causes the person distress and difficulty in functioning.

migraine: Headaches that are usually pulsing or throbbing and occur on one or both sides of the head. They are moderate to severe in intensity, associated with nausea, vomiting, sensitivity to light and noise, and worsen with routine physical activity.

mood disorders: Mental disorders primarily affecting a person's mood.

obsessive-compulsive disorder (OCD): An anxiety disorder in which a person suffers from obsessive thoughts and compulsive actions, such as cleaning, checking, counting, or hoarding. The person becomes trapped in a pattern of repetitive thoughts and behaviors that are senseless and distressing but very hard to stop.

panic disorder: An anxiety disorder in which a person suffers from sudden attacks of fear and panic. The attacks may occur without a known reason, but many times they are triggered by events or thoughts that produce fear in the person, such as taking an elevator or driving.

pharmacotherapy: Medication selection, dosing, and management. Pharmacotherapy for first episode psychosis typically involves a low dose of a single antipsychotic medication and careful monitoring for side effects.

phobia: An anxiety disorder in which a person suffers from an unusual amount of fear of a certain activity or situation.

physical therapy: Therapy aimed to restore movement, balance, and coordination.

postpartum depression: Postpartum depression is when a new mother has a major depressive episode within one month after delivery.

posttraumatic stress disorder (PTSD): An anxiety disorder that can occur after you have been through a traumatic event.

premenstrual dysphoric disorder (PMDD): A severe form of premenstrual syndrome, which causes feelings of sadness or despair, or even thoughts of suicide, feelings of tension or anxiety, panic attacks, mood swings or frequent crying, and other severe symptoms.

psychiatrist: A doctor (M.D.) who treats mental illness. Psychiatrists must receive additional training and serve a supervised residency in their specialty. They can prescribe medications.

psychosis: The word psychosis is used to describe conditions that affect the mind, where there has been some loss of contact with reality. When someone becomes ill in this way it is called a psychotic episode.

psychotherapy: A treatment method for mental illness in which a mental health professional (psychiatrist, psychologist, counselor) and a patient discuss problems and feelings to find solutions. Psychotherapy can help individuals change their thought or behavior patterns or understand how past experiences affect current behaviors.

psychotic depression: A mental health disorder that occurs when a severe depressive illness is accompanied by some form of psychosis, such as a break with reality, hallucinations, and delusions.

puberty: Time when the body is changing from the body of a child to the body of an adult. This process begins earlier in girls than in boys, usually between ages 8 and 13, and lasts 2 to 4 years.

resilience: Resilience refers to the ability to successfully adapt to stressors, maintaining psychological well-being in the face of adversity. It's the ability to "bounce back" from difficult experiences.

schizoaffective disorder: A mental condition that causes both a loss of contact with reality (psychosis) and mood problems (depression or mania).

schizophrenia: A severe mental disorder that appears in late adolescence or early adulthood. People with schizophrenia may have hallucinations, delusions, loss of personality, confusion, agitation, social withdrawal, psychosis, and/or extremely odd behavior.

seasonal affective disorder (SAD): A depression during the winter months, when there is less natural sunlight.

serotonin syndrome: Serotonin syndrome usually occurs when older antidepressants are combined with selective serotonin reuptake inhibitors. A person with serotonin syndrome may be agitated, have hallucinations (see or hear things that are not real), have a high temperature, or have unusual blood pressure changes.

sleep disorder: Sleep disorders are clinical conditions that are a consequence of a disturbance in the ability to initiate or maintain the quantity and quality of sleep needed for optimal health, performance and well being.

social phobia: Social phobia is a strong fear of being judged by others and of being embarrassed. This fear can be so strong that it gets in the way of going to work or school or doing other everyday things.

St. John's wort: St. John's wort is a plant with yellow flowers that has been used for centuries for health purposes, including depression and anxiety.

stimulants: A class of drugs that enhances the activity of monamines (such as dopamine) in the brain, increasing arousal, heart rate, blood pressure, and respiration, and decreasing appetite; includes some medications used to treat attention-deficit hyperactivity disorder (e.g., methylphenidate and amphetamines), as well as cocaine and methamphetamine.

suicide: Death caused by self-directed injurious behavior with any intent to die as a result of the behavior.

tolerance: A condition in which higher doses of a drug are required to produce the same effect achieved during initial use; often associated with physical dependence.

trauma: A life-threatening event, such as military combat, natural disasters, terrorist incidents, serious accidents, or physical or sexual assault in adult or childhood.

yoga: A combination of breathing exercises, physical postures, and meditation used to calm the nervous system and balance the body, mind, and spirit.

Chapter 71

Directory of Organizations That Help People with Depression and Suicidal Thoughts

Government Agencies That Provide Information about Depression

Agency for Healthcare Research and Quality (AHRQ)
Office of Communications and Knowledge Transfer (OCKT)
5600 Fishers Ln.
Rockville, MD 20857
Phone: 301-427-1104
Website: www.ahrq.gov

Centers for Disease Control and Prevention (CDC)
1600 Clifton Rd.
Atlanta, GA 30329-4027
Toll-Free: 800-CDC-INFO
(800-232-4636)
Toll-Free TTY: 888-232-6348
Website: www.cdc.gov

Resources in this chapter were compiled from several sources deemed reliable; all contact information was verified and updated in November 2016.

Healthfinder®
National Health Information
Center (NHIC)
1101 Wootton Pkwy
Rockville, MD 20852
Toll-Free: 800-336-4797
Phone: 301-565-4167
Fax: 301-984-4256
Website: www.healthfinder.gov
E-mail: healthfinder@hhs.gov

**National Cancer Institute
(NCI)**
9609 Medical Center Dr.
Bethesda, MD 20892-9760
Toll-Free: 800-4-CANCER
(800-422-6237)
Toll-Free TTY: 800-332-8615
Website: www.cancer.gov

**National Center for
Complementary and
Integrative Health (NCCIH)**
National Institutes of Health
(NIH)
9000 Rockville Pike
Bethesda, MD 20892
Toll-Free: 888-644-6226
Toll-Free TTY: 866-464-3615
Toll-Free Fax: 866-464-3616
Website: www.nccih.nih.gov
E-mail: info@nccih.nih.gov

**National Center for Health
Statistics (NCHS)**
3311 Toledo Rd.
Hyattsville, MD 20782
Toll-Free: 866-441-NCHS
(866-441-6247)
Phone: 301-458-4636
Website: www.cdc.gov/nchs
E-mail: nchsquery@cdc.gov

**National Center for
Posttraumatic Stress
Disorder (NCPTSD)**
U.S. Department of Veterans
Affairs (VA)
810 Vermont Ave. N.W.
Washington, DC 20420
Toll-Free: 800-273-8255
Website: www.va.gov
E-mail: ncptsd@va.gov

**National Institute of Mental
Health (NIMH)**
6001 Executive Blvd.
Bethesda, MD 20892
Toll-Free: 866-615-6464
Phone: 301-443-4513
Toll-Free TTY: 866-415-8051
TTY: 301-443-8431
Fax: 301-443-4279
Website: www.nimh.nih.gov
E-mail: nimhinfo@nih.gov

**National Institute on Aging
(NIA)**
31 Center Dr.
MSC 2292
Bethesda, MD 20892
Toll-Free: 800-222-2225
Phone: 301-496-1752
Toll-Free TTY: 800-222-4225
Fax: 301-496-1072
Website: www.nia.nih.gov
E-mail: nianews3@mail.nih.gov

National Institutes of Health (NIH)
9000 Rockville Pike
Bethesda, MD 20892
Phone: 301-496-4000
TTY: 301-402-9612
Website: www.nih.gov
E-mail: NIHinfo@od.nih.gov

National Women's Health Information Center (NWHIC)
Office on Women's Health (OWH)
200 Independence Ave. S.W.
Rm. 712E
Washington DC 20201
Toll-Free: 800-994-9662
Phone: 202-690-7650
Toll-Free TDD: 888-220-5446
Fax: 202-205-2631
Website: www.womenshealth. gov

Office of Disability Employment Policy (ODEP)
U.S. Department of Labor (DOL)
200 Constitution Ave. N.W.
Washington, DC 20210
Toll-Free: 866-ODEP-DOL (866-633-7365)
Toll-Free TTY: 877-889-5627
Website: www.dol.gov/odep
E-mail: odep@dol.gov

Office of Minority Health (OMH) Resource Center
P.O. Box 37337
Washington, DC 20013-7337
Toll-Free: 800-444-6472
Phone: 240-453-2882
TDD: 301-251-1432
Fax: 301-251-2160
Website: minorityhealth.hhs.gov
E-mail: info@minorityhealth. hhs.gov

Substance Abuse and Mental Health Services Administration (SAMHSA)
5600 Fishers Ln.
Rockville, MD 20857
Toll-Free: 877-SAMHSA-7 (877-726-4727)
Phone: 240-276-1310
Toll-Free TDD: 800-487-4889
Fax: 301-480-8491
Website: www.samhsa.gov

U.S. Department of Education (ED)
400 Maryland Ave. S.W.
Washington, DC 20202
Toll-Free: 800-USA-LEARN (800-872-5327)
Phone: 202-401-2000
Toll-Free TTY: 800-437-0833
Website: www.ed.gov

U.S. Department of Health and Human Services (HHS)
200 Independence Ave. S.W.
Washington, DC 20201
Toll-Free: 877-696-6775
Website: www.hhs.gov

U.S. Food and Drug Administration (FDA)
10903 New Hampshire Ave.
Silver Spring, MD 20993
Toll-Free: 888-INFO-FDA
(888-463-6332)
Website: www.fda.gov

U.S. National Library of Medicine (NLM)
8600 Rockville Pike
Bethesda, MD 20894
Toll-Free: 888-FIND-NLM
(888-346-3656)
Phone: 301-594-5983
Toll-Free TDD: 800-735-2258
Fax: 301-402-1384
Website: www.nlm.nih.gov
E-mail: custserv@nlm.nih.gov

Private Agencies That Provide Information about Depression

AIDS InfoNet
2200 Pennsylvania Ave. N.W.
4th Fl. E.
Washington, DC 20037
Website: www.aidsinfonet.org

Alzheimer's Association
225 N. Michigan Ave.
Fl. 17
Chicago, IL 60601-7633
Toll-Free: 800-272-3900
Phone: 312-335-8700
Toll-Free TDD: 866-403-3073
TDD: 312-335-5886
Toll-Free Fax: 866-699-1246
Website: www.alz.org
E-mail: info@alz.org

American Academy of Child and Adolescent Psychiatry (AACAP)
3615 Wisconsin Ave. N.W.
Washington, DC 20016-3007
Phone: 202-966-7300
Fax: 202-966-2891
Website: www.aacap.org

American Academy of Family Physicians (AAFP)
11400 Tomahawk Creek Pkwy
Leawood, KS 66211-2680
Toll-Free: 800-274-2237
Phone: 913-906-6000
Fax: 913-906-6075
Website: www.aafp.org
E-mail: aafp@aafp.org

American Academy of Pediatrics (AAP)
141 N.W. Point Blvd.
Elk Grove Village, IL 60007-1098
Toll-Free: 800-433-9016
Phone: 847-434-4000
Fax: 847-434-8000
Website: www.aap.org
E-mail: kidsdocs@aap.org

American Art Therapy Association (AATA)
4875 Eisenhower Ave.
Ste. 240
Alexandria, VA 22304
Toll-Free: 888-290-0878
Phone: 703-548-5860
Fax: 703-783-8468
Website: www.arttherapy.org
E-mail: info@arttherapy.org

American Association for Geriatric Psychiatry (AAGP)
6728 Old McLean Village Dr.
McLean, VA 22101
Phone: 703-556-9222
Fax: 703-556-8729
Website: www.aagponline.org
E-mail: main@aagponline.org

American Association for Marriage and Family Therapy (AAMFT)
112 S. Alfred St.
Alexandria, VA 22314-3061
Phone: 703-838-9808
Fax: 703-838-9805
Website: www.aamft.org
E-mail: central@aamft.org

American Association of Suicidology (AAS)
5221 Wisconsin Ave. N.W.
Washington, DC 20015
Phone: 202-237-2280
Fax: 202-237-2282
Website: www.suicidology.org

American Counseling Association (ACA)
6101 Stevenson Ave., Ste. 600
Alexandria, VA 22304
Toll-Free: 800-347-6647
Phone: 703-823-9800
TDD: 703-823-6862
Toll-Free Fax: 800-473-2329
Fax: 703-823-0252
Website: www.counseling.org
E-mail: webmaster@counseling.org

American Foundation for Suicide Prevention (AFSP)
120 Wall St.
29th Fl.
New York, NY 10005
Toll-Free: 888-333-AFSP
(888-333-2377)
Phone: 212-363-3500
Fax: 212-363-6237
Website: www.afsp.org
E-mail: info@afsp.org

American Medical Association (AMA)
330 N. Wabash Ave.
Ste. 39300
Chicago, IL 60611-5885
Toll-Free: 800-621-8335
Website: www.ama-assn.org

American Psychiatric Association (APA)
1000 Wilson Blvd., Ste. 1825
Arlington, VA 22209-3901
Toll-Free: 888-35-PSYCH
(888-357-7924)
Phone: 703-907-7300
Website: www.psychiatry.org
E-mail: apa@psych.org

American Psychological Association (APA)
750 First St. N.E.
Washington, DC 20002-4242
Toll-Free: 800-374-2721
Phone: 202-336-5500
TDD/TTY: 202-336-6123
Website: www.apa.org
E-mail: public.affairs@apa.org

American Psychotherapy Association
2750 E. Sunshine St.
Springfield, MO 65804
Toll-Free: 800-205-9165
Phone: 417-823-0173
Fax: 417-823-9959
E-mail: cao@
americanpsychotherapy.com

Anxiety Disorders Association of America (ADAA)
8701 Georgia Ave.
Ste. 412
Silver Spring, MD 20910
Phone: 240-485-1001
Fax: 240-485-1035
Website: www.adaa.org

Arthritis Foundation
1355 Peachtree St. N.E.
Ste. 600
Atlanta, GA 30309
Toll-Free: 844-571-4357
Phone: 404-872-7100
Website: www.arthritis.org

Association for Behavioral and Cognitive Therapies (ABCT)
305 7th Ave.
16th Fl.
New York, NY 10001
Phone: 212-647-1890
Fax: 212-647-1865
Website: www.abct.org
E-mail: clinical.dir@abct.org

Brain and Behavior Research Foundation
90 Park Ave.
16th Fl.
New York, NY 10016
Toll-Free: 800-829-8289
Phone: 646-681-4888
Fax: 516-487-6930
Website: www.bbrfoundation.org
E-mail: info@bbrfoundation.org

Brain Injury Association of America (BIAA)
1608 Spring Hill Rd., Ste. 110
Vienna, VA 22182
Toll-Free: 800-444-6443
Phone: 703-761-0750
Fax: 703-761-0755
Website: www.biausa.org
E-mail: braininjuryinfo@biausa.
org

Canadian Mental Health Association (CMHA)
2301-180 Dundas St. W.
Toronto, ON M5G 1Z8
Canada
Phone: 613-745-7750
Fax: 613-745-5522
Website: www.cmha.ca
E-mail: info@cmha.ca

Canadian Psychological Association (CPA)

141 Laurier Ave. W., Ste. 702
Ottawa, ON K1P 5J3
Canada
Toll-Free: 888-472-0657
Phone: 613-237-2144
Fax: 613-237-1674
Website: www.cpa.ca
E-mail: cpa@cpa.ca

Caring.com

2600 South El Camino Real
Ste. 300
San Mateo, CA 94403
Toll-Free: 800-973-1540
Phone: 650-312-7100
Website: www.caring.com

Cleveland Clinic

9500 Euclid Ave.
Cleveland, OH 44195
Toll-Free: 800-223-2273
Phone: 216-636-5860 (Info Line)
TTY: 216-444-0261
Website: my.clevelandclinic.org

The Dana Foundation

505 Fifth Ave.
6th Fl.
New York, NY 10017
Phone: 212-223-4040
Fax: 212-317-8721
Website: www.dana.org
E-mail: danainfo@dana.org

Depressed Anonymous (DA)

P.O. Box 17414
Louisville, KY 40214
Phone: 502-569-1989
Website: www.depressedanon.com
E-mail: depanon@netpenny.net

Depression and Bipolar Support Alliance (DBSA)

55 E. Jackson Blvd.
Ste. 490
Chicago, IL 60604
Toll-Free: 800-826-3632
Fax: 312-642-7243
Website: www.dbsalliance.org
E-mail: info@dbsalliance.org

Eating Disorder Referral and Information Center

2923 Sandy Pointe #6
Del Mar, CA 92014
Phone: 858-792-7463
Website: www.edreferral.com
E-mail: edreferral@gmail.com

Family Caregiver Alliance (FCA)

785 Market St.
Ste. 750
San Francisco, CA 94103
Toll-Free: 800-445-8106
Phone: 415-434-3388
Website: www.caregiver.org
E-mail: info@caregiver.org

Geriatric Mental Health Foundation (GMHF)

6728 Old McLean Village Dr.
McLean, VA 22101
Phone: 703-556-9222
Fax: 703-556-8729
Website: www.gmhfonline.org
E-mail: web@GMHFonline.org

International Foundation for Research and Education on Depression (iFred)
P.O. Box 17598
Baltimore, MD 21297
Fax: 443-782-0739
Website: www.ifred.org
E-mail: info@ifred.org

International OCD Foundation (IOCDF)
P.O. Box 961029
Boston, MA 02196
Phone: 617-973-5801
Fax: 617-973-5803
Website: www.iocdf.org
E-mail: info@iocdf.org

Kristin Brooks Hope Center (KBHC)
Toll-Free: 800-442-HOPE
(800-442-4673)
Website: www.hopeline.com/gethelpnow.html
E-mail: info@iamalive.org

Mental Health America (MHA)
500 Montgomery St.
Ste. 820
Alexandria, VA 22314
Toll-Free: 800-969-6642
Phone: 703-684-7722
Fax: 703-684-5968
Website: www.mentalhealthamerica.net

Mind
15-19 Bdwy.
Stratford, London E15 4BQ
United Kingdom
Phone: 020-8519-2122
Fax: 020-8522-1725
Website: www.mind.org.uk
E-mail: supporterservices@mind.org.uk

Multiple Sclerosis Association of America (MSAA)
375 Kings Hwy N.
Cherry Hill, NJ 08034
Toll-Free: 800-532-7667
Phone: 856-488-4500
Fax: 856-661-9797
Website: www.mymsaa.org
E-mail: msaa@mymsaa.org

National Alliance on Mental Illness (NAMI)
3803 N. Fairfax Dr.
Ste. 100
Arlington, VA 22203
Toll-Free: 800-950-NAMI
(800-950-6264)
Phone: 703-524-7600
Fax: 703-524-9094
Website: www.nami.org

National Association of Anorexia Nervosa and Associated Disorders (ANAD)
750 E. Diehl Rd.
Ste. 127
Naperville, IL 60563
Phone: 630-577-1333
Fax: 630-577-1323
Website: www.anad.org
E-mail: anadhelp@anad.org

National Association of School Psychologists (NASP)
4340 East W. Hwy
Ste. 402
Bethesda, MD 20814
Toll-Free: 866-331-NASP
(866-331-6277)
Phone: 301-657-0270
TTY: 301-657-4155
Fax: 301-657-0275
Website: www.nasponline.org
E-mail: center@naspweb.org

National Eating Disorders Association (NEDA)
165 W. 46th St.
Ste. 402
New York, NY 10036
Toll-Free: 800-931-2237
Phone: 212-575-6200
Fax: 212-575-1650
Website: www.
nationaleatingdisorders.org
E-mail: info@
NationalEatingDisorders.org

National Federation of Families for Children's Mental Health (NFFCMH)
12320 Parklawn Dr.
Rockville, MD 20852
Phone: 240-403-1901
Fax: 240-403-1909
Website: www.ffcmh.org
E-mail: ffcmh@ffcmh.org

The Nemours Foundation
1600 Rockland Rd.
Wilmington, DE 19803
Phone: 302-651-4828
Website: www.nemours.org
E-mail: info@kidshealth.org

Parkinson's Disease Foundation (PDF)
1359 Bdwy.
Ste. 1509
New York, NY 10018
Toll-Free: 800-457-6676
Phone: 212-923-4700
Fax: 212-923-4778
Website: www.pdf.org
E-mail: info@pdf.org

Postpartum Support International (PSI)
6706 S.W. 54th Ave.
Portland, OR 97219
Toll-Free: 800-944-4PPD
(800-944-4773)
Phone: 503-894-9453
Fax: 503-894-9452
Website: www.postpartum.net
E-mail: support@postpartum.net

Psych Central
55 Pleasant St.
Ste. 207
Newburyport, MA 01950
Website: www.psychcentral.com
E-mail: talkback@psychcentral.
com

Psychology Today
115 E. 23rd St.
9th Fl.
New York, NY 10010
Phone: 212-260-7210
Fax: 212-260-7566
Website: www.psychologytoday.
com

Suicide Awareness Voices of Education (SAVE)
8120 Penn Ave. S.
Ste. 470
Bloomington, MN 55431
Toll-Free: 800-273-8255
Phone: 952-946-7998
Website: www.save.org
E-mail: save@save.org

Suicide Prevention Resource Center (SPRC)
43 Foundry Ave.
Waltham, MA 02453-8313
Toll-Free: 877-GET-SPRC
(877-438-7772)
TTY: 617-964-5448
Website: www.sprc.org
E-mail: info@sprc.org

Index

Index

Page numbers followed by 'n' indicate a footnote. Page numbers in *italics* indicate a table or illustration.